Wake Up and Change Your Ways

How What You Consume Affects Your Life and the World

Johann Carolus

ebl

Wake Up and Change Your Ways
How What You Consume Affects
Your Life and the World

First Edition: 2022

ISBN: 9781524318321
ISBN eBook: 9781524328337

© of the text:
   Johann Carolus

© Layout, design and production of this edition: 2022 EBL

To my parents,
thanks for all your love.

Table of Contents

Introduction... 11

Chapter I And What Did We Eat Yesterday? 27

Chapter II And What Happened in the Last Century, the 20th
Century? 35

    Do you feel well? Do you feel healthy? 46

    You live with this killer, and you don't know it yet? 48

    We are not alone 51

Chapter III Beneficial Principles for Optimal Health and
Longevity... 61

    The fundamental principle 61

    Acidity vs. alkalinity 66

    The caloric principle..70

    Omega fatty acids: quality vs. qualities.......................................79

    Balanced intake 84

Chapter IV A Separate Chapter 91

    Ten reasons why you struggle to lose fat......................................91

    Slow food culture 95

    Overweight or not: we're swollen 100

    The great cholesterol hoax...100

    The truth about saturated fats 107

    Introduction 107

    The lipid hypothesis 108

    The "evidence" supporting the lipid hypothesis 109

    Studies challenging the lipid hypothesis 113

    To understand the chemistry of fats 118

    Classification of fatty acids by saturation 119

    Classification of fatty acids by length 121

The dangers of polyunsaturates 124

Too much omega 6..126

Too little omega 3 127

The benefit of saturated fats...128

What about cholesterol?...130

The cause and treatment of heart disease 134

Modern fat processing methods..135

Nutrients in butter 139

The composition of the different fats 145

Summary..150

Chapter V Learning to Eat 153

Breakfast is important 154

Trophology 158

The science of combining foods 159

Protein and tuber starch — cereal starch —................................163

Protein and protein 164

Starch — starches — and acid..165

Protein and acid..165

Protein and fat 166

Protein and sugar..166

Starch and sugar..167

Melon..167

Desserts 168

What an outburst! 169

A fair trial for the four white murderers 170

Milk...171

Pasteurized milk according to trophology 172

Refined flours 175

Sugar..182

Salt...197

Chapter VI Why People Get Sick 207
    Metabolism, the body, and the human self 219
    The self and my body: two distinct entities? 222
    How to proceed with self-healing 226
    Is healing the same as self-healing? 229
    Top seven tips to stop you from getting sick 241

Chapter VII The Genetic Factor 247
    DNA repair and more 247
    A bit of history..252
    GMO, transgenic, and genetically modified organisms 264

Chapter VIII Weight Loss 275
    How to tell if you are a carbohydrate burner or a fat burner......279
    Food groups 284
    The Hippocratic sandwich 288
    Salmon or trout sauce (dip)...289
    Basil pesto 290
    Chickpea hummus 290
    Fluid intake 292
    The hen's egg 297
    Oils for human consumption 301
    What about potatoes and white foods? 310
    The most important hormone you probably haven't heard of ..313
    Soups and rice dishes with everything 318
    Physical exercise 326

Chapter IX The Intelligent Consumer.................................... 335
    Synthetic coatings continue to be endocrine disruptors............348
    Recycling culture and other issues..354
    The power of one 365
    Final reflection 392

Introduction

Years ago, I realized that there was something wrong with people of all ages. Many of them are overweight, if not obese, irrespective of how much sport they may have done. We're not talking about the few extra pounds that come with age or a sedentary lifestyle, which many consider normal, but of weight that poses a risk to health. Some people, of course, are in denial about their weight, while others have become resigned to it. However, such acceptance or denial by society will have serious consequences in the western hemisphere where the problem of being overweight is now pandemic. "It's normal. Take these pills to lower your cholesterol; try going on a diet; do some exercise, and I'll see you in three months," many specialists tell their patients to justify their own karma. Being overweight or obese is, in fact, a major disease and not just a simple factor that triggers all manner of symptomatic conditions, some of which will prove lethal.

As I looked in the mirror, even though I was sporty in my youth, I realized that I had, like my father, also gained a lot of weight. This led me to think that there was something here, and if I didn't figure out what it was, I was inevitably going to get sick like he did. When hypertension and then diabetes spontaneously appeared, sustaining his life with conventional medicine came at a high cost. Worse still, I would also have the conviction that "things are still fine and under control. I feel healthy and I feel good, so I don't need to do anything. Besides, I carry it in my genes, and I will just have to get used to dealing with it for the rest of my days". I understood that something very bad was happening to everyone and that humanity is ignoring it.

This uneasiness led me to undertake a thorough investigation. And I am well aware that guides suggest doing a checklist of things. However, I ask you, in advance, to be patient. I can't help it: my macro vision as an architect urged me to include certain topics that do not seem to be closely related to nutrition and health, but rather to the title of the book. Ultimately, my main goal is to make you think.

The first thing I discovered is that we move between three realities: the first of which is the predominant reality that drives our daily lives; the second is its antipode, which I intend to scrutinize; the third is the spiritual reality. I know from experience that all this information will serve to open your mind, so that you can establish your own position, perhaps a very different one from the usual, so that you can successfully face this issue of being overweight or obese. Now, contrary to what the prevailing reality insists is due to genetic factors —which it tries to control with medication— what is really passed from generation to generation is bad eating habits, conflated by little, if any, education in nutrition. This was my first conclusion.

Not by coincidence, as I will illustrate below, I later discovered that everything is connected and that coincidences do not exist, because everything has a reason for being, even if we do not instantly understand it.

Before my very eyes, on the Internet, there was an eye-catching advertisement: "Lose weight without starving". Immediately, I asked myself: "What's so new about this and what's behind this ad?" It was a book. I found the book, *The Truth About the Six Pack Abs*, by Michael D. Geary, a nutritionist and personal trainer. Mike Geary (2006) has a cutting-edge way of thinking about nutrition and health issues; his view is distinctive and differs from the mainstream. I will repeatedly convey many of his concepts in this book, because science in the 21ST CENTURY has given us the tools to rediscover and refine concepts about nutrition and health.

I put Geary's concepts into practice and, in addition to losing weight gradually without starving myself, my life changed radically. Of course, I can't say for sure that it will continue like this, but since then I have not gotten sick at all. I don't remember the last time I caught the flu, and I have never been vaccinated against seasonal influenza —a vaccine which these days is given a different name each year. When something bad happens, I set out to investigate it. This didn't happen recently. Twice a year an alarm is triggered by the change of season that foreshadows extreme cold or heat. This fortunate beginning led me to immerse myself in topics that opened my mind to view life differently and, without even considering it, my cognitive processes over several years revealed to me other realities on different planes. Unexpected turns in a series of my own articles and those of health and nutrition professionals, closely related to the title of this book, revealed the parallels that I always suspected existed.

Thus, for example, in a world parameterized by numbers, time and money, statistics dictate life expectancies consistent with the bad habits promoted by the food and pharmaceutical industries. Also, in the media, the aims of alternative medicine are questioned and challenged by conventional medicine. Reality and truth differ. Being certain does not always mean being right. It is only right if it is supported by greater knowledge. That is why I propose we explore together the spectrum offered by a broader tripartite reality; perhaps it will lead us to different truths: the figures change.

From these first lines, I make it clear that the purpose of this book is to review history so that the readers can mitigate, reject, change, or mature any previous concept. And with the help of 21ST century technology and a deeper examination, they can establish clear educational notions to undertake the search for good health and, perhaps, also find the longed-for longevity.

Thanks to my research, I found my ideas fully coincided with the position of many people, among them Foster and Kimberly Gamble — Foster Gamble, heir to Procter & Gamble, and Kimberly Carter Gamble, his wife —, whom you can read in several languages, see, hear, and contact at www.thrivemovement. com. I say coincidence because, like them, during these years of processing my experience, I believe I have developed the ability to drive on this three-lane highway — as they describe it, usually navigating in the middle lane, parallel to the prevailing reality — and have achieved sufficient balance to fulfill my raison d'être. I emphasize that true judgment in these matters is only consolidated by personal experience. With this attitude you will avoid bland discussions with others; and, in the end, based on these novel concepts, you will enjoy resounding success; but above all, it will be thanks to your self-belief, your determination and your persistent educational effort.

In the world we live in, at least three realities coexist. If you face them, their sizes are proportionally based on acquired knowledge:

The first of these three realities — the dominant one — is perpetuated because it has everything going for it: it belongs to the world of the obvious and it is there so that you won't even try to go beyond what you see. And you couldn't anyway because you would be driving in the, high-speed lane. This daily experience, which the natural development of societies provides, is nothing more than a conforming reality, a great success in itself, because all the good things we obtain through its advances exist for our comfort and our best performance. But in exchange it has robbed us of the most precious thing in our daily lives: time for personal use and time for family in this mad race to attain its ruling value: money.

This reality is mainstream, and its speed does not allow us to stop and think about what is happening; we just accept the information we are given about ourselves. Again, in conformity, we assume that the big companies — especially the oil companies — do their best to give us alternative, safe, clean and cheap energy; that the pharmaceutical industry offers us all conceivable medicines, products of their research, to alleviate our physical ailments; and that we can fully trust the food and personal consumption products sold by supermarkets and stores because advertising assures us of the benefits of the products we need. But we forget that the main objective of all these is to sell.

In this first lane, trust is our companion on the road. We count on those who govern our destinies to have a certain suitability for the task but allow that they have no responsibility for the results or their consequences. We do this because we believe that our leaders, who are evolving and developing too, seek the common welfare of humanity at all costs. This dominant reality is presented every time you turn on the television, the radio or read the press, and it is based on the conviction that we were all born in the human paradigm of fear and ignorance. This paradigm is translated into the information media characteristic of this reality: television, press, radio, internet. The news always makes us alert, attentive and to feel constant fear and distrust of our neighbors, because this reality also maintains that war and hunger are inevitable and necessary; and, if you believe otherwise, you are naïve and innocent. Therefore, this reality also possesses the quality of calming or altering minds through dogmatic religious justification.

Reality is a very persistent illusion.

ALBERT EINSTEIN

Then there is the second lane, in which you decide how fast to go, and even stop to think. The reality of the first lane starts from the belief that violence is one of two resources to change things. It presents the violence as cyclically linked to the history of humanity, and for that reason, it makes use of force.

Contrary to this, education — the resource of the reality of the second lane — is the replacement for violence and has always been the way to change the world. Unfortunately, education has been manipulated in favor of doctrines in alliance with polities; many of which have manipulated it in order to trample democracy — the true resource of change — and favor vested interests.

Development should be measured by education and not just by numbers, productivity, and money, as is still claimed. Education that dignifies the being is the way forward; an education with free access to human knowledge that is already available on the Internet at the click of a mouse. The Internet — ironically in relation to the way we use it to navigate in either of the two lanes — became detached from the first reality because nobody visualized its reach. The reality of the second lane allows us, in many cases, to arrive at the truth and gives us access to all of history; to all the necessary information, but to disinformation as well. Contrary to its solid and successful impact as a tool of the mainstream, disinformation forces the second reality to investigate in depth and to scrutinize sufficiently to consolidate a true and proper criterion, which is part of an education that today can no longer be controlled. Such a criterion must be demanded and protected, because through it you can find out the reality that the first lane has never directly given you: an education that teaches you to think instead of an education that teaches you to obey.

The reality of the second lane, the lowest speed lane, is the reverse of the first lane which masks the enormous disparity of wealth. 80% of global financial resources are owned by 8% of the world's population. This reality motivated the Indignant Movement and its "we are the 99% of humanity governed and manipulated by the 1%". This slogan, however, does not do justice to those nations that manage their treasure honestly.

In fact, the reality of the second track exposes the failure of the first track, which is shown, paradoxically, in the success of the dominant reality: those who own most of everything want it all, and today they almost do own it all. That worldview believes it is okay for a small group to control the rest of us, since, no matter which area of the economy, banking, health, pharmaceuticals, energy, technologies or weapons, the same names and the same companies inevitably reoccur and intersect, as they do whatever it takes to keep things as they are.

This second reality makes for an uncomfortable discussion in social circles, since we have been taught that there are only two antagonistic political positions: the right and the left. The first is based on the protection of free enterprise and the right to private property. However, now, in the 21ST CENTURY, it requires imminent modification as it is displaying the errors which need to be corrected or eliminated. The other position had a valuable beginning, being founded on social sense, but ended up crashing and burning on the absurdity of communism, which castrates individual freedoms and conscience. In the first reality, when you question the establishment, you are either right or left; that is, being part of the paradigm fully justifies the signaling, and this is reason enough for discomfort.

In the second reality, which is open to the contribution that you can offer, it is not yet understood that paths focused on bringing novelty to what already exists are being freely developed in it; a novelty that is born from your own criteria provided you by education. Thus, positive changes and the redistribution of wealth arise from within the being, not in an imposing or authoritarian way as many believe, nor as others claim through the use of violence and wars. Accordingly, an attitude of positive and silent perception of things teaches you to observe whereas an attitude of negative and noisy perception simply will not let you see.

The third reality is intrinsic. It has no speed, no time, no place and is not directed by any lane. It is the reality of the spirit. Now, each of us has our own version of what spirituality is, and of all that supports and enriches the meaning of that version. The spirit is something inherent to the being, which goes beyond our rational mind, and definitely transcends the two previous realities.

We could not talk about spiritual reality without mentioning some basic definitions of the three main Eastern philosophical trends before Jesus.

Confucius: his philosophy says that man is born good, with the five virtues inscribed on his heart. Tolerance, kindness, benevolence, charity, and justice are virtues that — as an ideal — constitute a possibility which is open to all people but is then lost through apathy. It is all in the heart of man.

Buddha: in the search to overcome desires and to depersonalize the ego, *Siddhartha* talks about redeeming and teaching to change wrong behavior by example and personal work. He gives importance to emotion and affect in self-improvement.

Tao: *Lao-Tse* suggests that in the continuous search for self-perfection man should be spontaneous and natural, without laws or impositions, with an emphasis on an integrity that relies on its own strength and does not depend on the opinion of others. He stresses the courageous character that sacrifices himself for others without thinking too much about himself.[1]

When someone sets out to question the prohibitions or limits of thought — including dogmas — and fails to fully satisfy his concerns, he gives up the search for knowledge. He tends to settle in unjustified reiterative positions; does not test other paths; reaffirms and conforms to the mainstream. In its fixity, the paradigm has survived generation after generation, using the mainstream as the ideal environment to gain a foothold. These paradigms are the social response to impositions; "truths" that explained something at the time to the satisfaction of previous generations. In response to fear, paradigms are accepted without discussion in any era; but if they come from a religious authority, they easily become dogmas.

In my spirit and in my inner self, I find reasons to think that spirituality invites discovery. Because it does not invent, it frees the conscience and does not need rules because it is pure. I am sure that you, too, first heard the word "spirituality" in a religious setting. In their original objectives, religions were clothed in deep spirituality to deal with the great enigmas of existence. But later, in the midst of their institutionalization, doctrines turned those religions into structures that were inevitably contaminated by the vested interests of the different human groups, which, sheltered by ironically similar beliefs and the attachment to the sacred in a single book, have become intolerant and have become a reason for disunity rather than union. This is because they are, above all, human and so have NOT been able to remain exempt and oblivious to the great

---

[1]   Kuo Tsao, Carlos Bazterrica & Ricardo Bisignani (1998): *Vital energy in motion*, p. 16.

paradigm of fear and ignorance. Even so, spirituality persists, survives adversity, and tries to find the truth, including in the sacredness that may be within each book.

The attitude you take when solving this topic reveals the possibility of your falling (or not) into a deep religious fanaticism. Spirituality is not inculcated. It is not indoctrinated. It is your inner voice which you must always seek, and because you discover it, assume the consequences of your actions without accepting what anyone tells you it is or is not.

Each of us has a version of what spirituality is. I tend to find its nourishment deep in the love that emanates from the constant connection with the bipolar energy of the quantum universe. I feel a special bond with the positive energies that have transcended to the present day and sustain balance in my spirit.

According to scientists, there is a single inexhaustible source of energy that becomes powerful when transcended. In the Future World section of Ellen's Energy Adventure Pavilion (1996-2017) at the EPCOT (Experimental Prototype Community of Tomorrow) theme park, located in Central Florida, millions of people listened and learned in a didactic way — in the human context, according to Einstein — that this inexhaustible source is *brain power*, i.e., the "power of the mind".

Behold its immensity! That latent and inexhaustible source of energy that it creates by releasing — in the way of love that attracts or repels — in the midst of its gravity — for it too contains its opposite pole of repulsion —, was created by that Love which surrounds us today and invites mental development. Its power transcends because it comes from a human brain; the one that some time ago reminded the world of the unique ethical rule: "Do not do to others what you would not want them to do to you". And assured of feeling its great energy, without any religious connotation, it empowers my existence day by day. In fact, my spirit is more attached to the power and strength in Jesus between his twelfth and thirtieth year than to anything else written or interpreted by other people about him. But, as to his life in the intervening 18 years, we supposedly have no clue as to what happened to him. Today we know that, since the FIRST century, at least thirty documents were written — the good news, or the Gospels —, which together with the circumstances that arose due to the geopolitical crisis experienced by the emperor Constantine, who ruled the Roman Empire in the FOURTH century, only four were validated and recorded in the Bible after the first Council of Nicaea in 325 AD.

Attracting, binding, and repelling -reacting- is the fundamental gravitational characteristic of the creative forces that gave rise to the *big bang* theory. These creative forces may be related to indirectly observed dark matter and dark energy in the universe. And the *big bang* theory is, paradoxically — because of the eternal condemnation of paradoxes — the closest thing to the only credible dogma that is impossible to reveal. For this reason, and in spite of its chaotic approach, I consider the *big bang* to be a creationist theory as well. I find this theory very close to God (Allah, Yahweh or whatever you want to call the Creator), because around the world — despite the fact that many other words define him — Love will always be his name.

What a good time to implore that in my spirit, as I write, anxieties may not take precedence, and that I may then address reason with moderation and kindness. Now, to reiterate, the fact that education is summed up in a before and an after — a before in which you swim in ignorance, and fears are your limit; and an after in which knowledge presents consciousness as the basis to have an attitude that leads you to fulfillment and enlightenment. I know I am not the only one who shares the idea that eagerness

— provided by knowledge and an open mind, hand in hand with creativity — will be the only way for humanity to prepare itself to take the great leap and make the change that is coming.

Did I mention the word "enlightenment"?

Have you noticed that talking about "enlightenment", since 2012, is now an accepted topic in the social sphere and that, long ago, whoever risked pronouncing that word in public was branded as crazy?

On the metaphysical plane, a fact is passing unnoticed. Commercial science has ceased to refer to the most transcendental crossing in the universe that planet Earth and humans have experienced. This is the one the Mayans described in their prophecies as the change towards a new era, the crossing of the threshold of time and no time. Time, however, does not exist; it is a human invention to measure intervals and routes in spatiality; an illusion that, after ordering us, ended up limiting us. It also happened, for the better, that by crossing this threshold simultaneously, our senses — responding to an evolutionary adjustment — have concluded a phase of development and we have begun to focus, as theorized by Max Planck, on the perception of the total information and collective consciousness, which is found in a universal energetic whole communicated from the emotions. This goes beyond the scientific plane of the current limits of quantum physics that explain this phenomenon. As a science, its objective is to establish what is true when it is scientifically proven.

Have you ever experienced the feeling of knowing something unusual about certain topics? In other words, do you have knowledge about topics that you have not studied in any book or learned in any documentary or audiovisual media, about which you can speak with propriety in any circle or gathering? You are not the only one. Quantum physics scientists know it because this phenomenon has been already explained by several experiments. In one of them, they managed to split a photon — a particle of light, which is light itself — and to move its two halves seventeen kilometers apart; when certain stimuli were transmitted to one of the distanced and separated halves, everything that was imparted to one part caused exactly the same reaction in the other part, despite the lack of physical contact and, one assumes, their also being in a vacuum. This suggests and confirms that there is an intelligent and conscious energy that connects everything.

When the day comes that this reality has been assimilated and become part of common knowledge, it will no longer be argued that everything is connected; nor that the reason everything exists is in response to the natural balance posed by all connected energies, whose constant tendency is to verify their own balance. The irony lies in the human superego which requires us to be alive to verify it. In your today, past, present, and future are equivalent as every instant is the same; time literally does not exist.

Another good experiment that anyone can do at home is to put two plants in different pots, one with loud music and the other with classical music; the one stimulated with classical music grows beautiful and vigorous, while the one stimulated with loud music barely survives. The same happens with two glasses of water. Under the microscope, the molecules of water stimulated with loving feelings and harmonious music appear orderly and symmetrical; the opposite happens with water molecules exposed to noise and expressions of hate and disaffection, which appear disfigured and asymmetrical. This latter negative experience is also observed when water is boiled in a microwave oven. Conclusion: feelings and the environment directly affect the DNA of living organisms and living beings.

The macromolecule DNA, *deoxyribonucleic acid*, is a part of all cells and contains all the genetic information that actively or inactively has been involved in the development and functioning of known living organisms and, therefore, although it is responsible for their hereditary transmission, it can be affected, changed, or modified. The experiment also established that water — the most common and least studied compound — has feelings. In the East they have always understood this, which is why a good tea is not made with boiling water or burnt water; it is made with hot water, just before it reaches boiling point. For this reason, teakettles have a whistle that sounds when the first steam comes out of the spout and the water is removed from the heat source, so that its impulse offers the infusion its greatest potential.

The mainstream accustoms us to take explanations for granted only if they come from the scientific consensus on the prevailing reality. This leaves very little room for other hidden truths that you may well discover.

When, in 1900, Max Planck — the father of quantum physics, the science that studies the smallest particles; the unseen; the air and the light itself; which makes everything have order and sense; form and texture; color and location in space — theorized, he gave us the possibility of understanding subjects that in the past were only vaguely intelligible in the scientific, ecclesiastical, and intellectual spheres. Such matters could hardly be digested by the average reader and have always had a distinct taboo, due to the conceptual confrontation between the three positions.

His theory has been proven, thanks to current technology, and the writers and researchers who explain the science and real-life experiments that endorse its veracity. Gregg Braden, in his book *The Divine Matrix: Crossing the Barriers of Time, Space,*

Miracles and Beliefs (2007), details its scope and conclusions by describing them through easy-to-understand stories that demonstrate the truth, with scientific experiments about how "powerful" "emotions" are, and how they "connect us all in the same universal spiritual web". He also explains how the universe we see outside is a reflection of what is inside ourselves.

Are we heading towards a collective enlightenment? Evolution is bringing it to us. Shouldn't we go out to meet it? In facing the three realities, I must conclude that in most of us the only reason that limits us is latent: our stubborn persistence in continuing to cling to our beliefs.

So, *what are we going to eat today?* The answer to this daily question lingers in the family and, in principle, is a matter of habit and the natural instinct to satisfy a fundamental physical need. Some are fortunate enough to eat — between meals and snacks — at least five times a day, and out of habit have included vegetables, salads, and fruit all in moderate portions. To be sure, most of these people are unaware of why fruit — and especially citrus fruits — should be eaten only on an empty stomach to provide their benefits.

Let's get down to business. I hope you enjoy the book as much as I did reading, researching, and compiling the information to expand my knowledge. These articles are extremely innovative, and with them, you will also be able to help other people. I myself confirmed the facts through practice, through my feelings, in the mirror and with the scales; and, of course, I lost weight without starving myself. I connected with the body I inhabit and learned to listen to it until I understood what Mike Geary clearly defines: the human body is "a fat burning machine and not a fat storage machine".

In this book, I will try to recover something we have lost sight of: common sense. And with the application of new knowledge, I will try to break old schemas so that we will be able to deconstruct paradigms and beliefs. The simple right to doubt will give you sufficient pause to put it into practice and verify it for yourself.

"Those who dream by day are cognizant of many things which escape those who dream only by night." EDGAR ALLAN POE

Chapter I

And What Did We Eat Yesterday?

This question has a clear focus and the right educational perspective, because long before we developed our tastes, they were already ingrained in us before we were born. Later, anxiety, uneasiness and hunger caused us to put into our mouths anything in front of us that we identify as food. But is it really food? Today's animal instinct differs from the natural reason that motivated our ancestors to feed. They ate to live or, better, not to die; in their constant wandering, in search of green landscapes and better climates, they needed to kill their own food. Today, supposedly in safety, most of us have set the table to partake of food and our instinct has become governed by tastes, flavors, and smells.

There is evidence that the human species — with defined bipedal characteristics — has been walking upright on this planet for more than three million years. While it is true that humans died early and that many diseases decimated their life expectancy, we still have the idea that in the Stone Age — Paleolithic, Mesolithic, Neolithic — people had a rough time, were weak and barely survived in a hostile environment.

But Stone Age humanoids had to be first and foremost healthy, strong, and athletic to cope with nature and to be able to bring the best of their genetic traits with them to ensure evolutionary success.[2] Anthropology and other related sciences support the fact that Stone Age hunter-gatherers were physically fit and healthy. Wherever they lived, archaeological remains indicate that these people did not suffer from any of the chronic diseases that afflict us today and that all their medical parameters were better than those of today's sedentary man. These correlative facts are verifiable in the research carried out with the now almost non-existent indigenous populations in the different climates of the Earth.

We are what we consume. In fact, the diet of Stone Age man consisted of freshly gathered products, fruits, vegetables and wild vegetables, bee honey and other things that issue from the bark, such as the sap of the sugar maple; natural oils such as olive and coconut oil which were not fried; nuts, some grains that they found during their nomadic wanderings in search of a better climate; also, fish, mollusks and shellfish, naturally salted by the seas of the earth. From hunting — which, in fact, did not belong to the daily diet —, they enjoyed fresh eggs, without human intervention; poultry and lean meats of all kinds from which, before fire making was mastered, all the surrounding fat was removed. Lean meats were their source of the protein vital for brain development.

That's right, according to the theory of evolution, we were only genetically 1.7% away from having stayed in the trees rocking and consuming forage, the occasional insect, and the odd small animal on very rare occasions. Our stomachs, then, would have been 40% larger, like those of chimpanzees, and much bulkier, like those of horses and cows, with greater digestive activity in order to extract the nutrients from the fiber-laden vegetarian

---

[2] Hillard Kaplan, Kim Hill, Jane Lancaster & A. Magdalena Hurtado (2000): *A theory of human life history evolution: diet, intelligence, and longevity.*

diet. This difference was down to lean meat. The evidence of evolution from anthropological studies shows that as we became hunters, our stomachs and bellies became smaller in size in favor of our brains. That decisive change occurred when our ancestors realized that eating meat greatly increased their vital energy, and gradually the bellies became smaller because they no longer needed that extra volume; then all the energy previously required by the intestines was diverted to the brain, which doubled and then tripled in size.[3]

Today we know that meat acidifies the body, but this acidification is necessary to facilitate the metabolic and enzymatic processes of brain development. Despite its relevance, we must learn to manage this intake of meat, of protein, so that in the daily balance of our digestive process alkalinity prevails over acidity, which is synonymous with oxidation.

We can eat and process virtually all types of food, at least at this point in our evolution. However, it is a fact that our developing brains are leading us towards a different future in the centuries to come. If we heed evolution, in hundreds, or thousands of years — if we still exist as a species — the vegetarian dream of never eating animal foods again could be fulfilled.

For now, we are omnivores, we eat everything. Our body has omnivore, not ruminant, characteristics: first, we have only one stomach instead of the four-compartment stomach that evolution gave ruminants; cows need it to be this way to fully digest their singular diet of grasses, salt, and molasses. Secondly, our dental configuration presents the three dentitions that define omnivores — chimpanzees, bears, pigs, hedgehogs, coatis, mice, squirrels, skunks, turtles —, because in addition to molars similar to those of cows for ruminating, we have incisors at the front,

---

[3]   Loren Cordain (2011): *La dieta paleolítica*, pp. 52-53. Buenos Aires: Urano.

which are knives to cut with the lateral movement of the jaw — an exclusively human peculiarity — the meat that — if we did not use knife and fork — we would tear from the bones of the animals. Finally, we keep four canine teeth of good size to hold on to the prey during the bite, which are perfectly visible in any heated discussion between humans and during the occasional soccer game.

This Paleolithic diet is the one that has been consumed by mankind for practically its entire history. Today it has six basic rules:

Eat as much lean meat, fish, and seafood as you can.
Eat as many non-starchy fruits and vegetables as you can.
No cereals.
No legumes.
No dairy products.
No processed food.[4]

Let's take as a reference the finding of Lucy (*Australopithecus afarensis*), who lived about three million years ago, and let's do this mental exercise: three large boards, each one corresponding to one million years, and divide them into one hundred horizontal and one hundred vertical parts. On the last board, that last little square of the grid you drew represents the moment when everything changed during the Neolithic Age more than ten thousand years ago: with the beginning of the agricultural revolution, man went from hunting wild animals and gathering wild fruits to agriculture and abandoned nomadism to build permanent settlements. And the domestication of animals provided another product: milk. He then switched to eating pastured meats and concentrated on comfortably consuming

---

[4]   Loren Cordain (2011): *La dieta paleolítica*, p. 33. Buenos Aires: Urano.

foods derived from the cereals he began to cultivate, but which his ancestors had not eaten regularly: wheat, barley, soybeans, rice and much later, from America, corn, and starchy tubers such as potatoes, the universal accompaniment. Finally, at the beginning of the 19TH century, refined sugar. Refined sugar and salt are the ideal additives to captivate the consumer; in the 20TH CENTURY, almost the entire food industry focused on these six or seven generic foods and their derivatives, already processed, modified, and loaded with sugar or salt to preserve them.

In short, cereals, grains and milk became essential in the last second of food history, although they never were, and never are, essential to the human diet. We make them an everyday food and repeat portions several times a day; cereals are poor in fat, a food trend of the 20TH CENTURY; industrially loaded with sugar, they lean heavily towards omega-6 fatty acids, which are above all inflammatory. We will see later how this aversion to fats — ill-founded — favored the propagation of these products.

The mental exercise we did illustrates how this radical change in our diet occurred from one moment to the next. Having loaded ourselves with artificial calories and preservative chemicals in the food we eat is an abuse that compromises our genetic structure: we are destroying the DNA, which translates into the spontaneous appearance of previously unknown diseases.

And what happens when we consume these new things? The DNA does not recognize them easily and we are exposed to toxins. This does not mean that we suddenly become seriously ill, but it does mean that our immune system gradually deteriorates and, for example, we get frequent flus.

I would like to say congratulations to those who have submitted to the rules of the Paleolithic diet that many would be unwilling to follow. Research has advanced and found that in the nomadic wanderings they ate grains, flowers and even breads with wild cereals and reed roots, so it would not be fair to dismiss out of hand the last ten thousand years of human gastronomic history. I know well that there are other ways to lose weight, it is your decision, but we will see how prolonged fasting, and diets are not advisable.

Next, and in contrast, let's look at the typical daily intake of a young working person in North America — the variations in the menu are minimal — whose excuse is not having time to take care of his need to eat as he should and not knowing what is really going on in the body he inhabits:

For breakfast, he eats a Danish pastry — puff pastry filled with pastry cream and fruit; two cups of cereal — genetically modified... but he doesn't know it — with 8 fl oz of pasteurized and homogenized cow's milk, with a tablespoon of refined sugar or with a natural or artificial sweetener to avoid calories; and drinks a cup of coffee with a tablespoon of cream or creamer and one or two servings of sugar. Given the large amount of refined simple carbohydrates in this breakfast, which contain sugar, your blood sugar level soon drops due to the immediate release of insulin to control it, and you feel hungry again mid-morning; additionally, you feel the need for more cereals and sugar: therefore, you eat a glazed donut and drink another cup of coffee with cream and sugar or a soda.

At noon, he feels hungry again. He goes to the fast-food place near his office and orders a quarter-pound hamburger, a small portion of French fries and a 12 fl oz cola drink, this time diet and loaded with artificial sweetener to help him out a bit.

Mid-afternoon, during the break, he eats a packet of *chips* — dehydrated potato chips — of any brand, accompanied by another carbonated beverage.

For dinner, either from a supermarket on the way home or from his freezer, he gets two slices of cheese *pizza* and a small salad of iceberg lettuce with half a tomato with thousand island dressing, and all this he once again washes down with a cold 12 fl oz soda drink — this time, for a change, lemon-lime flavored.[5]

No comment.

---

[5]   Loren Cordain (2011): *La dieta paleolítica*, pp. 43-44. Buenos Aires: Urano.

Chapter II

And What Happened in the Last Century, the 20th Century?

September 11, 2014.
Grief, anger, shame.

And today only silence cries out for humanity to find the path that offers us the light capable of healing the wounds of time; a silence that today in the distance continues to walk in the minutes and days, because thirteen years after what happened, only the pain of so many families who lost their dear ones, their beloved, stands legitimate in the hopelessness of perpetuity.

Years ago, when I noticed that date on the calendar, I realized that fourteen years of this 21ST century had already passed, in the third millennium of our era, and that it was time enough to pause and objectively examine the mistakes we made in the last century in order to learn from them.

And what happened in the 20TH CENTURY? That century brought together all the development of our history. It caught up with us and we started the crazy race we are in today. Socially and economically, we had the opportunity to try conflicting policies: from the right and left axes. And with two world wars under our belts, it proved something: competition was conducive to development.

However, it is time to review history, to correct the constant that led us to extremes. The perennial mistake we have made as a society, the consequences of which are not only political, is not giving import to the education of the populace; hence the polarization of society has worsened in the 21ST CENTURY. A good example from health and nutrition, when it comes to extremes, has been salt: "From daily overdosing with its refined industrial form, we went on to develop a phobic complex against it and the myth of hypertension and salt consumption arose".[6] The same with cholesterol in relation to coronary heart disease, and with sugar and cancer. It turns out that without salt, cholesterol and sugar-minerals, fats, and glucose — just like society without education — the organism loses its vital balance.

From riding horses, we progressed to crossing the planet by plane. When industrialization began to consolidate, at the end of the NINETEENTH century, we made the great leap to the convenience of the industrial revolution. Telegraphs, telephones, ocean liners and airplanes arrived, and we began to connect to a network that produced and gave meaning to globalization. Instant communication made the world more dynamic and connected humanity through an infinity of cables and ducts that practically covered the Earth. Suddenly, at the end of the 20TH CENTURY, we got rid of the cables and connected wirelessly, at a greater distance and without touching each other. Change and progress were so rapid that smartphones appeared as useful tools, but in the process of assimilating them, anxiety was fostered, because not only do they provide information but also misinformation.

We have been dependent on fossil fuels since the 18TH CENTURY, but we have now discovered that we can exchange this non-renewable source of energy for clean and renewable sources. Humanity has gradually come to understand the urgency of

---

[6] nestorpalmetti.com/books/la-sal-saludable-nestor-palmetti/

supporting companies committed to the health of the planet, that is, those which take advantage of wind, sunlight, ocean waves, magnetism. This provides a glimpse of where we are headed.

Development allowed us to venture into outer space; and that established in our minds the concept of conquest and total dominion over this small speck in the universe, which is as borrowed and alien as our children; for their children and their children's children, this single contract is transferred as a successive loan. Therefore, the privilege of owning private property consists in taking care of the environment: protecting the flora, the fauna, the aquifers and letting the land rest, so that, when we depart, we leave it as healthy and valuable as when we acquired it to bring us prosperity. This goes beyond a simple sense of belonging, exploitation, and ego.

Land is not a gift from your parents, but a loan from your children.

MAASAI PROVERB

The true conservationist is someone who knows that the world is not an inheritance from his fathers but borrowed from his children.

JOHN JAMES AUDUBON

From there we misunderstood and began to misuse the word "globalization", focusing on quality as a sales standard. We have overlooked whether the mass consumer products, which we acquire for novelty, possess real qualities. Without a real projection of their consequences on human health, we offered these products and devices to be tested by the masses. And globalization, which became a fierce competition that crossed the fine line of common interests in the seats of government, has, today, clearly been invaded by the vested interests of the *corporatocracy* that governs us.

Corporatocracy — a neologism accepted in English, but not in Spanish — was coined by the Global Justice Movement to call attention to the role of private enterprise (and other states) as the principal creditors of national governments. Without foreseeing the consequences, governments issued bonds and other papers, as a repeated source of financing, to service the decades of enormous public debt, which inevitably caused national bankruptcy. And that fine line of common interests — the interests of the people — is violated by those unpayable debts in favor of a self-interested few. It is not in vain that for some time sociologists, journalists and economists have been warning that we must learn to live in a "permanent economic chaos".[7] Objective or consequence? The truth is that they aim to get us used to the term in order to normalize this reality.

Could they have been referring to the practice of quantitative easing which has undermined the credibility of each banknote being backed by gold? Beyond its objectives, what would happen could not be foreseen, because the risk was incalculable; and, within a short time, since it was decided to free its price, gold has achieved a value high enough to reach its equivalence in dollars. Many light-weight dollars awakened greed in people who pursue this mirage of wealth. These people, with their own hands, have dedicated themselves to the daily task of wounding and bleeding the earth to death.

---

[7]   Cornelius Castoriadis (1988): *Political and social writings*, v. 3, 1961-1979, p. 252. David Ames Curtis (trans. and ed.). Minneapolis: University of Minnesota Press.

Or do they mean that the economic recovery that would rekindle the flame of the dream has ceased to exist? No one is saying that. The widespread unemployment of almost 200 million people globally confirms another mirage. This figure is on the rise, according to the International Labor Organization (ILO). Unilaterally, the States announce their success in tackling unemployment, but those who got tired of looking for a job are no longer counted; the statistics exclude them *de facto* because their unemployment insurance does not cover them anymore and they uncomfortably passed to unreliability. in many countries, forced by circumstances, people simply disappeared off the face of the earth and, without looking back, emigrated, abandoning their homes.

The time has come to pause! We only have this one chance and, even if we don't want it, there is this frenetic urge to become involved in every awakening. Destiny has given us this vital moment in history to correct errors of principle and to discover their true origins, which have, frighteningly, been reengineered by the reality of neoliberal thinking. Along the way, we tend to cloak errors and continue to try to remedy the consequences with temporary solutions from the extremes.

Are they also asking us to accept predatory zeal? Apparently so, as we purport to reject the wisdom of nature, which has taught us so much: great discoveries, which have led to technological advances in various fields of knowledge, have been brought about through our observing it. Nature that today we strive to make disappear. The World Wildlife Fund (WWF) report in 2018 assures us that in the last forty years, because of human activity, there has been a 60% decrease in the populations of mammals, birds, fish, reptiles, and amphibians.

I know that you must be feeling uncomfortable now, not necessarily with me, because I have already been there when

I looked everywhere for someone to blame. We were taught to compete ruthlessly in order to win, to be "successful", and they turned us into human beings who don't know how to lose and who don't accept second place. This principle drove development with efficacy and rapidity, but due to our nature, competition ceased to be healthy. Today, with the persistence of educational errors, and the compulsion to win, corruption has resurged stronger than ever. So, now we must look within ourselves for the real causes of our common mistakes and, before proceeding, facilitate mutual forgiveness.

This successful career has also left us with a lot of wear and tear. When are we going to recognize what it is that prevents us from realizing the mistakes that we must correct, the ills from which we are already suffering, whose immediate result is that society has become sick or almost relieved?

We live day by day without worrying about a symptomatology and, although we are comforted by the news that the global average life expectancy at birth has increased from 71.4 in 2015 to 72 years in 2016, this claim has a big flip side. Support for that assertion, as scored by pharmaceutical companies, laboratories, and the practice of conventional medicine, which counts as success in the first lane — the prevailing reality — would lack relevance were we to remove from every person who claims to feel healthy the medications they regularly consume, and the average would drop substantially. Especially since this regular and periodic medication is given to younger and younger patients.

On the other hand, alternative medicine, in all its branches, is focused on preventing and curing as soon as symptoms appear in order to give dynamic changes of direction to the body, balance it and to stimulate self-healing. This natural medicine was already practiced by the Greek Hippocrates, the father of medicine, who enunciated: "Let your food be your medicine, let medicine be your food". Naturopathic medicine translates into eating natural and as far as possible, organic food, i.e., food that has been grown and ripened without any contact with pesticides, fungicides, or industrial herbicides. Natural medicine — misnamed alternative medicine — should be prioritized and at the forefront, but someone in the media managed to label it as "alternative"; this word has demeaned the healing power of nature. Ironically, let us cite the case of a poorly managed diabetes that worsens causing gangrene, and the harm is done: conventional medicine offers the patient antibiotics and anti-inflammatory drugs, injects him with painkillers and offers the optional — *alternative* — of successfully amputating and repairing the damage with a smart prosthesis.

So, in order to vindicate their coexistence, shouldn't we give alternative medicine the place it deserves as an ideal complement to conventional medicine? I do not mean to discredit conventional medicine, but it is not designed to cure; under the right conditions, the human body always heals and regenerates itself.

Why is it that almost every day you learn that someone you know, and seemingly at a younger and younger age, suddenly has developed a rare disease?

Simple. The industrial revolution led us to accept the fast-food industry — 1945 to the present —, which is harmful to our health, because with it, heart disease grew alarmingly. With the limited scientific resources of a few decades ago and the logic of the mainstream, that of the first lane, doctors and scientists concluded that cholesterol caused deaths through the clogging of the arteries, which, in fact, occurred. Therefore, up to the present day, cholesterol has been the villain. This is disturbing because they also knew that the body produces it naturally and the liver regulates it to displace and heal the internal inflammations that have been increasing due to the consumption of all kinds of processed meats and cereals present in fast foods; breaded foods accumulate hydrogenated and refined oils that fill the body with free radicals. The charge against cholesterol was quite well received and settled in the minds of several generations.

In time, this charge provided the enormous opportunity to provide the precise solution to the cholesterol problem and, since the mid-1970s, created another line in the economy: the diet food industry. A little earlier, in the same decade, science achieved the genetic manipulation of soybean and corn crops to make them resistant to pests and grow vigorous, larger kernels and to optimize harvests in adverse climates, which saved regions from the famine that threatened millions of people in Africa. Scientists at the time did not suspect the extent of this *success* and the consequences of greedy genetic engineering.

The *fat-free* diet industry — 1975 to the present — was the answer to the villainous cholesterol. Thus came the labels "zero cholesterol" and the most attractive for the consumer: "Zero sugar - zero calories, with our products you will lose those extra pounds and you will be able to regain your alluring figure! With the problem now solved, the fear of consuming fast-food was removed. Because the complementary solution was dietetical, a very successful alliance was established between the two industries, which increased the consumption of products from both and took almost all of us out of the kitchen. This solved another big problem: we now had more time to work and make more money.

However, industrial processes that require extremely high temperatures, for example, in the process to obtain 1% and 2% fat dietary milk, from which up to 99 and 98% of healthy fats are removed to produce other products, leave residues that become a burnt cholesterol full of free radicals that are impossible to filter. These residues do not appear on food labels because their amounts in the products of the family shopping basket are minimal — the standard of the Food and Drug Administration, FDA, contemplates that 0.05 or less is equal to 0. For decades, we have "digested" this daily dose of 0.05 free radicals.

What happens when foods are industrially stripped of their naturally balanced fats and sugars, what would their taste and composition be like?

Linked to the flow of money, the sensation of a demographic explosion that occurred in the second half of the 20TH CENTURY, which in reality corresponded to the exponential growth of humanity, was due to the fact that, seduced by industry, rural people migrated to the cities, which grew very fast. This labor force satisfied the needs of industry and filled the vacancies in the industrial plants that had arisen out of the manufacture of supposedly healthy alternatives to the saturated fats of real butter and lard. Then came the appearance of highly polyunsaturated vegetable oils from corn, soybean, canola — mostly from genetically modified seeds, GMO —, sunflower and cotton, among other crops; in addition to all their derivatives, such as spreads and dressings.

And the taste? It was invented and manufactured. Starting in the 1970s, trans hydrogenated fatty acids appeared; margarines and refined vegetable oils are rich in omega-6, inflammatory fatty acids. Most dehydrated soups and broths combine artificial sugar, salt with excess sodium, and potentially carcinogenic flavorings. Monosodium glutamate (MSG) also appears in most seasonings. Since then, sausages have contained industrial preservatives, nitrites and nitrates, colorants, emulsifiers, and additives created in the laboratory. High Fructose Corn Syrup is a reconcentrate of residual sugars obtained from genetically modified corn and, because of its low cost, has been very successful in the food industry as a replacement for cane and beet sugar; this sugar has given an exaggerated sweet taste to everything and has been established in our brains since birth; even baby milk formulas — which are supposed to replace the irreplaceable mother's milk — contain absurd amounts of this sweetener or other similar sweeteners. Today the industry is withdrawing this fructose from its products.

When this goal of offering the best quality products at the lowest price was set up this great surge included pastry and bakery products, which end up metabolized as simple absorption carbohydrates. Cereals could supply the daily fiber intake, but bread in the Western diet is poor in fiber, being manufactured in vast quantities in an industrial way: the artisan bakery has practically disappeared. Some bakers are making valiant efforts to "innovate": they are baking breads from old recipes and have decided to rescue the traditional so that their breads guarantee the fiber content provided by fresh, natural, and organic ingredients.

Once the majority had adopted the dietary habit of fast food, the solution to the damage caused by cholesterol made packaged food and industrial diet food irresistible. As a result, the constant consumption of toxins is imperceptible, though it does not lead to immediate death, which explains why many people — including doctors and scientists — who have spoken out and openly confronted the mainstream, have been removed from their professions, had their professional licenses cancelled in obscure circumstances, had their research budgets withdrawn or decimated, and their names sullied. We owe it to them to attest to our own experiment and expound the research that supports their arguments.

There has also been a constant physical weakening due to the direct effects on the DNA that is transmitted from generation to generation. This macromolecule has been affected, and is already beginning to remember this genetic factor, which is manifested in the birth of apparently healthy human offspring, who succumb more and more quickly to the same diseases as always, because they have less resistance to them. Diseases have become stronger, and have put us at a disadvantage, because their genes have mutated in face of the artificial chemical battle, we have put them through over the three previous generations; and they are becoming increasingly aggressive. This battle is led by antibiotics, hormones, and all kinds of chemicals from today's pharmaceuticals which are present in food.

In addition to this, we have been ingesting medications by the bucketload; chemicals that advertising has sold us as an indispensable product for the family shopping basket; drugs that compromise the powerful human immune system in the daily battle. We need to learn how to nourish ourselves; we need to learn how to eat, really knowing what we consume in order to find the ideal way to face and avoid the real reason for current diseases.

Inflammation is the true cause of many other diseases, especially heart disease. It does not show up in routine laboratory tests because these do not pinpoint the clues to inflammations. For example, even if cholesterol — which the liver produces naturally and in a controlled manner — were at levels above or around 200 mg/dl in the tests, providing the arteries are not inflamed internally, it would flow without risk of clogging the blood vessels. However, the valuable recommendation is to be careful with what we consume and learn to know how to keep high-density *lipoprotein* (HDL), or good cholesterol elevated and reduce low-density *lipoprotein* (LDL) or bad cholesterol.

Because of the constant attacks on our DNA, which result in the weakening of the immune system, in combination with our bad eating habits, our lack of education, our emotions and the ambient environment in which we live, we are on the verge of the manifestation of any disease from the flu to the worst cancer; and neurological, endocrinological, psychological and sexual problems could appear at any time. Oh! I forgot the obvious, although our society has not acknowledged it, the accumulation of abdominal fat, being overweight or obese, is by definition a swelling, and in itself a serious disease — an additional inflammation — which is not a simple problem.

Do you feel well? Do you feel healthy?

If you are already taking prescription medication, the answer is NO, you are not healthy, even if you feel healthy. Face it: you have to do something.

We tend to answer that question mentally as follows:

"To tell you the truth, I don't have any pain. Well, a little headache occasionally, when my children or my partner drive me crazy with questions. A feeling of weakness or tiredness? It's normal; it's reasonable that when I get home in the evening with the natural stress of work that I take a painkiller from the medicine cabinet and that's it, problem solved. Do I shake when I walk? Not much. Yesterday, I had to walk just to my brother's to get some papers because I'd lent the car to my son, who is crazy about buying those energy drinks — comparable to swallowing a fragmentation grenade which nobody knows when it will detonate — that he is going to take to this party tonight, and I got a little shaky, nothing special. What are we going to do with this tummy? It's not so big. Besides, I'm not eighteen anymore. It's normal with the routine that I have that doesn't allow me to exercise — yeah, I'm lazy —, and besides, it comes with age. But if I walked more, *would I shake* as much? I don't know. I don't remember the last time. Ah! I remember, it was on that trip to the beach with the family; we had a fantastic time, and nobody got sick, as far as I know — evading the question — and what does it matter anyway? Why do I have to walk when that's what I have a car or a motorcycle for. And you know what? The last time I had full screen tests, the ones the doctor sent me about four or five months ago, the levels were fine. The doctor told me to eat less fat because my cholesterol is a little high and he told me to take something to lower it — statins — for a few months; not to stop taking the medication for hypertension; and to try to eat less and earlier at night; he also recommended a good antacid for reflux; he suggested I try to do some exercise. What's more, I don't even smoke! At the end of the day: as long as I can walk, breathe, don't hurt and can go to work, I'll be fine.

That's the average response, the automatic reflection, when anyone under normal circumstances is asked if they feel healthy, if they feel well.

Since mid-2010, when I became fully involved in these issues, several people around me and those close to me were diagnosed with type two diabetes or high blood pressure; three of them were found to have tumors that had to be removed. Another suffered from leukemia and the doctors gave up hope for him. He refused his doctors' invitation — with no guarantees — to have chemo and radiotherapy. Given his life-or-death condition, he heeded a couple of my recommendations and began a personal battle with a severe natural detoxification plan: his platelet count has risen, from where it was near zero, to near-normal levels; also, the symptoms that had gradually appeared and, according to his doctors, would increase, ceased. Now, he is well past the predicted time.

I'll let you now read a free article from the team of nutritionists at Prograde Nutrition, a laboratory that, in addition to selling, also generates interesting and informative articles that invite you to investigate. Thanks to this, I chose them to provide me with a supplement that I needed initially as an essential part of my healing process. I recommend it because we need to add it to the system, due to its deficiency in relation to the fatty acids that we consume and that the Western diet does not sufficiently supply: the anti-inflammatory omega 3 fatty acid.

You live with this killer, and you don't know it yet?

Jayson Hunter, RD, CSCS

Are you one of the forty-seven million Americans affected by this health problem? If you are, you are probably also one of the many who had never heard of metabolic syndrome before their doctor told them they have it.

The lack of awareness about this problem is worrisome because metabolic syndrome is avoidable and preventable. It is a condition that arises from many different risk factors, so it is vital that you learn more about it.

Statistics suggest that metabolic syndrome may be one of the most prevalent diseases in our country — the U.S. Japan already considers it one of its priority health concerns.

One third of Americans have symptoms of this disease and sooner or later another third will also be diagnosed.

According to the American Heart Association, metabolic syndrome is classified as a group of metabolic risk factors that includes:

Abdominal obesity — excessive fat around the abdomen

Dyslipidemia — high triglycerides, low HDL cholesterol and high LDL cholesterol.

Arterial hypertension

Insulin resistance or glucose intolerance

High C-reactive protein in the blood — this symptom warns of internal inflammations and infections.

Several research studies are currently underway to help combat this disease. A recent study at Tufts University indicated that vitamin C and vitamin E deficiencies may be partly responsible for this syndrome. The study, however, showed that metabolic syndrome was more prevalent in overweight people.

I still don't know what we are overlooking in the causes of this deficiency, but we know for a fact that excessive abdominal fat leads to glucose intolerance and insulin resistance. This has already been well documented.

Actually, all of these symptoms are reduced if you lose excess fat and increase your exercise. These two things have the greatest impact on reversing metabolic syndrome. They are also powerful decisions you can make to reduce the effects of metabolic syndrome if you have already been diagnosed.

Thermogenesis is one of the keys to increasing your metabolism. If you are able to increase your metabolism, you will immediately activate fat loss and burn more calories — thermogenesis consists of eating foods that the body requires more energy to process than they provide and, therefore, burns more calories. An apple provides sixty calories, and the body spends eighty calories digesting it.

When you lose fat, you have less abdominal fat; this lowers your blood pressure and can even improve your insulin sensitivity. If you use muscle toning and other higher intensity workouts after weight loss, you will increase your metabolism, increase your HDL cholesterol and you can also regain your insulin sensitivity.

Losing 5 to 10% of your body weight can reduce blood pressure according to the American Heart Association. If you change your eating habits and try to decrease or even get rid of the simplest carbohydrates such as potatoes, rice and added sugars, your triglycerides will be reduced.

Simple changes like these can prevent you from most of the causes of metabolic syndrome so you won't be affected by it and can stay away from an eventual diagnosis of diabetes.

If you are one of the forty-seven million Americans already affected by this, you obviously know you need to make these changes right now. If you are overweight but have not yet been officially diagnosed with this disease, it's only a matter of time before you are.

Make the decision now to decrease these risk factors, eat more lean protein and less simple carbohydrates and sugars, build muscle with higher intensity and consistent exercise to burn more calories and create new toned muscle mass. Finally, and most importantly, lose weight, which will begin to correct many of these risk factors immediately.

Why should you follow these tips? Although I am not a nutritionist, doctor or scientist, my simple answer is that my perseverance in the search for information led me to certain reflections and revelations that I wish to share.

Information is just a click away. In the last century, the patient "belonged" to the doctor and there were filters against achieving improvement and prosperity, related to the cost of education. This concept made us believe that education was the privilege of a few and that we should only believe in someone with a professional degree certificate hanging on the wall. For this reason, we could not even give an opinion on subjects other than our profession.

Nowadays, with an investment of will and minimal costs, we can acquire online accurate information and the education we need. At the same time, you can get rid of what they convinced you and, not only that, since you know more, you will be able to charge more for your work. Don't do it just to know more; do it to unknow less.

How about you? Is it your time to break out of the stagnation in which humanity finds itself? Stick with me with the goal of focusing on good health, or learning how to regain it if necessary, and you will find that losing weight will be just a corollary.

We are not alone

What is the largest organ in the human body? That's right, the skin. The skin — which includes the scalp — is the membrane that covers almost the entire large cell that is the body. Due to its permeability, this strong and delicate lining interacts with the environment and serves as both a filter and a receptor, as its extraordinary sensors allow us to feel.

In the last century, development has brought us skin care products that are easy to apply. Industry has perfected and developed all those products with which we come into contact: soaps, shampoos, conditioners and hair dyes, sunscreens, makeup, shaving creams, depilatories, toothpastes, mouthwashes, cleansers, and moisturizers. And in indirect contact, products used in the home, such as disinfectants, air purifiers, fragrances, soaps for the kitchen, floors, carpets, glass, curtains; there are also soaps and fabric softeners of all forms and colors for washing clothes.

These industries developed their products using chemical ingredients obtained in the laboratory and tested on animals for certification by the US Food and Drug Administration (FDA). But today's technology has shown that the animal research that established the safety parameters for human utilization of these ingredients was almost in vain.

Although that observation phase is over, we are still in the trial and time has shown that we all participate in these experiments on a daily basis. We are subjected to the constant emission of radio waves and, when we sleep with our cell phones on, we do not perceive the damage they do to our brains, or to our reproductive system when we carry them in our pockets for long periods of time. Something similar happens with the microwave oven that is one of the appliances in the modern kitchen. We can educate ourselves to have a preventive attitude without doing without them.

The Environmental Working Group (EWG), founded by Ken Cook and Richard Wiles, is a non-profit, donation-driven organization. Since its foundation in 1993, this interdisciplinary group of scientists has analyzed bottled water and products already on the market to identify the ingredients in their formulas, the radiation emissions of cell phones by brand and model and ranks them on a scale of 0 to 10 in relation to their toxicity to humans, other living creatures and planet Earth. The EWG focuses on cosmetics, cell phones, agro-industrial products and everything that affects human beings and the environment.

Constituted as the FDA's counterpart in the second lane, on its website www.ewg.org you can choose — among more than three hundred companies — brands that, in addition to respecting the planet, have chosen to list the chemicals they do NOT contain and that we should avoid, with healthy products that they try to position in low-cost stores. People do not massively buy these products because they are not of a known brand. But we can stop buying specific brands and focus on learning to buy ingredients.

Since 1972, soaps have been advertising the great wonder: "Now with triclosan! EWG research found that triclosan belongs to the group of mutagenic and carcinogenic hormone disrupters, like parabens and BPA (bisphenol-A) present in plastic containers and canned goods, which merits a separate article below. It should be noted that, after forty years, the FDA banned the sale in the United States of soaps containing triclosan and triclocarban on September 2, 2016.

We come into contact with all these products several times a day. That's why we should learn to read labels and know if exactly what we are putting on our hair, mouth, eyebrows and eyelashes, nails or skin contains potentially hazardous ingredients.

Below, I will introduce you to some of these toxic ingredients. Let's start with the easiest one to remember in deodorants: aluminum in the form of aluminum hydrochloride. A study published in the *Journal of Applied Toxicology* has shown that aluminum is not absorbed by the body, but is deposited in breast tissue and concentrated in the nipple as a liquid that descends from the breast duct tree. The researchers determined that this concentration was very high in women with breast cancer compared to levels in healthy women and may suggest that elevated aluminum levels serve as a biomarker to identify those at increased risk of developing breast cancer.[8]

---

[8] Ferdinando Mannello, Gaetana A. Tonti, Virginia Medda, Patrizia Simone & Philippa Darbre (2011): '*Analysis of aluminium content and iron*

On the back labels of products, among the ingredients, you will find up to three different types of parabens — methylparaben, propylparaben and butylparaben — in deodorants, shampoos, depilatory creams, soaps, or shower gels, which are also used as preservatives in frozen and packaged foods. Multiple studies indicate that the methyl, propyl, and butyl forms of parabens interfere with the functioning of the endocrine system and are stored in body tissue and interfere with glandular activity and hormone production because they increase estrogen production. Closely related to breast cancer in both women and men, molecular biologist Philippa Darbre of the University of Reading and colleagues claim that the type of paraben esters found in breast tumors come from their application on the skin by the use of deodorants, creams or underarm *sprays.*[9] Researchers at Kyoto Prefectural University of Medicine in Japan found that methylparabens in sunscreens increase sensitivity to sun damage, i.e. when you are exposed to ultraviolet rays, skin cells die at a much faster rate than normal and aging is accelerated. By the way, avoid deodorants with artificial fragrances, which are usually allergenic.[10]

Hair straightening keratins and many shampoo formulas contain formaldehyde, which has been linked to a specific form of leukemia and is genotoxic in animals and humans, meaning it

---

homeostasis in nipple aspirate fluids from healthy women and breast cancer-affected patients'. Journal of Applied Toxicology, 31 (3), 262-269.

[9] Philippa Darbre, Adil Aljarrah, William R. Miller, Nick G. Coldham, Maurice J. Sauer & Gerald S. Pope (2004): *"Concentrations of Parabens in Human Breast Tumours". Journal of Applied Toxicology, 24* (1), 5-13.

[10] Osamu Handa, Satoshi Kokura, Sakoto Adachi, Tomohisa Takagi, Yuji Naito, Toru Tanigawa, Norimasa Yoshida & Toshikazu Yoshikawa (2006): *"Methylparaben potentiates UV-induced damage of skin keratinocytes". Toxicology, 227* (1-2), 62-72.

directly affects DNA, and is already considered carcinogenic by the World Health Organization (WHO).[11]

As for makeup with mineral ingredients, some contain iron oxide, nickel, or lead, banned since 1989 in various industries — toys, paints, construction — for being highly carcinogenic. Hypoallergenic cosmetics do not contain them.

Synthetic fragrances containing oxybenzone-benzophenone-3 — present in soaps, shampoos, sunscreens, skin creams and laundry detergents are allergenic and produce adverse hormonal reactions. You can avoid them if you look for the *phthalates-free* label on these products: "More than 2,500 fragrance ingredients are used in perfumes and scented consumer products, such as cosmetics, detergents, fabric softeners and other household products to impart a specific, usually pleasant scent. As these ingredients can cause skin irritation or allergic reactions, there has been a list of twenty-six substances that must be identified in products to inform consumers since 1999".[12]

Propylene glycol, a strong chemical solvent used as an antifreeze, is also used as a humectant in pharmaceuticals, cosmetics, food, and tobacco products and as an ingredient in intimate genital lubricants. Make sure that products in contact with the skin do not contain propylene glycol or other petroleum derivatives, such as mineral oil, liquid kerosene, petrolatum, ozokerite, ceresin and microcrystalline wax. Specialists say that

---

[11] Robert G. Liteplo, R. Beauchamp, Mary Elizabeth Meek & Richard Chénier (2002): *Concise international chemical assessment document 40, Formaldehyde.* Geneva: World Health Organization. http://www.who.int/ipcs/publications/cicad/en/cicad40.pdf?ua=1

[12] European Commission, Health & Consumers, Scientific Committee on Consumer Safety, SCCS (2012): *OPINION on Fragrance allergens in cosmetic products, SCCS/1459/11,* The SCCS adopted this opinion at its 15th plenary meeting, 26-27 June 2012. http://ec.europea.eu/health/scientific_committees/consumer_safety/docs/sccs_o_102.pdf

many toxins are not harmful in small quantities, but they are if used daily... BPA (bisphenol-A) is also present in most ordinary sex toys.

Nanoparticles in lotions, anti-aging creams and sunscreens with a sun protection factor higher than 50 disrupt the normal growth of the skin and could cause the opposite effect: the appearance of wrinkles. The ingredients of these sunscreens are extremely strong, e.g., toxic titanium dioxide prevents the sun radiation necessary for any living being. In February 2020, the European Union classified titanium dioxide ($TiO2$), one of the most common white pigments used in the textile industry, as a suspected "category 2 carcinogen by inhalation".[13] It is preferable to expose ourselves to sunlight at the right times: early morning and late afternoon. Sunlight synthesizes and activates vitamin D, which allows the absorption of calcium by the bones and strengthens the immune system; it is difficult to replace with the version synthesized in laboratories.

That's not all: retinol — vitamin A — in some sunscreens may also cause cancer if exposed to the sun's rays. The EWG claims that nearly half of the five hundred most popular sunscreen products may actually increase the rate at which malignant cells develop and spread skin cancer because they contain vitamin A and its derivatives, retinol and retinyl palmitate.[14]

---

[13] European Union, EC Regulation 1272/2008: https://eur-lexeuropa.eu/legal-content/EN/TXT/?uri=uriserv%3AOJ.L_2008. 353.01.s003.01. ENG&toc =OJ%3AL%3A2008%3A353%3ATOC
and its technical update:
https://eur-lex.europa.eu/legal-content/EN/TXT/?uri=CELEX%3A02020R0217-20200218

[14] Environmental Working Group (2020): *EWG's Sunscreen Guide: a decade of progress, but safety and marketing concerns remain.* https://www.ewg.org/sunscreen/report/executive-summary/

And in industrially produced foods, colorants with numbers — such as blue 1, yellow 5, yellow 6, red 40, the caramel color used in some colas and Stout, Bock or Pale Ale style beers to give them darker tones —, combined with ammonium, and in chocolates and candies with the super-addictive high fructose corn syrup (HFCS), have generated many concerns in relation to the grams/kilogram amount of weight allowed for daily human consumption.[15] Several studies have already established that they can have harmful effects on health and have even link them to different types of cancer.

My father's question is valid: "If all these products are so bad for our health, why are they still letting them be sold freely instead of banning them?" The answer is simple: the research and development process for these products took years and considerable investment even before safety testing in the laboratory. It will be many years before these products are withdrawn from the market; not until the conceptual clash of the two lanes, the two realities, is resolved in the legal and bureaucratic realms. In practice, when these products are officially banned, for many it will already be too late, which provides space for another business: lawsuits against manufacturers.

Although bloggers who stand up to companies — such as Vani Hari of Foodbabe.com — are challenged by the mainstream in the first lane, they have already succeeded in getting fast food companies — such as Kraft, Starbucks and Chick-Fil-A — to remove one or more of these chemicals, which are harmful to human health, from their ingredients, and with popular support they continue to pressure companies to purchase purely organic

---

[15] http://www.fao.org/gsfaonline/docs/CXS_192s.pdf
https://www.who.int/news-room/fact-sheets/detail/food-additives
https://www.ecoportal.net/paises/oms-advierte-efectos-cancer-igenos-en-colorantes/

ingredients. For example, the Subway sandwich chain removed azodicarbonamide, a chemical used in the production of plastic rubber and registered as mutagenic, which can affect genes and whose toxic effects include damage to the kidneys and respiratory tract, from white bread and other products.

With human health at stake, reading labels and understanding ingredients is urgently needed to stop being naïve and to avoid using toxic products. Although the body gives you the feeling that you are used to dealing with these harmful chemicals and, because you ingest them daily, that it demands these carcinogenic preservatives, the truth is that your immune system remains low. Persevering with detoxification until the immune system is corrected will prevent any relapse into disease and, once you begin the detoxification process, in just two to three weeks, the body will assume that it will no longer receive those chemicals it was struggling with, and it will thank you for it.

The human reaction to all this information can be anger, disenchantment, indignation, rejection... When processing my anger, I decided to change direction and target myself. You change your attitude; everything changes, and you start to see other positive things. The challenge is to look objectively at the past and to amend our mistakes. Starting from individual common sense, interesting social phenomena also arise. For example, out of the economic crisis of 2008, in different areas of the planet, in face of the prevailing chaos, a new social class was born: unemployed professionals, who returning to the countryside with education that updated their knowledge, discovered that it allowed them to reinvent themselves and "turn the tables", as happened in Spain. And it happened again, across the whole world, in 2020 as a result of the pandemic. Thus, I understood that what happened in the 20TH CENTURY

also belonged to the development of societies. Caroline Myss'
perspective helped me to use all that outrage to my advantage;
to believe and grow.

Becoming aware means changing the rules by which we live
and the beliefs we hold.

CAROLINE MYSS

Chapter III

Beneficial Principles for Optimal Health and Longevity

To lay a clear foundation regarding the subject that concerns us, I include these principles, which were also the objectives and my conclusions at the beginning of the book. Keep them in mind as they are key, given that you will repeatedly encounter these same concepts, which corroborate my synthesis, in the articles referred to by 21ST century experts in nutrition and health.

But for now, I would like to contribute what in my opinion is the fundamental concept required to adapt the mind for this educational challenge to form a solid base. This practice, a pedagogical exercise, will mark a "before" and an "after" on the approach that education should consolidate in the fields of health and nutrition. Therefore, I present you:

The fundamental principle

— Son, who is do you see over there?

— It's me in the mirror, Daddy.

— And when you speak, who do you hear? Where do the words come from, you or him?

— Well, I think from me: my voice comes from me.

— And when I give you a kiss, mwah, who is feeling it, you, or him?

— Woohoo, I'm feeling it, woohoo.

— Son, I present to you..." Pointing to the mirror. The body in which you live. It simply imitates you; it cannot speak or think or feel, because you are the one who really does that. That is the human body in which you will live forever, as long as you know how to take care of it, because if you get sick it is not you; it does it because of your carelessness, but you will feel it. If you persist with carelessness, the day will come when it will most probably not allow you to live in it anymore.

— So, if I don't take care of it, will I die? Then, where will I go?

— Son, we will all only know that answer on the day it happens. People have many theories about that, and I would like you to study them all. But don't think about that anymore. What I can assure you is that, with what I have just told you, you will live many, many years, right?

— Yes, Daddy, I'm going to live forever!

Did you know, son, that the body works non-stop while you sleep at night? The heart keeps beating but much slower so that the energy saved can be used to process what you ate during the day; the body nourishes itself and takes from your food the energy you need to recharge and wake up the next day. It is the body that, as you program it with your thoughts, will wake you up in the mornings to go to school, just as on Sunday, it lets you get up later.

— Why don't I have school?

— Because you don't have school on Sundays, son. I love you!

— I love you too, Daddy.

Did you notice that I almost invariably referred to "the" body rather than using a possessive, "your" body, "my" body, or "our" bodies, during the reading? This surely raised some questions in your mind. I have been inviting you to think about it and the time has come to clarify it.

The above dialogue is a pedagogical way of avoiding, from an early age, attachment to the ego, which is itself attachment to appearances. In fact, it is an exercise of ego dissolution that should be given to children at the age of six, which is the age when the brain begins to store data, to create awareness and to naturally consolidate learning through observation. And that would also save us the embarrassment of checking in the mirror the reality of what we are and what we have become through simple carelessness. Although the body does NOT speak, we must learn to read its messages to understand it and take care of it, instead of worshiping it or, worse, hating it. We still have a lot to learn in order to know how to inhabit this marvelous container called the human body, which we insist on calling "my body".

Perhaps we will discover that the correct path to eternal youth involves, at least, reaching longevity with full faculties and without taking any prescription drugs. This is a second lane truth that has always been there, but of which we lost sight during the 20TH CENTURY, because of the illusion that others could offer it at any price, without ever thinking that the answer has always been within us.

Now, religions and even science — quantum physics — assure us that at death the body is discarded, and energy is released almost immediately. Matter and essence. Therefore, being aware that the dilemmas related to beliefs could arise from the subject of death, I feel certain in my spirit that I am NOT going to offend anyone with the following statement: each human body, being at the peak of evolution, is able to be plural or identical to another, and without requiring any rest, it always tends to function continuously as the perfect creation in which we have come to exist. Thus, imperfection occurs as an immense and inherent motive for a constant overcoming — and it is the being in each body that requires total, absolute, and periodic rest.

While having dinner at a friends' house, someone asked me if there is a special food, an elixir that restores health and postpones or delays aging; or, in the case of a specific food, would its frequent consumption prevent us from ever getting sick again. It sounds like something out of a fantasy movie, and yet it is closer to us than we can imagine. And no, I don't know of any creams, drops or pills, much less a potion; neither is there a specific food. But there is a clue: superfoods such as lemon, apple, ginger, turmeric, soursop, guava, cinnamon, kiwi, garlic, asparagus, aloe, almonds, flaxseeds, chia seeds, nori and wakame algae — a source of iodine —, quinoa, broccoli... are part of this elixir.

From Caroline Myss, PhD, I learned about holistic medicine (from the Greek *holos*, the 'whole'), i.e., the whole and each of the parts are linked through constant interactions, — this happens fully in the body —, and the energizing concept, which is also included in the whole, that is obviously harbored in this science.[16]

The true elixir is a three-part or three-step concept, because holistically speaking, if one part is missing, any chance of success is compromised. The first step is that before ingesting any naturopathic medication, superfood, or natural supplement — conventional medicines also work better this way — we must detoxify. For this, we must at least stop the consumption of toxic ingredients.

Before describing the next step, which is the core of any self-healing process, I want to mention the third step, which is the

---

[16] Caroline Myss (2006): *Anatomy of the spirit. The healing of the body comes through the soul*. Buenos Aires: Zeta Bolsillo.

culminating one; the one that reaches the peak of the objective of regaining health, which is also part of the methodology we will use to lose weight without starving ourselves. I will return to this topic later and expand on it. By the time we have achieved it, without realizing it, our lifestyle will have changed completely: it consists of accelerating the metabolism so that it works at the right speed, burns fat for energy and evacuates waste at least once, twice, or even three times a day.

Superfoods have one thing in common: in their chemical balance, they all lean toward the alkaline and therefore provide the body with alkalinity and attract oxygen, help the cells to store it, breathe it and are beneficial because they are loaded with antioxidants. Red fruits such as cherries and blackberries, dried fruits, green tea and *kombucha* tea, to name a few.

To achieve fullness of health and perhaps longevity as well, we must keep the pH tilted toward alkaline in the daily or weekly balance of what we consume and not toward *acidic*. Lemon tastes acidic but produces alkaline reactions; therein lies the miracle of fruits. The opposite of alkaline is acid, which rejects oxygen.

Holistically, the three simultaneous steps are: detoxification, which begins when we stop consuming toxic ingredients at our table and in our bathroom. By eating a higher proportion of alkaline foods, the ideal balance is achieved naturally, and the metabolism is accelerated so that the body works optimally. All this keeping in mind the fundamental concept: it is not my body; it is the body I inhabit — visible and verifiable yesterday and today in the mirror — that will allow me to live fully in direct proportion to the way I pay attention to it and take care of it. This total concept will restore your health, if you have lost it, by enabling your immune system and DNA to restore themselves, and you will lose weight and achieve wholeness.

Although other authors I quote have done so, you will notice that I do not mention physical exercise and sport. It is clear that they should be included and are absolutely necessary in the formative and growth stage, but this is not the time to mention them here, because their importance in adults is conceptually misplaced by the predominant trend; the first lane, the high velocity lane, links them to diets without first attending to being overweight, so we will take charge of the pertinent comments.

When comparing the effects of the intake of various foods in different places on Earth, it is clear that the holistic concept of applied alkalinity is the core from which optimal health and longevity are derived. And in this regard, the work of Otto Heinrich Warburg, Nobel Laureate in Physiology and Medicine in 1931, merits recognition.

Acidity vs. alkalinity

Honored in 1931 with the Nobel Prize in Physiology and Medicine for his discoveries on the nature and mode of action of respiratory enzymes, the German physiologist Otto Heinrich Warburg (1883-1970) broke new ground in the study of cellular respiration and metabolism. His subsequent research led him to present his theory on the primary cause and prevention of cancer during his speech at the Nobel Laureates' meeting in Germany in 1966.

Warburg discovered that cancer cells are anaerobic — they do not breathe oxygen — and do not survive in the presence of high levels of oxygen. On the contrary, they survive thanks to glucose, as long as the environment in which they are found lacks oxygen. Therefore, cancer would be nothing more than a "defense mechanism" that certain cells, present in the organism, have in order to continue living in an acidic and oxygen-free environment. This can be summarized as follows: healthy cells live in an alkaline and oxygenated environment, which allows them to function normally, but cancer cells live and reproduce in an extremely acidic environment devoid of oxygen. According to Warburg, cancer is the consequence of an unphysiological diet and lifestyle.

The human body is a wonderful machine. One of its most important functions is to regulate its pH levels. The pH, or hydrogen potential, is the measure of the concentration of hydrogen ions which, according to their proportion, defines the level of acidity or alkalinity that a substance may have. It is expressed on a scale from 0 to 14, and at pH 7, the solution is neutral. Between pH 7 and pH 14, the substance is alkaline, it is called a base and has the capacity to neutralize acids; the closer it is to 14, the more alkaline it is. Cells only function normally within relatively narrow pH limits. In the body, it is measured in the blood in a very narrow range from 7.35 to 7.45. If it deviates from this range, the body will become sick begin to show symptoms of illness; if it falls below 6.8 or rises above 7.8, cells stop functioning and death quickly follows. So, keeping the body functioning properly prevents cancer and many other diseases. With the body's ability to heal itself, an alkaline diet frees it from the possibility of getting sick. While doctors could educate us about this because their doctrine allows them to do so, what I'm going to explain below has more to do with the personal aspect.

Most of what we eat is acidic and only some foods are more alkaline than others. The body regulates pH through physiological processes, such as kidney function, and only you — depending on what you eat — can determine whether you add or subtract time to the body: when you eat foods with an acidic pH, you expose it to oxidation. Every time you breathe, these acids oxidize and corrode in the presence of oxygen. A body in acid imbalance is a magnet for disease, aging, and cancer.

Without leaving home, you can check your urine pH on an empty stomach with the test strips sold in pharmacies because it gives you a clue as to the state of acidity or alkalinity when you went to bed. To stay healthy, your daily intake should contain 60% alkaline foods and 40% acidic foods. If you are looking to regain your health, increase your alkaline food intake to at least **80%.**

Due to the high consumption of refined sugar, meats and processed cereals, the Western diet is fundamentally acidic. Meat, which is alkaline, becomes acidic due to the environment that the gastric juices create in order to metabolize it. Although citrus fruits taste acidic in the mouth, when ingested they become part of the alkaline elixir. Processed cheeses, animal milk, cereals, fruits in syrup, tobacco, alcohol, almost all processed foods and yogurts with dead or inactive bacilli are acidic. Also acidic are products made with refined flours and oils, that is, white bread and bakery products. Most pharmaceutical products — except for a few, such as sodium bicarbonate —, and sodas and energy drinks, are closer to dangerous drugs which could have serious and unpredictable effects when mixed with alcohol, or any other substance you ingest, and, especially, drugs.

The following fruits are very alkaline: apples, peaches, avocados, bananas and plantains, blackberries, coconut, harvested cherries — not those preserved in syrup —, dates, figs, pears, oranges, pineapple, grapes, and prunes — without added sugars —, grapefruit, melon, lemons, tangerines, strawberries and raspberries, tomato, watermelon, and tropical fruits. Most green vegetables are high in alkaline. Vegetables with high alkalinity include asparagus, dandelion, alfalfa, seaweed, watercress, broccoli, spinach, celery, fresh green beans, string beans, kidney beans, potato, or sweet potato — boniato —, squash, peas, peppers, onions, lettuce, mushrooms, Brussels sprouts, eggplant, garlic, curly lettuce, endive, cucumber, cabbage, carrots, fennel, *sweet* or *roman fennel*, beets, chestnuts, almonds, chili, tamarind, ginger, cinnamon. Some foods with high or medium alkalinity are fermented soy cheese — choose organic corn, soy, or wheat products, since at least 87% of the world's soy and corn has been genetically modified —, organic soy milk and almond milk, both without added sugar, pure or mineral water without gas, homemade vegetable broth, fresh vegetable juice, lemon water and most clear teas, such as green and white. The only alkaline whole grain cereal is millet. Infusions of aromatic and medicinal herbs provoke alkaline reactions that displace acids. You are sure to find many more alkaline foods when you do your own research.

Regarding the alkaline concept, nutritionist Theodore Alexander "Ted" Baroody (1950-2020) comments the following in his book *Alkalize or Die*: "It doesn't really matter how many names there are for diseases. What does matter is that they all stem from the same cause: too much acidic waste in the body."

The people who have written the following sentences have been right:

"The struggle of life is against acid retention." Henry Louis Mencken (1880-1956), American journalist, editor, and critic.

"Aging, lack of energy, bad temper and headaches, heart disease, allergies, eczema, hives, asthma, stones and arteriosclerosis, and even multiple sclerosis, are nothing but the accumulation of acids." Fereydoon Batmanghelidj (1931-2004), internationally renowned Iranian writer and researcher, advocate of the healing power of water, graduated from St. Mary's Hospital Medical School, University of London.

Although these authors and many others have expressed it, alkalinity is still a concept discordant with the mainstream.

Holistic medicine and the concept of alkalinity are often discredited in articles that highlight the personal mistakes of some practitioners and the cases of people who have died after trying it. This practice is unequal, because if all the cases of patients who die after undergoing chemo and radiotherapy were exposed, the result would be dramatic. However, belief has always been the preponderant placebo for making a decision in both realities.

The caloric principle

Overweight people, and the parents of children and adolescents with obvious signs of obesity, tend to believe that their volume is directly proportional to the amount of food they need to stay well and, therefore, consume the wrong portions and meals. With what they eat, they continue to compromise their body's oxygenation, steadily gain weight, and get sick. Parents should check their cupboard and refrigerator to see what food they have made available to their children and make a radical change.

We tend to believe that the number of calories to be ingested should be directly related to daily energy expenditure — measured in kilocalories — according to age, sex or physiological state; and that, if physical activity is greater, the caloric supply should also be higher. But when it comes to health, in the West we have disregarded the nutritional value of food and, in order to provide us with energy, we have been forced to consume a higher proportion of carbohydrates — 45-65% — to the detriment of fat consumption. In its documents, the FAO (Food and Agriculture Organization of the United Nations) says: "People who are sedentary or lightly active expend less energy than those who are intensely active".[17] And it recommended reducing fat consumption to between 15 and 35% of daily food intake.

In the same document, FAO also said that vitamins and minerals essential for good nutrition help the body to function properly and stay healthy, but they are needed in much smaller amounts than proteins, fats, and carbohydrates.[18] Almost everyone associates vitamins and minerals with vegetables and fruits for inclusion on the dinner plate, but many people supplement this need with vitamin tablets. However, vegetables and almost all fruits are slowly absorbed complex carbohydrates that are low in calories, rich in fiber, antioxidants, and other essential micronutrients. Without a clear message, we assumed that the suggested carbohydrates should be cereals — sugared —, white rice, corn flour and its products, such as tortillas[19] and arepas, grains, cooked or in soups, pasta, starches such as potatoes, plantains, and cassavas. And on a daily basis, we must also include bakery and pastry products — simple, fast-absorbing, high-calorie carbohydrates —, which metabolize into more sugars and accumulate as fat if we do not burn the calories they provide.

---

[17] Food and Agriculture Organization of the United Nations, FAO (2003): *Food and Nutrition Education for Basic Education. Modules of contents. Module 2, Nutritional needs*, p. 31. Santiago de Chile: Food and Agriculture Organization of the United Nations, FAO. http://www.fao.org/docrep/014/am401s/am401s00.htm, http://www.fao.org/docrep/014/am401s/am401s03.pdf

[18] FAO (2003): Module 2, p. 54.

[19] 1. f. Food prepared with beaten egg, curdled with oil in the frying pan and of round or elongated   form to which sometimes other ingredients are added (RAE). 2. Food of circular and flat form that is made with a dough of pressed corn or wheat flour, or by hand, that is cooked on fire and eaten alone or stuffed with various ingredients; it constitutes an essential element in the diet of various countries of America, especially in Central America and Mexico (Google).

Excluding fats and proteins, rapidly absorbed simple carbohydrates are the foods that contribute the most calories. Among them is refined sugar, and its artificial substitutes, which are full of empty calories; and alcoholic beverages which, due to the excess energy they provide with little or no nutritional contribution, favor appetite and fat storage.

And the slow-absorbing complex carbohydrates that have the highest nutritional qualities are also those with the lowest calorie content: it is the nutritional values of foods that make the difference.

In the 20TH CENTURY, the plate of food was established with simple and fixed parameters that were contrary to the history of gastronomy. This is how we have accepted it and how 21ST CENTURY nutritionists demonstrate it. For example, ancestrally, *sumō* wrestlers have had a diet very high in simple fast-absorbing carbohydrates, with large portions in order to maintain their large body volume, which means a lot of weight, so that they won't lose their next fight as their opponents will not be able to pull them out of the *dohyō*. Although they are coached, their hearts tend to fail, and they die young. We are not *sumō* wrestlers, but with the Western fast-food habit we have been becoming burners of carbohydrates that do not contain healthy fats. We have made the wrong choice of energy fuel.

Let us examine another assertion of the FAO module. A person who requires the optimal supply of nutrients and energy from her food, without becoming overweight, manages to develop a special metabolism: i.e., the pregnant woman. "It is recommended that women of childbearing age consume a diet with adequate amounts of folic acid".[20] It explains: "Folic acid is contained in oranges, strawberries, kiwis, mangoes, guavas, melon, bananas, avocadoes, broccoli, cauliflower, asparagus,

---

[20]   FAO (2003): Module 2, p. 58.

beets, corn, tomatoes, green leafy vegetables, legumes (beans, chickpeas, peas, lentils, soybeans), liver, oats, whole grains".[21] The irony is that all or almost all of the other necessary macro and micronutrients are included in these same foods. Liver provides a high dose of "saturated" fat and healthy calories. So, any variable based on these foods is an extraordinary diet that would not exceed 1800 calories for a woman of average height to maintain an ideal weight of 130 lbs. and, most importantly, a healthy body.

As for the distribution on the food plate, the studies of the last century analyzed the nutritional constitution or bromatology of foods and yielded a full range of tabulations applicable to the energy expenditure corresponding to the height, age, sex, and physiological state of each individual. But today, 21ST CENTURY nutritionists propose a personalized approach that emphasizes having two complementary tools that combine information about yourself: first, you need to establish as a reference your basal metabolic rate (BMR), which calculates the daily number of calories you require, at rest, to carry out vital physiological functions; and second, find your body mass index (BMI), which represents the ideal range of weight in relation to your body mass. These two parameters will help you determine whether you need to lose, maintain, or gain weight.

21ST century nutritionists have discovered how to optimize the energy acquired from food that the body uses as potential calories for regular metabolism and as kinetic calories for physical exercise. Michael Geary, having tested it on his body, proposes: "To begin with, it is vitally important for your overall health to eat an adequate supply of healthy fats in the regular diet. Fats are one of the major components in all cell membranes throughout the body. If you eat enough healthy natural fats,

---

[21]   FAO (2003): Module 2, p. 58.

your cellular processes will proceed normally."[22] They have also developed a modern method of exercise that focuses on toning rather than "building muscle," combining the oxygenating aerobic — jogging, swimming, biking, walking — and the intense anaerobic — weights, short runs with fast sprints, i.e., exercises that require great effort in a short time — none of which require the long hours in the gym as in the previous century.

Conclusion: nutritionists in this 21ST century recommend increasing the consumption of healthy fats between 20 and 40 % and proteins up to 30 %: that is, approx. 0.04ozs. per pound per day of the ideal weight — which is obtained by calculating the BMI — and that the rest of the calories come from unrefined carbohydrates, preferably low glycemic ones. This implies an increase in the consumption of complex carbohydrates — fruits, fresh vegetables, and greens — to ensure the natural supply of vitamins, minerals and, above all, valuable antioxidants. In order to keep the body healthy and wholesome, an ideal diet is that of the pregnant woman with some nutritional variations and adapted to each individual.

We get to the point: when overweight people use the enormous energy potential, in the form of fat that they have accumulated, and burn that net fuel — without starving or exercising yet — they are more easily oriented towards the desired health. In the 21ST CENTURY, the following caloric principle has been established:

Regardless of your height, mass and weight, the human body needs a daily intake of food to provide it with the calories or energy vital for its functioning. The general rule of thumb when it comes to weight loss is that the sum of daily

---

[22]   Michael D. Geary (2004-2016): *The shocking truth about dietary fats and saturated fats.* http://www.truthaboutabs.com/dietary-fat-article.html

calorie intake should never be below 1200 calories for women or below 1600 for men to avoid losing muscle and causing hormonal imbalance.[23]

I will explain what this caloric principle means with a financial example, relevant to many of us because it is about saving:

At the moment you are born, you stop depending on your mother's metabolism and, at that very moment, Mother Nature opens a current account for you with an amount that corresponds to the calories you need to maintain a healthy metabolism in a body that has the capacity to build muscle without accumulating fat. From the time you are born — under normal conditions —, your parents must take care of the administration of this account that nature will adapt with age, until you acquire the awareness and capacity for good management. Of course, as it is an account for daily spending and consumption, it must become an intelligent investment in healthy fats, proteins, fruits, vegetables, and greens to ensure your good health so that it can give you its best utilities; an investment that invites moderation, balance, and the verification of the good daily functioning of things in what you call "my body". It consists of a long-term saving in you and differs greatly from the concept of accumulating. The same does not happen with this account that Mother Nature gives us at birth: humans do not need to accumulate fat to live, and we do NOT need to save calories in the account.

It is different for bears, who overfeed and accumulate calories in the form of fat to endure hibernation, because nature endowed them with a metabolism that allows them to sleep peacefully for five or six months during the winter months. During their deep sleep, their metabolism gradually uses its "savings" of calories every day to sustain their vital functions and, like clockwork,

---

[23] Geary (2006), p. 44.

precisely wakes them up, during the thaw at the beginning of spring. After drinking water, ingesting worms, berries, roots, replenishing themselves with a diet high in healthy fats and proteins provided by salmon, they enjoy the mating season. On the contrary, overweight humans have a slumber that is not sleep. They suffer a serious alteration due to cellular toxins and lack of oxygen in the blood that manifests as apnea, a transient suspension of breathing during sleep.

In humans, the average daily number of calories — 1200 to 1800 in women and 1600 to 2200 in men — should never be below the benchmark: 1200 in women and 1600 in men. In the past, the guideline for weight loss was to avoid consuming calories and, of course, more gym and exercise. Today, that thinking is obtuse. First, because the suppression of calories destroys the body by denying it the energy necessary to function normally and, second, it excludes the person because it subjects him to an unsustainable condition: after an absurd sacrifice, he loses weight, but gains it later in greater quantity and at greater speed by the simple law of action and reaction; the physical claim is such that the demand for calories necessary to subsist will arise at any time, whether you want it or not. For now, you don't have to go around counting the calories you consume. For the time being, do not exceed the lower limit — anorexia, bulimia — or the upper limit — gula —, because in both cases you begin to suffer a decrease in physical and mental capacities.

So, how do you lose weight and get rid of that stubborn abdominal fat? Of course, with your change of habits and beliefs you will be able to intelligently and properly invest your calorie count in healthy foods. And most importantly, your metabolism and psyche will continue to function properly until you fully embrace the changes you intend for your body and your being. To do this, ask yourself if that piece of cake full of empty calories provides you with any nutrients; if your body absorbs the high fructose corn syrup that accompanies the refined flours of that cheese pie — a very high-calorie but fiber free cheesecake — and turns them into sugars and more harmful fats; or, worse yet, if the toxic chemicals in the refined oils or margarines that donut was fried in, or that irresistible Danish pastry you wash down with diet cola, are going to immediately accumulate in your abdomen, hips or arms.... In the end, they will only make you more anxious and, because of the empty calories and excess sugar, your pancreas will immediately secrete insulin to counter the high blood glucose load you have given it, but which, in a short while, it will be asking for more of the same.

Will this be a good investment of your calorie budget? Any other healthy selection will provide you with a greater variety of nutrients and great value for a very low caloric price: an apple, half a bowl of raw mixed nuts, two slices of pineapple. How about an open-faced sandwich on a slice of artisanal whole wheat bread with basil pesto, anchovies, salmon, or a sardine on top — to guarantee protein and omega 3 — and a slice of farmer's cheese. Or a similar bread with raisins, cream or curd cheese, a couple of spinach leaves, *prosciutto* or bacon without nitrites or nitrates, defatted with heat, topped with slices of onion, tomato, basil leaves and oregano. Any of these options with the infallible drizzle of olive oil, a pinch of sea salt or Himalayan salt, pepper and chia seeds or flaxseed or toasted sesame seeds. Or an unsweetened yogurt, but with some stevia and crunchy almonds. In fact, if a couple of hours before lunch or eating, mid-morning or mid-afternoon, you can take something as a snack, you will feel satisfaction, fullness and real nutrition and you are not going to polish off everything when it is finally mealtime: you will know how to choose or to say NO, which sums up the real benefit of snacks or snack time. In terms of numbers, you consumed the same calories and, if not, for you to reach the amount of calorie investment of donuts, eat another slice of pineapple and it's solved. If you still believe that healthy foods don't equal the calories of donuts, you're right: the two donuts add up to far more calories than the three slices of pineapple or the apple. But if you ate the two slices of pineapple or the yogurt with nuts, the feeling of fullness is the same and during the day, at meals, you can invest the remaining calories in healthy fats, proteins, fiber, and other nutrients.

The caloric principle is like a bank account that is spent in full every day and is automatically renewed at each sunrise. By consuming more or less than the necessary calories, the body starts charging you — with high doses of stress — a very expensive maintenance fee. This is ironic and quite similar to what happens with finances; the entity becomes unbalanced, and, because of your excesses, the body makes you suffer for lack of vital energy or money. In conclusion, in order to function and exist harmoniously in the environment, body and being have to maintain these parameters on a daily basis so as not to get sick and not to go crazy.

Thus, you will see these substantial savings in the long term when they become wealth, free time, and a good retirement, full of health — without depending on medications, to enjoy and share with your partner, your children, and your grandchildren. And never forget that...

Medications will not be able to correct the consequences of bad eating habits throughout life.

JOEL FUHRMAN, MD

Omega fatty acids: quality vs. qualities

Another beneficial principle for *optimal health* is to know how to choose the fats we consume. Fats are a subgroup of lipids, monoglycerides, diglycerides and triglycerides which, in turn, have simpler structures: omega-3, 6 and 9 fatty acids. Unlike excess glucose, which is a harmful source of energy that creates an extremely acidic cellular environment capable of altering the mechanisms that regulate its burning and cause rapidly absorbed simple sugars to accumulate in the form of fat, fatty acids provide us with energy. However, the body does not produce them; that is why they are essential and must be consumed.

The required omega fatty acids, which we can consume, are contained in foods that have some type of fat or oil. For example, salmon, avocado, flax, and chia seeds provide us with omega-3. Vegetable oils can be extracted by a simple cold-pressing processes, whereby the resulting oil is called virgin or extra virgin, which has a pleasant natural flavor, and they are suitable for direct human consumption; or they can be extracted by a more complex processes involving high temperatures to facilitate blending and other additional refining processes, such as purification — which includes chemical solvents — or hydrogenation. With the aid of a catalyst, a hydrogen molecule is injected into them to solidify them and produce spreadable mixtures such as margarine, an industrial product, as opposed to butter, a natural product, which is obtained by churning the cream from cow's milk.

When refined oils are subjected to high temperatures for a long time and reused several times, dangerous and toxic trans fats are obtained. In refined oils — even if the label says "heart-healthy" and they contain omega-3, during cooking, the omega-6 content in the food shoots up to the detriment of omega-3. All omega fatty acids are necessary for the functions of the body, but the big problem in consuming them lies in their disproportion in food: processed food, and the Western diet, are loaded with inflammatory omega-6 fatty acids. In other words, refined oils tend to lose the specific qualities that favor nutritional benefit and health.

The body acquires the anti-inflammatory omega-3 and 9 fatty acids from fish and seafood, algae, olive oil, flaxseed oil, nuts and seeds, green leafy vegetables such as lettuce, spinach and purslane, cereals such as oats, quinoa... And as a source of saturated fat, the Iberian pig — raised in open fields among olive groves —, whose basic diet consists of acorns from oaks and cork oaks that contain these healthy omegas. That is why it is said that "the Iberian pig is an olive tree with legs". Omega-9 from olive oil and omega-3 from fish are anti-inflammatory.

When buying olive oil, eggs, and fish, be sure to verify certain specific conditions that guarantee the qualities of these products. When purchasing oil for raw consumption, make sure it is extra virgin in dark glass containers and first *cold pressed, i.e.,* without blends obtained in a high temperature process. Store it in a dark, cool place, as light will spoil it within eight or nine months after extraction. This date used to be printed on the shoulder of the best quality bottles; today, to make it easier to read, it is printed on the labels. Make sure, because the oils with dubious qualities only have on the label the expiration date of the product, not the extraction date. Extra virgin olive oil is to be consumed daily without heating, adding it to salads or on top of an open sandwich with a single piece of bread or whatever you can think of. The point is not to stop consuming unsaturated oils.

For decades we have been told that the best oils must be clear and almost transparent. This is NOT true: due to the industrial processes to which they are subjected, in clear oils — refined — or in margarines, the inflammatory omega-6 fatty acids could reach a ratio with anti-inflammatory omega-3 fatty acids of up to 25:1 (twenty-five parts to one part).

The same is true for eggs and other products of the poultry industry. Organic eggs have an ideal maximum ratio of 4:1 or less of omega-6 and omega-3 fatty acids. Factory-farmed eggs come from captive birds and reach a ratio of 19:1. But even *cage-free* eggs cannot guarantee the origin of the food consumed by these birds, as they are usually fed concentrates based on *genetically modified organism* (GMO) grains. Nor does the guarantee of origin exclude eggs from birds that the market calls "vegetarian" — this is hard to believe, because they are omnivorous, and some insect or worm must be captured. As they are not 100% organic — without disregarding that they could have received hormones and antibiotics during breeding —, chemical fertilizers and pesticides could have been used in the growth of these vegetables that the birds consume, which radically change the products that you consume. That is why, in the chemical balance of the eggs of these birds — unlike the organic ones —, the ratio of inflammation/anti-inflammation — omega 6/omega 3 — is maintained in ranges of 19:1 or more.

Resulting from industrial mass production, something similar happens with cattle and meat products: their chemistry varies. In cattle that walk and graze with a more delicate and probably more compassionate breeding, the final product — organic, which is still expensive — is clearly natural. At some point, I heard the Spanish biochemist and molecular biologist, Carlos López-Otín, say that local food is the cheapest and most environmentally friendly because it leaves a smaller carbon footprint.

It's the same with fish. The food consumed during their life by the fish you eat can affect the proportion of omega fatty acids in their fats and flesh; fish provide high and very good amounts of omega 3. In oily fish, such as tuna, sardines, anchovies, salmon, swordfish, mackerel, bonito or *mahi mahi*, all of them with a V-shaped tail, depending on the season, the fat content of polyunsaturated omega 3 reaches up to 10%. However, in the supermarket, the qualitative aspect to take into account is that the packaging guarantees that they are wild caught, or their meat tends to lose quality, that is, at least, until the farms find a solution to feed the fry better. Similarly, there have already been advances in regard to sedentarism in the cages through the introduction of a small shark that stalks these fish, which has considerably improved the final product.

Cereals, even though the packaging says they contain omega-3s and are an important source of fiber, in reality do not exceed the fiber content of a whole fruit with pulp and everything. When the industry processes the grains — which usually come from genetically modified seeds — it saturates them with sugar and thus turns them into acidifying foods. Consumers have the right to know what each product contains and to have the producer mention it on the label, since the genetic modification of industrially cultivated grains involves toxins in the soil and has repercussions on our health.

In summary, although omega-3 and 9 improve blood chemistry and reduce the risk of many chronic diseases, perhaps more out of ignorance than taste, when choosing foods, we insist on giving priority to the consumption of inflammatory omega-6.

Unsaturated fats, present in avocados, dried fruits, nuts, raw seeds, and virgin oils that you can consume directly, should not be missing in your daily intake because they are the broom that sweeps toxic waste and burnt cholesterol residues from your body. The fat that surrounds that delicious fillet of sirloin cap, haunch tip or rump steak which gives it that wonderful roasted flavor is the one that could contain burnt cholesterol and free radicals. The important thing is to learn to eat, to choose and to understand when to eat a food. For example, red meats, which provide iron and coagulation factors, are not to be consumed daily, but weekly. You can increase your consumption of fish, shellfish, seafood, chicken, turkey, rabbit, lamb, and other meats, including pork and some insects, which provide a variety of nutrients and enzymes that red meat does not. However, one day a week you can also abstain from consuming animal products and enjoy a vegetarian day; which is a form of light fasting recommended by the European Medical Institute of Obesity (IMEO):[24] "It consists of eating little, basing your diet on vegetables and avoiding foods of animal origin and meals that are too solid, abundant or heavy"; "in what can be considered a less strict and restrictive version of fasting, more of our days — which includes light broths, fruits and lots of liquid — that can be done on a weekly basis and favors longevity".

Since the second post-war period, with fast-food and diet food, saturated fats have been in constant controversy. In this issue of quality versus qualities, they have been a dubious subject since the last century: we demean their quality, we associate them with the villainous cholesterol, and we are unaware of their qualities. Present in meats, dairy — and almost all products derived from these industries —, and in fruits such as coconut, consuming saturated fats is strictly necessary because their enzymes strengthen cell walls, favor the absorption of minerals, facilitate neuronal functions, and protect the brain.

We must have balance and moderation with foods; that is why we are studying them. It is not a matter of prohibiting, but of enlightening and educating, because prohibitions pinch curiosity and, in most cases, we end up succumbing to temptations. We have given priority to saturated fats and foods with inflammatory

---

[24] https://www.prensalibre.com/vida/salud-y-familia/comer-menos -a-few-days-to-live-longer/

omega-6, present in what we call "snacks" and in most pastry and bakery products. But it is NOT a question of prohibiting; for me it would be unthinkable to abstain from all of these and not enjoy some delicious Andalusian tapas.

Eat saturated and unsaturated fats in the same day in a 1:1 ratio. Choose healthy fats because they are the right fuel the body needs. Cholesterol can be a constant concern, but recent discoveries have proven the contribution and benefits of saturated fats. Meats should correspond to a quarter of the plate — a portion no larger than the thickness of a deck of cards, and at least half of your plate should be dominated by green and bright colors as an accompaniment — vegetables and greens over the brown of the meats. Potatoes, pasta, and white rice should not be eaten daily, as they are NOT essential and help to accumulate abdominal fat. And don't forget to eat fruits, which are like cheesecloth, the scouring pad that cleans the intestines. The predominance of green and bright colors and the restraint in the white recall the Mediterranean diet. On Icaria, a beautiful Greek island, longevity is ten years longer than the average population.

Balanced intake

It is also known as the balanced diet. In both lanes — you read the introduction — the term balance is referred to as the equilibrium we should seek in the body and in the self. Equilibrium, which is obtained by having equal weight on both sides, corresponds to a place. Not so the balance, which indicates the tendency towards the side where there is more weight. If it is constant — depending on gravity —, at some point, that movement is reversed generating a pendulum and, due to the weight, it passes the point of equilibrium to the opposite side. The same thing happens between body and being, which, because they are tied together, affect each other by the force of action and reaction. To be healthy, in health and nutrition, the balance must tend to the alkaline and it is not easy to keep it that way. However, if you set your mind to it and assimilate the concept of alkalinity, your body will thank you and, given this constant desire to educate yourself, your mind and being will always tend to balance.

To clarify the relationship between balanced diet and weight loss diet, I prefer to use the term from the second lane, balanced intake, proposed by cutting-edge nutritionists in the 21ST CENTURY, because it encompasses what the body ingests not necessarily through the mouth: the skin is permeable, and you also ingest through the skin. Unlike the diet or eating pattern, which is restricted only to food, in the new concept of nourishing, intake includes everything that is absorbed by the body.

Now, a balanced intake also corresponds to a balanced diet that does not omit any meal and controls portions and, when it comes to balance or equilibrium, proportion is important. To establish it and wake up your metabolism, discard the idea of three main meals a day and divide your intake into five or six separate meals, including snacks, as our grandparents used to do. If you distribute foods in groups and combine them as they should be, you will be able to eat more nutrients with a wise caloric investment. The food groups are the proteic: meats, fish, crustaceans, mollusks, eggs, dairy and leguminous — fruits and seeds in pods like beans and lentils — ; the starchy — starches, cereals and derivatives — : flours, pasta, bread, oatmeal, potatoes, corn, cassava, banana and rice — these two groups should not be mixed in the same intake; and the neutral: vegetables, nuts and seeds or dried fruits, including oils, teas and aromatic herbs — the foods of this group can be combined with each other or accompany any of the other two. Fruits also belong to the neutral group, and it is advisable to consume them on an empty stomach and without mixing them with other solids in order to take advantage of their alkalinity.

Drinking wine has enormous advantages. Chilled white wine, refreshing and exquisite, contains a high dose of quercetin that prevents arteriosclerosis; and red wine, which is recommended to be drunk at room temperature, also contains acetylsalicylic acid — the active principle of aspirin — and antioxidants such as resveratrol — present in red grapes, peanut butter, dark chocolate, and blueberries — and tocopherol, polyphenol flavonoids that take care of the heart. Now, regarding the pandemic and SARS-CoV2 causing COVID-19, in late 2020, U.S. researchers demonstrated *in vitro* that antioxidant polyphenols present in grapes and wine alter the way the virus replicates and spreads, and a medical group at Taiwan University that had been studying the effects of tannic acid on the SARS 2003 virus with promising results recently discovered that tannins present in red wine, green tea, bananas and other vegetables effectively inhibit the activity of two key enzymes of the virus, which can then no longer enter cell tissue.[25] Although this conclusion caused controversy, it makes sense: vegetables use tannins and specifically tannic acid as a defense mechanism against insects. Because they can interfere with the body's ability to absorb vitamins or minerals, it is said that these vegetables are anti-nutrients. And it is precisely these phytonutrients and antioxidants which act against obesity,

---

[25] https://www.vitisphere.com/actualite-93368-Une-nouvelle-etude-etaye-lhypothese-dun-effet-protecteur-des-composes-du-vin-contre-la-covid-19-modifie-.htm

diabetes, pain, inflammation and protect against cancer. For all these reasons, it is advisable to drink a glass of wine a day, at least three times a week.

It should be said that if you are diabetic and radically change your eating habits, you could once again enjoy that vine that has been out of your reach due to the high dose of fructose in grapes — and ripe bananas —, because diabetes is reversible, especially type 2 diabetes. In fact, a Look AHEAD Research Group study of type 2 diabetic patients who voluntarily underwent clear changes in dietary habits established that 90% of them were already able to stop taking their prescribed medications.[26]

In summary, repeat fruits, vegetables, and greens, as many times as you wish during the day, but do not mix foods from the protein and starch groups in the same intake: do not mix meat and potatoes, for example.

Healthy snacks become relevant, as they can be the complement or replacement meal. So, open your mind and your palate: taste other things. Hummus based on *tahini* — sesame paste — and chickpeas with celery or carrot sticks or the traditional Arabic bread will give you a lot of nutrients. I will give you some recipes later on.

In the balanced intake you do not need to become a slave to the scales, calories, or precise measures of what you are supposed to consume, because adopting and applying the proposed changes will be enough for you to experience the benefits and

---

[26] Edward W. Gregg, Haiying Chen, Lynne E. Wagenknecht, Jeanne M. Clark, Linda M. Delahanty, John Bantle, Henry J. Pownall, Karen C. Johnson, Monika M. Safford, Abbas E. Kitabchi, F. Xavier Pi-Sunyer, Rena R. Wing, Alain G. Bertoni, Look AHEAD Research Group (2012): *"Association of an intensive lifestyle intervention with remission of type 2 diabetes"*. *Journal of American Medical Association, JAMA, 308* (23), 2489-2496. doi:10.1001/jama.2012.67929. https://jamanetwork.com/journals/jama/fullarticle/1486829.

become aware of what was missing: think before you eat. This translates into the right mixes or combinations, NOT a little bit of everything served on the same plate, as we used to do.

Practicing the segmentation and distribution of food groups invites you to think about the desirable alkaline balance. Once you apply these concepts, the attitude that is required for you to become fully involved in the design of a healthy intake that is unique to each individual will emerge. After all, it is difficult for someone to bathe, smear on their skin, exactly the same things as another person, or for both to eat exactly the same things on the same day.

Thus, with the answers that your body gives you, you will learn to eat; you will establish your own "diet"; you will lose weight; and eating will become instinctive again. The most important thing is that all this will allow you to start, or restore, the natural and mental process of the body: the body is "a machine to burn fat, NOT to accumulate it".[27] Among other mistakes, we have the idea that exercise burns fat and it does not: the body burns fat with or without exercise.

You are now in a position to judge, check the bathroom, go to the kitchen, bathroom, open the pantry and the refrigerator: evaluate what to take out and get what you need. You have at your disposal thousands of edible or ingestible vegetable and animal species and minerals that you can prepare and sample in a thousand ways, so that your daily diet consists of something different from white rice, bread — wheat —, corn or soy products, pasta, potatoes, or denatured cow's milk; the usual food options. And in your bathroom, there are plenty of products that have not removed from their formulas the harmful ingredients you now know about.

---

[27] Michael D. Geary (2006): *The truth about the six-pack abs.* Springville, Utah: Vervante.

Your perspective on other foods and meals begins to open up. When you go to the restaurant, the entrée can be the main course; share portions; order a large salad; swap in roasted bell peppers, asparagus or scallions for that usual side of fries; rice or stuffed potato with cheese sauce for that succulent meat; or pair it with organic wild rice of different colors, quinoa, broccoli or cauliflower sautéed with garlic and bacon (back bacon or streaky bacon in the South American); or tabbouleh, an Arabic salad made with couscous and vegetables. Before or after, not during meals, drink tea — without milk —, aromatic water or water with lemon. Trophology is the science that advises on the proper combination of foods. Its scientific support is relatively new, but, thanks to technological advances in microscopy and research, it now offers reliable scientific bases. In the chapter on learning to eat, we will consider its basic concepts. Perhaps at the restaurant you are also willing to access the usual house menu, from appetizer to dessert. Hmm, you could be on your cheat day. Keep this term in mind for when you come across its explanation.

In the communication between the body and the self, the scales are only an instrument of control, i.e., where the encounter with yourself takes place. The bodily adjustments that you propose to yourself will be optimized as the communication with the body improves. We tend to silence the body. For this reason, at first, you will misperceive some of the messages that the body transmits to you, but little by little you will pay attention to them and learn to interpret them. To be close to balance, the above is not enough; you need to learn to master the unconscious factor. To achieve this, I suggest you start exploring a relaxation technique: something as simple as walking invites you to meditate. In meditation, reflection gives you the attitude you need to break bad habits and, as a consequence of meditating, you will find the tranquility you need to avoid the anxiety and stress that lead you to eat excessively.

You must find the place within yourself where nothing is impossible.

DEEPAK CHOPRA

Chapter IV

A Separate Chapter

Let nothing be called natural, in an age of bloody confusion, ordered disorder, planned caprice, and dehumanized humanity, lest all things be held unalterable.

Kevin DiDonato is the owner and director of the Human Performance Lab and Wellness Center and is among the elite of cutting-edge health professionals in the 21ST century. Kevin is a sports medicine graduate of the University of Southern Maine, who then earned a Master of Science degree, with a specialization in health promotion and rehabilitation sciences, from Penn West California.

Ten reasons why you struggle to lose fat

By Kevin DiDonato, MS, CSCS, CES

As I walk around the gym while working with clients, I notice a trend. Today's typical gym clients and people who want to get the svelte look of defined abs (*six pack*) have extra weight around the abdomen. What is the reason behind this weight gain and why is it so hard to lose those extra pounds?

Here are the top ten reasons why people continue to gain weight.

10. Medications

There are an increasing number of people who are depressed or on medication for depression. These medications slow metabolism regardless of dietary changes and can change hormone levels in the body. This affects our ability to lose weight and keep the weight off.

9. Latent diseases/chronic diseases

An increasing number of people have persistent conditions, such as thyroid disease, diabetes, and Cushing's syndrome — increased cortisol production in the body. These people end up gaining weight and medical treatment is necessary to help them lose weight or control it. Due to decreased hormone levels, the body is unable to increase metabolism to burn additional calories.

8. Genetics

Research shows that genetics may play a role in weight gain. Evidence shows that some people may be more likely to gain weight. Although genetics may play a role in weight gain, environmental factors and individual choices are more important determinants of whether a person becomes overweight than genetics.

7. Stress

Our natural defense against stress is the fight or flight system: in the face of increased stress, our body prepares to fight or flee. When stress levels increase, cortisol is released into the bloodstream and causes changes in the body. Cortisol helps release sugar stored in the muscles and liver into the bloodstream for instant energy. This hormone is responsible for the accumulation of fat in the abdomen, but it is difficult for the body to get rid of it. Cortisol suppresses the immune system, making it harder to fight infections. Stress will always be there so our cortisol levels will always be high.

6. Portion sizes

Do you always overload your plate at a fast-food chain or buffet? I'm sure most of us do. Portion control is a major factor in weight gain. We constantly tend to overeat high-fat, high-calorie foods. We have lost control over our portions. Plates and cups today are bigger, so taking in extra calories is even easier.

5. Cutting meals/skipping meals

Depriving yourself of a meal is just as bad as not controlling portions: it slows down your metabolism because of the lack of calories and nutrients in your body. When we skip a meal, nine times out of ten we overindulge at the next meal. Food choices are usually affected, and portion sizes become monstrous. This translates into lots of calories, lethargic moods and those calories being stored as fat.

4. The "low fat" label

How many of us have been fooled into thinking that low fat is low calorie? The label "low fat" means three grams of fat or less. Just because a label says "low fat" does not mean lower in calories. So, before you buy that low-fat product, remember to read the label, and see how many calories, what type of sweetener it uses and what the serving size is. We tend to buy and consume more low-fat products because we think low-fat means low calories. Sometimes, the real *deal* may be better for you because of the portion size.

3. Lack of exercise

Vigorous exercise and cardio help increase the number of calories we burn. But we are exercising less and less and consuming more and more calories. The combination of lack of exercise and high calorie intake causes us to gain weight. The more vigorous the exercise, the more muscle we have: this speeds up metabolism and helps us burn more calories at rest and during exercise.

2. Slower metabolic rate

A slow metabolic rate helps weight gain. Muscle is metabolically more active-meaning it burns more calories-than fat, so we need more muscle than fat. A common myth is that as we age, we lose more muscle. If we stay active, this is not true. Continuing to do cardio and strength exercises will maintain muscle tone in our body, which will keep the metabolism working on burning fat. After this and after that, we can continue to eat those extra calories — the cravings — without worrying about getting fat.

And the number 1 reason why people gain weight is...

1. An unhealthy diet

Let's face facts: our diets are generally not good. Our diets are full of processed foods that are easy to prepare and probably not very good for us. Portions are out of control and meals lack essential foods such as fruits, vegetables and complex carbohydrates that help nourish our bodies. Fast-foods, canned, and packaged foods can cause us to gain that extra weight around the waist due to their high amount of fat and extra calories.

Diet and exercise help us monitor our weight as we age. Making better food choices, portion control and not skipping meals will help you lose weight. A healthy snack or meal replacement will help you avoid skipping meals and leave you satisfied and full of nutrients until your next meal.

KEVIN DIDONATO

But for most of us, "it's my body and I'll do what I want with it". This haughty and natural response trumps any argument and shuts up anyone who suggests anything, let alone asks what we are eating today. Nevertheless, from my perspective, I am going to expound what I think about subjects that seem to be unrelated. You will realize that, although they seem unrelated, they are an inescapable part of the three lanes in which we all drive.

Slow food culture

There is no magic anymore in economies where working families have been forced to include foods with few qualities in the basic food basket: industrialized and packaged, frozen or precooked, instant fast-food. Over several generations they have dedicated their time and themselves to work more and, incidentally, they didn't know the pleasure of cooking their own food. In the last century, after World War II, a dream of freedom and opportunity arose in the United States that swept much of the globe, reaching its peak in the late 1980s. The prize: a stable job and salary, enough to purchase a home and vehicles for each member of the family. And it was a success because it boosted development and for many the "American dream" was fulfilled. But this mirage ended, and we fell asleep.

Awakening from this dream will allow us to correct fundamental errors: monetary savings and work time have gone up in smoke and have played a large part in the generalized loss of our families' health. The basis of the American dream has survived as a cultural mandate to leave our children a prosperous, promising future with clear accounts, but it does not match the bankruptcy and global chaos we are inheriting. The result has been a huge public debt; a negative balance that has us at the mercy of the pharmaceutical and health sector, insurance companies and other industries to close the circle: it is increasingly difficult to access money and a job with a stable salary commensurate with the chosen profession or work that allows us to live, at least, at ease and with dignity.

Faced with this, in Italy in 1989 the non-profit Slow Food movement was founded, an antagonistic ideal that has gained strength in recent years and proclaims: "It is a growing idea, a way of living and a way of eating". Its objective is sustainable plural development, in addition to economic profit; protecting biodiversity and food security; its symbol is a snail that identifies restaurants, local markets, farmers' associations, fishermen and traders related to this philosophy "[to] prevent the disappearance of local gastronomic traditions and combat society's loss of interest in food, its origin, its taste and the consequences that each of our food choices has on the world".[28]

But you have to work hard and dedicate a lot of time to it.

Contrary to what people think of a leisurely attitude, working less does not mean being less productive; it is about paying attention to detail in order to give the final product or service a much higher added value. It has been proven: based on this philosophy of life, in Northern European countries, productivity has increased by 12 to 20% with reduced working hours.

When we talk about quality, we associate it with paying more: the higher the quality, the higher the price. But the truth is different: there are already competitive brands that take into account the origin of the product, its ingredients, consistency with sustainable production and care for the environment. The quality of life and the quality of the product must be human achievements. Slow Food emphasizes

> The notion of food quality is defined by three interrelated principles: good, clean, and fair. Good: tasty, fresh, seasonal food that satisfies the senses and is part of the local culture. Clean: production and consumption of food that does not harm the environment, animal welfare or human health. And fair: affordable prices for consumers and fair rewards for producers.[29]

As a result, today these formerly poor communities offer excellent quality and enjoy prosperity.

Eating and drinking calmly is beneficial and a right we all have. Life since March 2020, due to the pandemic, reminds us of its great lesson: it is not necessary to have too much to live well;

---

[28]   www.slowfood.com, "Who we are".
[29]   www.slowfood.com, "Who we are".

it is enough to have products and services of sufficient quality. Quantity is valued in the quality of life, which is achieved and translated into human qualities: the indispensable attribute of avoiding attachment to excesses and the vice of accumulating.

Let's recover our common sense and build a different dream with the experience left by the American dream of the last century. Where, with such haste, has development without pause and attending obediently to the doctrine of *"do it now"* led us? Do we not realize that depredation is the consequence of producing only quantity, NOT quality; single use and throw away? These goods and services generate huge monetary flows enjoyed by only a few. Yes, of course, they have also generated employment everywhere. But in pursuing this dream, many workers — to the detriment of their health — sacrificed time with their families and in every other activity.

People fear change because it implies readjustment. For this new dream to be attainable for all without intensifying environmental deterioration and social conflict, we can make changes that alleviate the economic disparity, as many workers' associations wish, as opposed to others who continue in the inertia of those who want to keep things as they are, even if they do not work. Recovering the planet's health begins with renewing the infrastructure of services, such as transportation. For example, the United States has been slow to adopt high-speed rail systems for freight and passenger transportation. In 2016, a *Fortune* report said, "Over the next decade, the United States must spend $3.32 trillion to keep its infrastructure of ports, roads, bridges, trains, water and electrical facilities up to date"; this investment "could generate 2.5 million jobs and contribute $4 trillion to gross domestic product."[30] Today it

---

[30] *Fortune* (May 10, 2016). *"Both republicans and democrats want more infrastructure spending now"*. https://fortune.com/2016/08/09/

still has no bullet train line. And in individual habits, it would not be unreasonable to increase the consumption of locally produced goods of extraordinary quality.

It is clear: natural resources are running out and it is NOT possible to maintain economic growth based on infinite consumption at the expense of a delicate and finite biosphere. Moreover, in this mad race of depredation, people are also deteriorating. This reality has led to an adhesion to the Slow Food movement of the second lane (www.slowfood.com).

We are not alone in this endeavor to heal the planet. Archaeologists and historians argue that other non-terrestrial, or older brothers, hidden out there in an interdimensional space have been watching our short history to protect us from ourselves and have subtly intervened to prevent our childish follies from jeopardizing human existence, so that we can overcome this passage through humanity's adolescence and head towards true maturity of being. Just listen to the news: our behavior as a species is evidence enough of our immaturity. The irony is that, if they were to appear, many would not hesitate to call them gods or God, because the *what of God* is still unresolved.

For now, it is about something earthly: promoting food diversity, valuing, supporting, and caring for its richness. There are different ways to achieve the new dream of social and economic prosperity: the development models presented in universities, among other things, rule out monocultures. The mere fact of acquiring in our local environment fresh food that guarantees nutritional qualities would commit us directly and positively to regional development and prosperity. This is an intelligent way to contribute individually to the redistribution of wealth.

---

republicans-democrats-infrastructure-spending/

Overweight or not: we're swollen

Consuming carbonated beverages that bloat and produce gas, and resorting to industrialized food with excess salt, sugar and hydrogenated fats and refined oils guarantee constant inflammation of the body.

The great cholesterol hoax

People make mistakes and, at some point in life, others may take advantage of that to call them into question. We tend to flatly disqualify those whose contribution and intellectual or scientific testimony may affect the interests of the *establishment*. This is the case of Dr. Dwight Lundell, a Yale graduate, founder of the Healthy Humans Foundation and chief of the Coronary Surgery Service at Banner Heart Hospital, Mesa, Arizona. After practicing cardiovascular surgery for more than twenty-five years, the Arizona Medical Board investigated him (between 2000 and 2008), and he was forced to resign and retire in 2004 when they revoked his license.

In the two lanes, the realities are disparate, unequal, and address the same issue differently. While the first lane holds that cholesterol is responsible for heart disease, the second clarifies that the real cause is internal inflammations. In 2016, Joseph A. Hill, MD, PhD, chief of cardiology at UT Southwestern Medical Center, Dallas, and editor of American Heart Association News, wrote, "In the United States, there were 167.1 deaths per 100,000 population in 2015 compared with 166.7 in 2014," and said, "Cholesterol-lowering statins and artery-opening *stents* have allowed people to live longer." He added: "Many are living with heart failure, which creates new challenges for physicians facing rising rates of obesity and diabetes." But Dr. Lundell, author of the books *The Cure for Heart Disease: Truth Will Save a Nation* and *The Great Cholesterol Lie*, four years earlier, in 2012, had stated:

We physicians, with all our training, knowledge, and authority, often acquire a huge ego that makes it difficult for us to admit that we have been wrong. So, I freely admit to being wrong... As a heart surgeon with twenty-five years of experience, with over five thousand open heart surgeries performed, today is my day to rectify the error with medical and scientific facts.

Along with other prominent physicians, labeled as "opinion makers," I have for many years trained other physicians. With a barrage of scientific literature and continuing education seminars, we opinion leaders have insisted that coronary heart disease is the result of simply having elevated blood cholesterol levels.

The only accepted therapy has been to prescribe cholesterol-lowering drugs and a severe diet restricting fat intake. The latter, of course, we insisted, could reduce cholesterol and coronary heart disease. Any deviation from these recommendations was considered heresy and quite possibly could result in medical malpractice.

This does NOT work!

These recommendations are not scientifically or morally defensible. For some years now, the discovery that inflammation in the arterial wall is the real cause of heart disease is gradually leading to a paradigm shift in the way we treat heart disease and other chronic ailments.

Since long ago, established dietary recommendations have created the obesity and diabetes epidemics, the consequences of which dwarf any other historical plague in terms of mortality, human suffering, and serious economic effects.

Despite the fact that 25% of the population takes expensive statin drugs and that we have reduced the fat content of our diet more than ever before, many Americans will die this year from heart disease.

American Heart Association statistics indicate that today seventy-five million Americans suffer from heart disease, twenty million have diabetes and fifty-seven million have pre-diabetes. These disorders are affecting younger and younger people in greater numbers each year. Simply put, without inflammation in the body, there is no way for cholesterol to build up on the walls of blood vessels and cause heart disease and stroke. Without inflammation, cholesterol would move freely throughout the body as nature intended. Inflammation is the cause of cholesterol becoming trapped.

Inflammation is not a complex process: it is simply a natural defense of the body against invaders such as bacteria, toxins, or viruses. The inflammatory cycle is perfect because the body protects itself against bacterial and viral invaders. However, if we are frequently exposing our body to toxins or foods that the body was not designed to process, a condition called chronic inflammation occurs. Chronic inflammation is as harmful as acute inflammation is beneficial.

What sensible person would intentionally expose themselves repeatedly to foods or other substances known to cause harm to the body? Well, maybe smokers, but at least it is a voluntary decision. The rest of us have simply followed the mainstream recommended diet: low in fat and high in polyunsaturated fats and carbohydrates, unaware that we have been causing repeated damage to our blood vessels. This repeated assault produces chronic inflammation that leads to heart disease, stroke, diabetes, and obesity.

Let me repeat: the injury and inflammation of our blood vessels is caused by the low-fat diet that has been recommended for years by conventional medicine.

What are the biggest culprits of chronic inflammation? Simply put, an overload of highly processed simple carbohydrates — sugar, flour, and all products from them — and overconsumption of omega-6s in vegetable oils such as soybean, corn, and sunflower oils, which are in many processed foods. Take a moment to visualize scrubbing with a stiff brush repeatedly on soft skin until it becomes red and bleeds; keep doing this several times a day every day for five years. If this painful brushing could be tolerated, you would have bleeding and swelling in the infected area, which would get worse and worse with each new injury. This is a good way to look at the inflammatory process and is what might be going on in your body right now.

Regardless of where the inflammatory process occurs, whether internal or external, it is the same. I have compared the inside of thousands and thousands of arteries. A diseased artery looks as if someone had taken a brush and rubbed it several times against its walls. Several times a day, every day, the food we eat produces small lesions and upon these other lesions are produced, so that our body responds continuously and appropriately with inflammation.

As we savor a sweet bread roll, our bodies respond alarmingly, as if an invader is declaring war. Foods loaded with sugars and simple carbohydrates, processed with omega-6 oils used for long shelf life, have been the mainstay of the American diet for six decades. These foods have been slowly poisoning us.

Why does eating a simple sweet bread create a cascade of inflammation that makes you sick?

Imagine spraying your keyboard with fructose syrup; this is a visual representation of what happens inside the cell. When we consume simple carbohydrates such as sugar, blood sugar levels rise rapidly. In response, the pancreas secretes insulin, whose primary mission is to drive the sugar to reach each cell where it is stored as energy. But if the cell is full and does not need any more glucose, the excess is rejected to avoid dysfunction of the processes taking place inside the cell. When the cells reject the excess glucose, blood sugar levels rise, which produces more insulin, and the glucose is converted into fat that is stored.

How does all this relate to inflammation? Blood sugar is controlled in a very narrow range. The extra sugar molecules attach to a variety of proteins that, in turn, injure the blood vessel wall. This repeated injury to the blood vessel walls triggers inflammation. When the blood sugar level rises repeatedly, every day, it is like rubbing sandpaper on the delicate interior of the blood vessels.

While you can't see it, you can be sure it happens. I saw it in more than five thousand surgical patients over twenty-five years and they all shared a common denominator: inflammation of their arteries.

Let's go back to the sweet bread roll. Underneath its innocent appearance, not only does it contain sugar, but it is also made with one of many omega-6 oils, such as soybean oil. French fries and *chips* are fried in soybean oil; processed food is manufactured with oils high in omega-6 fatty acids to achieve a longer shelf life. While omega-6 fats are essential as they form part of the cell membrane and thus control what enters and leaves the cell, they must be in proper balance with omega-

3s. If this balance is disrupted by excessive consumption of omega-6 fatty acids, the cell membrane produces chemicals called cytokines, which directly cause inflammation.

Today, the diet often produces a very large imbalance between these two types of fatty acids. The imbalance ratio can be around 15:1 or even 30:1 in favor of omega-6 fatty acids. This turns into a huge number of cytokines that cause inflammation. The ideal ratio would be 3:1 to be optimal and healthy.

To make matters worse, being overweight leads to an overload of fat cells that shed large amounts of pro-inflammatory chemicals, adding to the injury caused by high blood sugar levels. The process that started with the sweet bread roll has become a vicious cycle that eventually generates heart disease, elevated blood pressure, diabetes, and ultimately Alzheimer's disease if the inflammatory process does not abate.

There is no escaping the fact that the more processed foods are consumed, the more inflammation gradually increases each day. The human body cannot process nor was it designed to consume packaged foods, overloaded with sugars and omega-6 oils.

To decrease inflammation, there is no other solution than to consume foods as close as possible to their natural state. To build muscle, consume more protein. Choose very complex [slow-absorbing] carbohydrates such as fruits and colorful vegetables. Reduce or eliminate consumption of omega-6 fats, such as corn and soybean oil, and processed foods that have been made with these oils.

One tablespoon of corn oil [each tablespoon equals 15 grams, 15 cm3 or 15 ml] contains 7280 mg of omega-6 fatty acids; soybean 6949 mg [7.2 grams and 6.9 grams of omega-6]. Instead, use olive oil or butter from grass-fed cows. Animal fats contain less than 20% omega-6 and are much less likely to produce inflammation than oils labeled as polyunsaturated, which are said to be supposedly healthy. Forget the "science" that has been drummed into your head for decades. The science that says saturated fats alone cause heart disease does not exist. The science that says saturated fats increase blood cholesterol is vague. Now we know: cholesterol is not the cause of heart disease, the concern about saturated fats is even more absurd today.

The cholesterol theory led to the recommendation of low or fat-free foods, which brought about the consumption of these foods that have now caused this epidemic of inflammation. Conventional medicine made a tremendous mistake when it advised people to avoid saturated fats in favor of foods rich in omega-6 fatty acids. We now know that we have an epidemic of inflammation of the arteries, leading to heart disease and other silent killers.

What you can do is eat whole foods, the kind your grandmother knew about, not the aberration mom got by grabbing them from the isles of stores crammed with processed foods. Eliminating the inflammation-producing foods and adding the essential nutrients present in fresh, unprocessed foods would reverse the deterioration that for years has been caused in your arteries and throughout your body by the typical American diet.

DR. DWIGHT LUNDELL

The truth about saturated fats

The article below, *The Skinny on Fats*, is one of the two scientific pillars of my book. It is written by Mary G. Enig, MS, PhD, and Sally Fallon Morell. Enig and Fallon Morell are also co-authors of *Eat Fat, Lose fat — the Healthy Alternative to Trans Fats*.

***

The Skinny on Fats, excerpt from *Nourishing Traditions: The Cookbook that Challenges Politically Correct Nutrition and the Diet Dictocrats, Nourishing Traditions: The Cookbook that Challenges Politically Correct Nutrition and the Diet Dictocrats*.

Written by Mary G. Enig, MS, PhD,
and Sally Fallon Morell

Introduction

Fats from animals and vegetables provide a concentrated source of energy in the diet; they also provide the building blocks for cell membranes and a variety of hormones and pseudohormones. As part of a meal, fats slow down absorption, which makes it take longer for us to feel hungry. In addition, they act as carriers of important fat-soluble vitamins, such as A, D, E and K. Dietary fats are necessary for the conversion of carotenes into vitamin A, mineral absorption and as a host for other processes.

Politically correct nutrition is based on the assumption that we should reduce our intake of fats, especially saturated animal fats. Animal fats also contain cholesterol, presented as the evil twin — with saturated fats — the villain of the civilized diet.

The lipid hypothesis

In the late 1950s, the researcher Ancel Keys proposed the lipid theory or hypothesis, according to which the amount of saturated fats and cholesterol in the diet have an impact on coronary heart disease. Several subsequent studies have questioned his data and conclusions. However, Keys' articles received much more publicity than those presenting alternative views. The food and vegetable oil processing industries — the main beneficiaries of any research that found fault with traditional food, their competitor — began to promote and fund more research designed to support the lipid hypothesis.

Nathan Pritikin was the most prominent advocate of the low-fat diet. In fact, Pritikin advocated the elimination of sugar, refined white flours and all processed foods from the diet and recommended the consumption of fresh raw foods, whole grains, and a strenuous exercise program; but in his regimen, the aspect that received the most media attention was that of being low in fat. His followers lost weight and lowered their blood pressure and blood cholesterol levels. The success of Pritikin's diet was probably due to a number of factors that had nothing to do with reducing dietary fat — for example, weight loss alone precipitated a reduction in blood cholesterol levels — but Pritikin soon discovered that the fat-free diet presented many problems, not least of which was the fact that people could not stay on it for long.

Those who possessed enough willpower to remain fat-free for some time developed a number of health problems, such as low energy, difficulty concentrating, depression, weight gain and mineral deficiencies.[31] Pritikin may have saved himself from coronary heart disease, but his low-fat diet did not save him from cancer. He died, in the prime of his life, from suicide when he realized that his Spartan regimen was not curing his leukemia. We should not die of heart disease, and we should not die of cancer — nor should we eat a diet that depresses us.

When the problems of the fat-free regimen became apparent, Pritikin introduced a small amount of vegetable-source fat to his diet-something like 10% of total caloric intake. Today, dietary dictates advise limiting fats to 25-30 % of caloric intake, which is nearly two 1/2 ounces or five tablespoons a day for a 2400-calorie diet. They say the key to perfect health is careful calculation of fat intake and avoidance of animal fats.

The "evidence" supporting the lipid hypothesis

These "experts" assure us that the lipid hypothesis is supported by incontrovertible scientific evidence. Most people would be surprised to learn that there is in fact very little evidence to support the argument that a diet low in cholesterol and saturated fat reduces death from heart disease or increases our lifespan.

Consider the following:

Prior to 1920, coronary heart disease was rare in the United States; so rare that when the young internist Paul Dudley White presented the German electrocardiograph to his colleagues at

---

[31] Ann Louise Gittleman (1988): *Beyond Pritikin*. New York, NY: Bantam Books.

Harvard University, they advised him to concentrate on a more profitable branch of medicine.

The new machine revealed the presence of arterial blockages, allowing early diagnosis of coronary heart disease. But in those days the presence of arterial blockages was a medical rarity, and White had to seek out patients who could benefit from his new technology.

However, over the next forty years, the incidence of coronary heart disease increased dramatically, so much so that by the mid-1950s, heart disease was the leading cause of death among Americans. Today, heart disease causes at least 40% of all deaths in the United States. If, as we have been told, heart disease is the result of saturated fat consumption, one would expect to find a corresponding increase in animal fat in the diets of Americans. In fact, the opposite is true.

During the sixty years between 1910 and 1970, the traditional proportion of animal fat in the American diet declined from 83 to 62%, and annual butter consumption per person plummeted from eighteen pounds to four pounds. During the past eighty years, dietary cholesterol intake has increased by only 1%. During the same period, the percentage of dietary vegetable oils in the form of margarine, shortening and refined oils increased by 400%, while the consumption of sugar and processed foods increased by almost 60%.[32]

The Framingham Heart Study is often cited as evidence for the lipid hypothesis. This study began in 1948 and involved some six thousand people from Framingham, a town in Massachusetts. Two groups were compared at five-year intervals: those who

---

[32]   Mary G. Enig (1995): *Trans Fatty Acids in the Food Supply: A Comprehensive Report Covering 60 Years of Research*, 4-8. 2nd ed. Silver Spring, Maryland: Enig Associates, Inc.

consumed little cholesterol and saturated fats and those who ingested large amounts.

After forty years, the study director had to admit: "In Framingham, Massachusetts, the more saturated fat you ate, the more cholesterol you ate, the more calories you consumed, the lower the person's serum cholesterol [serum cholesterol or serum cholesterol is the level of total cholesterol in the blood]...We found that people who ate more cholesterol, more saturated fat and more calories weighed less and were physically more active."[33] The study showed that those who weighed more and had abnormally high blood cholesterol levels had a slightly increased risk of future heart disease; but weight gain and cholesterol levels had an inverse correlation with dietary fat and cholesterol intake.[34]

In a multi-year UK study of thousands of men, half of them were asked to reduce saturated fats and cholesterol in their diets, stop smoking and increase the amount of unsaturated oils, such as margarine and vegetable oils. After one year, among those on the "good" diet, there had been 100% more deaths than among those on the "bad" diet, even though the men on the "bad" diet continued to smoke! But in describing the study, the author ignored these results in favor of the politically correct conclusion: "The implication for UK public health policy is that a preventive

[33] William P. Castelli (1992): "*Concerning the Possibility of a Nut...*," *Archives of Internal Medicine, 152* (7), 1371-1372. http://www.survivediabetes. com/Essay/On%20the%20possibility%20of%20a%20nut.html.

[34] Helen B. Hubert, Manning Feinleib, Patricia M. McNamara & William P. Castelli (1983): *Obesity as an Independent Risk Factor for Cardiovascular Disease: a 26-Year Follow-Up of Participants in the Framingham Heart Study. Circulation, 67* (5), 968-977. http://citeseerx.ist.psu.edu/viewdoc/ download?doi=10.1.1.613.3378&rep=rep1&type=pdf. Russell Lesley Smith & Edward Robert Pinckney (1991): *Diet, Blood Cholesterol and Coronary Heart Disease: A Critical Review of the Literature*, Vol 2. Sherman Oaks, California: Vector Enterprises.

program such as the one we evaluated in this trial is likely to be effective."[35]

The U.S. Multiple Risk Factor Intervention Trial (MRFIT), sponsored by the National Heart, Lung, and Blood Institute, compared mortality rates and dietary habits in more than 12,000 men.

Those with "good" dietary habits — reduced saturated fat and cholesterol, less smoking, etc. — showed a marginal reduction in total coronary heart disease, but their mortality rate from other causes was higher. Similar results have been obtained in other studies. The few studies that show a correlation between fat reduction and a decrease in CHD mortality also report a concurrent increase in death from cancer, stroke, suicide, and violent death.[36]

The Lipid Research Clinics Coronary Primary Prevention Trial (LRC-CPPT), which cost one hundred and fifty million dollars, is the study most often cited by experts for the sake of justifying low-fat diets. In reality, dietary cholesterol and saturated fat were not tested in this study, as all subjects were given a low-cholesterol, low-saturated fat diet. Instead, the study tested the effects of a cholesterol-lowering drug. Statistical analysis of the results implied a 24% reduction in the rate of coronary heart disease within the group taking the drug compared to the placebo group. However, death from non-heart-related diseases increased in the drug group — death from cancer, heart attack,

---

[35] Geoffrey Arthur Rose, Hugh D. Tunstall-Pedoe & Richard F. Heller (1983): UK Heart Disease Prevention Project: Incidence and Mortality Results. *Lancet, 1* (8333), 1062-1066.

[36] No author (1982): "*Multiple Risk Factor Intervention Trial. Risk Factor Changes and Mortality Results*" [study sponsored by National Heart, Lung, and Blood Institute, National Institutes of Health, Bethesda, Maryland]. *Journal of the American Medical Association, JAMA, 248* (12), 1465-1477.

violence, and suicide.[37] The conclusion that lowering cholesterol reduces heart disease is still in doubt. Independent researchers who tabulated the results of this study found no statistically significant difference in the CHD death rate between the two groups.[38] Nevertheless, the popular press and medical journals touted the LRC-CPPT as the long-sought proof that animal fat is the cause of heart disease-America's number one killer.

Studies challenging the lipid hypothesis

While it is true that several researchers have induced heart disease in some animals by giving them extremely large doses of oxidized or rancid cholesterol — amounts ten times that of an ordinary human diet —, several population studies directly contradict the connection between cholesterol and heart disease. A follow-up of 1700 patients with hardening of the arteries by renowned heart surgeon Michael DeBakey found no relationship between blood cholesterol level and the incidence of atherosclerosis.[39] Research among South Carolina adults found no correlation between blood cholesterol levels and "bad" eating habits, such as consumption of red meat, animal fat, fried foods,

---

[37] No author (1984): "*The Lipid Research Clinics Coronary Primary Prevention Trial Results. I. Reduction in Incidence of Coronary Heart Disease*" [study sponsored by National Institutes of Health]. *Journal of the American Medical Association, JAMA, 251* (3), 351-364, 359.

[38] Richard A. Kronmal (1985): "*Commentary on the Published Results of the Lipid Research Clinics Coronary Primary Prevention Trial*". *Journal of the American Medical Association, JAMA, 253* (14), 2091-2093.

[39] H. Edward Garrett, Evan C. Horning, Billy G. Creech & Michael de Bakey (1964): "*Serum Cholesterol Values in Patients Treated Surgically for Atherosclerosis*". *Journal of the American Medical Association, JAMA, 189* (9), 655-659.

butter, eggs, whole milk, bacon, sausage and cheese.[40] A Medical Research Council study showed that men who ate butter had half the risk of developing heart disease compared to those who used margarine.[41]

Breast milk provides a higher proportion of cholesterol than almost any other food. It also contains more than 50% of calories as fat, much of it saturated fat. Both cholesterol and saturated fat are essential for growth in infants and children, especially for brain development.[42] But the American Heart Association is now recommending a low-cholesterol, low-fat diet for children!

Commercial formulas are low in saturated fat and soy formulas are cholesterol-free. A recent study links low-fat diets to developmental delays in children.[43]

Several investigations of traditional populations have yielded information embarrassing to dietary dictators. For example, a study comparing Jews, whose diets contained only animal fats while living in Yemen, with Yemeni Jews living in Israel, whose diets contained margarine and vegetable oils, revealed little heart disease or diabetes in the former group, but high levels of both diseases in the latter group.[44] — The study also showed that

---

[40]   Daniel T. Lackland & Frances C. Wheeler (1990): "*The Need for Accurate Nutrition Survey Methodology: The South Carolina Experience*". *Journal of Nutrition, 120* (11S), 1433-1436.

[41]   Gary Farr (1991): "*What are Fats?*". *Nutrition Week, 21* (12), 2-3.

[42]   Roslyn B. Alfin-Slater & Lilla Aftergood (1980): "*Lipids.*" In Robert S. Goodhart & Maurice E. Shils (eds.). *Modern Nutrition in Health and Disease; Dietotherapy*, 131. 6th ed. Philadelphia: Lea & Febiger.

[43]   Melanie M. Smith & Fima Lifshitz (1994): "*Excess Fruit Juice Consumption as a Contributing Factor in Nonorganic Failure to Thrive*". *Pediatrics, 93* (3), 438-443.

[44]   Aharon M. Cohen (1963): "*Fats and Carbohydrates as Factors in Atherosclerosis and Diabetes in Yemenite Jews*". *American Heart Journal, 65* (3), 291-293. http://www.ahjonline.com/article/0002-8703(63)90001-2/pdf.

Yemeni Jews consumed no sugar, but those in Israel consumed amounts equivalent to 25-30% of total carbohydrate intake. A comparison between populations in northern and southern India revealed a similar pattern. People in northern India consumed seventeen times more animal fat but had an incidence of coronary heart disease seven times lower than people in southern India.[45] In Africa, the Maasai and related tribes subsist largely on milk, blood, and beef. They are free of coronary heart disease and have excellent blood cholesterol levels.[46] Eskimos eat generous amounts of animal fats from fish and marine animals. In their native diet, they are disease-free and exceptionally strong.[47] An extensive study of dietary patterns and disease in China found that, in the region where large amounts of whole milk were consumed, the population had half the rate of heart disease compared to several districts where only small amounts of animal products were consumed.[48] Several Mediterranean societies have low rates of heart disease despite the fact that fat — including highly saturated fat from veal, sausages and goat cheese

---

[45] S. L. Malhotra (1968): *"Studies in Blood Coagulation, Diet, and Ischaemic Heart Disease in Two Population Groups in India". Indian Journal of Industrial Medicine, 14,* 219. Editor's note: The text was also published in the *British Heart Journal, 30,* 303-308. https://www.ncbi.nlm.nih.gov/pmc/articles/PMC487621/pdf/brheartj00320-0013.pdf

[46] Kang-Jey Ho, Kurt Biss, Belma Mikkelson, Lena A. Lewis & C. Bruce Taylor (1971). Lewis & C. Bruce Taylor (1971): *"The Maasai of East Africa: Some Unique Biological Characteristics". Archaeological Pathology, 91* (5), 387-410. George V. Mann, Anne Spoerry, Margarete Gary & Debra Jarashow (1972). Atherosclerosis in the Masai. *American Journal of Epidemiology, 95* (1), 26-37.

[47] Weston A. Price (1945): *Nutrition and Physical Degeneration,* 59-72. San Diego, California: Price-Pottenger Nutrition Foundation.

[48] Junshi Chen (1990): Diet, *Lifestyle and Mortality in China: A Study of the Characteristics of 65 Chinese Counties.* Ithaca, New York: Cornell University Press.

— constitutes up to 70% of their caloric intake. For example, the people of Crete are noted for their good health and longevity.[49]

A study of Puerto Ricans has revealed that, although they consume large amounts of animal fat, they have a very low incidence of colon and breast cancer.[50] Research on the long-lived inhabitants of Soviet Georgia revealed that those who consume the fattiest meat live the longest.[51] In Okinawa, where life expectancy for women is eighty-four years — the longest in Japan — the inhabitants eat generous amounts of pork and seafood and prepare their food with lard.[52]

Those who advise saturated fat restriction do not mention any of these studies.

---

[49] Walter C. Willett, Frank M. Sacks, Antonia Trichopoulou, Greg Drescher, Anna Ferro-Luzzi, Elisabet Helsing & Dimitrios Trichopoulos (1995): *"Mediterranean Diet Pyramid: A Cultural Model for Healthy Eating"*. *American Journal of Clinical Nutrition, 61* (6S), 1402S-1406S. Francisca Pérez-Llamas, Marta Garaulet, Pedro M. Nieto, Juan Carlos Baraza & Salvador Zamora (1996): *"Estimates of Food Intake and Dietary Habits in a Random Sample of Adolescents in South-East Spain"*. *Journal of Human Nutrition and Dietetics, 9* (6), 463-471. Adalberta Alberti-Fidanza, C. Alunni Paolacci, M. P. Chiuchiù, R. Coli, Daniela Fruttini, G. Verducci, Flaminio Fidanza (1994): *"Dietary Studies on Two Rural Italian Population Groups of the Seven Countries Study. 1. Food and Nutrient Intake at the 31st Year Follow-Up in 1991"*. *European Journal of Clinical Nutrition, 48* (2), 85-91.

[50] Nelson A. Fernández (1975): *"Nutrition in Puerto Rico"*. *Cancer Research, 35,* 3272-3291. http://cancerres.aacrjournals.org/content/canres/35/11_Part_2/3272.full.pdf. Isidro Martínez, Raquel Torres & Zenaida Frías (1975). Cancer Incidence in the United States and Puerto Rico. *Cancer Research, 35,* 3265-3271. http://cancerres.aacrjournals.org/content/35/11_Part_2/3265.full-text.pdf

[51] G. Z. Pitskhelauri (1982): *The Long Living of Soviet Georgia*. New York, New York: Human Sciences Press.

[52] Deborah Franklyn (1976): *"Take a Lesson from the People of Okinawa"*. *Health, September,* 57-63.

116

The relatively good health of the Japanese, who have a longer life expectancy than any other country in the world, is generally attributed to a low-fat diet. Although the Japanese eat little dairy products, the notion that their diet is low in fat is a myth; rather, it contains moderate amounts of animal fat from eggs, pork, chicken, beef, seafood, and offal. With their taste for fish and seafood casserole, which they consume daily, the Japanese probably ingest more cholesterol than most Americans. What they do not consume is much vegetable oil, white flour or processed foods-although they do eat white rice. Japanese life expectancy has increased since World War II with the increase in their diet of animal fat and protein.[53] Those who point to Japanese statistics to promote the low-fat diet fail to mention that the Swiss live almost as long on one of the world's fattiest diets. Tied for third place in longevity are Austria and Greece, both with high-fat diets.[54]

As a final example, consider the French. Anyone who has eaten in France has observed that the French diet is full of saturated fats in the form of butter, eggs, cheese, cream, liver, meat, and pâtés. Yet the French have a lower rate of coronary heart disease than other Western countries. In the United States, 315 out of every 100 000 men of average age die of heart attack each year; in France, the rate is 145 per 100 000. In the Gascony region, where goose and duck liver are the basis of the diet, the rate is notoriously

[53] Yoshinori Koga, Ryuichi Hashimoto, Hisashi Adachi, Makoto Tsuruta, Hiromi Tashiro, Hironori Toshima (1994): *"Recent Trends in Cardiovascular Disease and Risk Factors in the Seven Countries Study: Japan"*. In Ancel Keys, Hironori Toshima, Yoshinori Koga & Henry Blackburn (eds.) *Lessons for Science from the Seven Countries Study. A 35-Year Collaborative Experience in Cardiovascular Disease Epidemiology*, 63-74. New York, New York: Springer.
[54] Thomas J. Moore (1990): *Lifespan: What Really Affects Human Longevity*. New York, New York: Simon and Schuster.

low at 80 per 100,000.[55] This phenomenon has recently attracted international attention as the French Paradox. — However, the French do suffer from many degenerative diseases. They consume large amounts of sugar and white flour and in recent years have succumbed to the temptation to save time with processed foods.

A chorus of *establishment* voices, including the American Cancer Society, the National Cancer Institute and the Senate Committee on Nutrition and Human Needs, argue that animal fat is linked not only to heart disease, but also to several types of cancer. However, when researchers at the University of Maryland analyzed the data used in those arguments, they found that vegetable fat consumption was correlated with cancer and animal fat was not.[56]

To understand the chemistry of fats

Something is wrong with the theories we read in the press — and which are used to bolster sales of low-fat, cholesterol-free foods. The concept that saturated fats *per se* cause heart disease is not only simplistic, it is simply wrong. But it is true that some fats are bad for us. To understand which ones are, we need to know something about the chemistry of fats.

Fats — or lipids — are a type of organic substance that are not soluble in water. In simple terms, fatty acids are chains of carbon atoms with hydrogen atoms filling the available bonds. Most of the fat in our bodies and in the food we eat is in the form of

---

[55] Molly O'Neill (November 17, 1991): "*Can Foie Gras Aid the Heart? A French Scientist Says Yes*". *NY Times*, World Section, November 17, 1991. http://www.nytimes.com/1991/11/17/world/can-foie-gras-aid-the-heart-a-french-scientist-says-yes.html?pagewanted=all

[56] Mary G. Enig, Robert J. Munn & Mark Keeney (1978): "*Dietary Fat and Cancer Trends — A Critique*". *Federation Proceedings*, *37*(9), 2215-2220.

triglycerides, that is, three fatty acid chains connected to a glycerol molecule. Elevated triglycerides in the blood have been positively linked to the likelihood of heart disease; but these triglycerides do not come directly from dietary fats; they are formed in the liver by excess sugar that has not been used for energy. The source of this excess sugar is any food containing carbohydrates, particularly refined sugar, and white flour.

Classification of fatty acids by saturation

Fatty acids are classified as follows:

Saturated: A fatty acid is saturated when all available carbon bonds are occupied by a hydrogen atom. They are highly stable because all the carbon atom bonds are filled — or saturated — with hydrogen. This means that they do not normally go rancid even when heated for cooking. They are in their pure form and, therefore, come together easily to form solid or semi-solid fat at room temperature. Your body produces saturated fatty acids from carbohydrates; saturated fatty acids are found in animal fats and tropical oils [palm oil and coconut oil].

Monounsaturated: Monounsaturated fatty acids have a double bond in the form of two carbon atoms double bonded together and therefore lack two hydrogen atoms. Your body produces monounsaturated fatty acids from saturated fatty acids and uses them in various ways. Monounsaturated fats have a bend or fold at the site of the double bond so that they cannot come together as easily as saturated fats and, therefore, tend to be liquid at room temperature. Like saturated fats, they are relatively stable. They do not go rancid easily and thus can be used in cooking. The most common monounsaturated fatty acid found in our foods is oleic acid, the main component of olive oil, almond oil, pecan nuts, cashews, peanuts, and avocado.

Polyunsaturated: Polyunsaturated fatty acids have two or more pairs of double bonds and, therefore, lack four or more hydrogen atoms. The two polyunsaturated fatty acids most frequently found in our food are double unsaturated linoleic acid, with two double bonds — also called omega 6 — ; and triple unsaturated linoleic acid, with three double bonds — also called omega 3. The omega number indicates the position of the first double bond. Your body cannot produce these fatty acids and, therefore, they are called "essential". We must get our essential fatty acids or EFA (Essential Fatty Acid) from the foods we eat.

Polyunsaturated fatty acids have bends or folds at the double bond position and, therefore, do not join together easily. They are liquid even under refrigeration. Unpaired electrons in the double bonds make these oils highly reactive. They go rancid easily, particularly omega-3 linoleic acid, and must be treated with care. Polyunsaturated oils should never be heated or used in cooking. In nature, polyunsaturated fatty acids are normally found in the cis form, which means that both hydrogen atoms in the double bond are on the same side.

All fats and oils, of both animal and vegetable origin, have the same combination of saturated fatty acids, monounsaturated fatty acids and polyunsaturated linoleic acids and linoleic acid. Generally speaking, animal fats such as butter, lard and tallow contain between 40% and 60% saturated fat and are solid at room temperature. Vegetable oils from northern [or southern and mid-latitude] climates contain a preponderance of polyunsaturated fatty acids and are liquid at room temperature. But vegetable oils from the tropics are highly saturated.

For example, coconut oil is 92% saturated. These fats are liquid in the tropics, but hard like butter in northern — or southern and mid-latitude — climates. Vegetable oils are more saturated in hot climates because the higher saturation helps them to maintain the rigidity of plant leaves — coconut, palm —. Olive oil with its preponderance of oleic acid is a product of a temperate climate. It is liquid at hot temperatures but hardens when refrigerated.

Classification of fatty acids by length

Researchers classify fatty acids not only according to their degree of saturation, but also by their length.

Short-chain fatty acids have four to six carbon atoms. These fats are always saturated. Four-carbon butyric acid is found mostly in dairy fat from cows and six-carbon capric acid is found mostly in dairy fat from goats. These fatty acids have antimicrobial properties — this means that they protect us against viruses, yeasts, and pathogenic bacteria in the intestine. They do not need to be activated by bile salts but are directly absorbed for quick energy. For this reason, they are less likely to cause weight gain than olive oil or commercial vegetable oils.[57] Short-chain fatty acids also contribute to the health of the immune system.[58]

Medium-chain fatty acids have eight to twelve carbon atoms and are found primarily in dairy fat and tropical oils. Like short-chain fatty acids, these fats have antimicrobial properties, are directly absorbed for quick energy, and contribute to immune system health.

Long-chain fatty acids have fourteen to eighteen carbon atoms and can be saturated, monounsaturated, or polyunsaturated. Stearic acid is an eighteen-carbon saturated fatty acid found mainly in meat and mutton tallow. Oleic acid is an eighteen-carbon monounsaturated fat and the main component of olive oil. Another monounsaturated fatty acid is sixteen-carbon palmitoleic acid, which has strong

[57] María del Puy Portillo, Francisca Serra, Edurne Simón, Antonio S. del Barrio & Andreu Palou (1998): *"Energy Restriction with High-Fat Diet Enriched with Coconut Oil Gives Higher UCP1 [Uncoupling Protein] and Lower with Fat in Rats"*. International Journal of Obesity Related and Metabolic Disorders, 22 (10), 974-979. https://www.researchgate.net/publication/13480850_Energy_restriction_with_high-fat_diet_enriched_with_coconut_oil_gives_higher_UCP1_and_lower_white_fat_in_rats, http://www.nature.com/ijo/journal/v22/n10/pdf/0800706a.pdf. Abdul G. Dulloo, Nouri Mensi, Josiane Seydoux & Lucien Girardier (1995). *"Differential Effects of High-Fat Diets Varying in Fatty Acid Composition on the Efficiency of Lean and Fat Tissue Deposition during Weight Recovery after Low Food Intake"*. Metabolism, 44 (2), 273-279.

[58] Jon J. Kabara (1978): *"Fatty Acids and Derivatives as Antimicrobial Agents — A Review"*. In *The Pharmacological Effects of Lipids*, 1-14. Champaign, Illinois: The American Oil Chemists' Society. Leonard A. Cohen, Diane O. Thompson, Keewhan Choi, Rashida A. Karmali & David P. Rose (1986): *"Dietary Fat and Mammary Cancer. II. Modulation of Serum and Tumor Lipid Composition and Tumor Prostaglandins by Different Dietary Fats: Association with Tumor Incidence Patterns"*. Journal of the National Cancer Institute, 77 (1), 43-51.

antimicrobial properties. It is found almost exclusively in animal fats. The two essential fatty acids also have a long chain, each is eighteen carbons long. Another important long-chain fatty acid is gamma-linolenic acid (GLA), which has eighteen carbons and three double bonds. It is found in *evening primrose oil*, borage, and blackcurrant. Your body can produce GLA from omega-6 linoleic acid and use it for the production of substances called prostaglandins, hormones located in certain tissues that regulate many cellular processes.

Very long fatty acids have twenty to twenty-four carbon atoms. They tend to be highly unsaturated with four, five or six double bonds. Some people can produce these fatty acids from EFAs, but others, particularly those with ancestors who ate a lot of fish, lack the enzymes to produce them. These "obligate carnivores" must obtain them from animal foods such as offal, egg yolks, butter, and fish oils. The most important very long-chain fatty acids are *dihomo-gamma-linolenic acid* (DGLA) with twenty carbons and three double bonds; arachidonic *acid* (AA) with twenty carbons and four double bonds; eicosapentaenoic acid (eicosapentaenoic acid) with twenty carbons and four double bonds; eicosapentaenoic *acid* (EPA) with twenty carbons and five double bonds; and docosahexaenoic *acid* (DHA) with twenty-two carbons and six double bonds. All of these, with the exception of DHA, are used in the production of prostaglandins, tissue-specific hormones that direct many cellular processes. Additionally, AA and DHA play important roles in the functioning of the nervous system.[59]

---

[59] Pierre Guesry (1998): "*The Role of Nutrition in Brain Development*". *Preventive Medicine, 27* (2), 189-194. Peter Willatts, J. Stewart Forsyth, M. K. DiModugno, Sonal Varma & Mark Colvin (1998): "*Effect of Long-Chain Polyunsaturated Fatty Acids in Infant Formula on Problem Solving at 10 Months of Age*". *The Lancet, 352* (9129), 688-691. Good

The dangers of polyunsaturates

The public has been fed a great deal of misinformation about the virtues of saturated fats versus polyunsaturated oils. The politically correct diet gurus say that polyunsaturated oils are good for us and that saturated fats cause cancer and heart disease. As a result, the Western diet has undergone fundamental changes. At the turn of the century (from the 19TH to the 20TH), most of the fatty acids in the diet were saturated or monounsaturated, coming mainly from butter, lard, tallow, coconut oil and small amounts of olive oil. Today, most fats in the diet are polyunsaturated and come from vegetable oils derived from soybean, corn, safflower, and canola (rapeseed).

Modern diets may contain up to 30% of calories from polyunsaturated oils, but scientific research indicates that this amount is too high. The best evidence indicates that our intake of polyunsaturates should be no more than 4% of total calories, in portions of approximately 1.5% omega-3 linoleic acid and 2.5% omega-6 linoleic acid.[60] This EFA consumption rate appears in native populations of temperate and tropical regions, whose intake of polyunsaturated oils comes from small amounts in legumes, grains, nuts, green vegetables, fish, olive oil and animal fats, but not from commercial vegetable oils.

Excessive consumption of polyunsaturated oils has been shown to contribute to a host of diseases, including increased cancer and heart disease; immune system dysfunction;

Fats Help Children's Behavioral Problems, *Let's Live*, September 1997, 65 (9), 45.

[60] Manon Lasserre, François Mendy, Danièle Spielmann & Bernard Jacotot (1985), "*Effects of Different Dietary Intake of Essential Fatty Acids on C20:3ω6 and C20:4ω6 Serum Levels in Human Adults*". *Lipids*, 20 (4), 227-233.

damage to the liver, reproductive organs, and lungs; digestive disorders; poor learning ability; poor growth; and weight gain.[61]

One reason why polyunsaturates cause so many health problems is that they tend to oxidize and become rancid when exposed to heat, oxygen and moisture, as happens in processing and cooking. Rancid oils are characterized by free radicals — that is, single or cluster atoms with an unpaired electron in an outer orbital. Chemically, these compounds are extremely reactive. They have been characterized as "marauders" in the body because they attack cell membranes and red blood cells and cause damage to DNA and RNA components, triggering mutations in tissues, blood vessels and skin. Free radical damage to skin causes wrinkles and premature aging; free radical damage to tissues and organs sets the stage for tumors; free radical damage to blood vessels initiates plaque buildup.

---

[61] An overview of the literature for problems related to polyunsaturated intake is found in Edward R. Pinckney & Cathey Pinckney (1973): *The Cholesterol Controversy*, 127-131. Los Angeles: Sherbourne Press. Research showing the correlation between polyunsaturated oils and learning disabilities is found in Denham Harman, Shelton Hendricks, Dennis E. Eddy & Jon Seibold (1976): *"Free Radical Theory of Aging: Effect of Dietary Fat on Central Nervous System Function"*. *Journal of the American Geriatrics Society*, 24 (7), 301-307. F. Z. Meerson, L. S. Katkova & Yu. P. Kozlov (1983), *"Prevention of Disturbances of Cardiac Contractility during Long-Term Stress by Preliminary Adaptation to Short-Term Stress"*. *Bulletin of Experimental Biology and Medicine*, 96 (6), 1675-1678. With respect to weight gain, linoleic acid levels in adipose tissue reflect the amount of linoleic acid in the diet. Daniel Valero-Garrido,-Magdalena López-Frías, Juan Llopis-González & María López-Jurado (1990): *"Influence of Dietary Fat on the Lipid Composition of Perirenal Adipose Tissue in Rats"*. *Annals of Nutrition and Metabolism*, 34 (6), 323-327. Carl V. Felton, David Crook, M. J. Davies & M. F. Oliver (1994): *"Dietary Polyunsaturated Fatty Acids and Composition of Human Aortic Plaques"*. *The Lancet*, 344 (8931), 1195-1196.

Is anyone surprised that tests and studies have repeatedly shown a high correlation between cancer and heart disease with polyunsaturated intake?[62] New evidence links free radical exposure to premature aging, autoimmune diseases such as arthritis and Parkinson's disease, Lou Gehrig's disease, Alzheimer's disease, and cataracts.[63]

Too much omega 6

The problems associated with excess polyunsaturates are compounded by the fact that most of the polyunsaturates in commercial vegetable oils are in the form of doubly unsaturated omega-6 linoleic acid, with very little of the vital triple unsaturated omega-3 linoleic acid. Recent research has revealed that too much omega-6 in the diet creates an imbalance that can interfere with the production of important prostaglandins.[64]

This interference may result in an increased tendency to produce blood clots, inflammation, high blood pressure,

---

[62] Edward R. Pinckney & Cathey Pinckney (1973): *The Cholesterol Controversy*, 130. Los Angeles: Sherbourne Press. Mary G. Enig, Robert J. Munn & Mark Keeney (1978): "*Dietary Fat and Cancer Trends — A Critique*". Federation Proceedings, *37* (9), 2215-2220.

[63] Lawrence J. Machlin & Adrianne Bendich (1987): "*Free Radical Tissue Damage: Protective Role of Antioxidant Nutrients*". FASEB Journal, The Official Journal of Federation of American Societies for Experimental Biology, *1* (6), 441-445.

[64] John E. Kinsella (1988): "*Fish and Seafoods: Nutritional Implications and Quality Issues*". Food Technology, *42* (5), 146-150. Manon Lasserre, François Mendy, Danièle Spielmann & Bernard Jacotot (1985): "*Effects of Different Dietary Intake of Essential Fatty Acids on C20:3ω6 and C20:4ω6 Serum Levels in Human Adults*". Lipids, 20 (4), 227-233.

irritation of the digestive tract, depression of immune function, sterility, cell proliferation, cancer, and weight gain.[65]

Too little omega 3

Several researchers have argued that, in addition to an excess of omega-6 fatty acids, the American diet is deficient in omega-3 linoleic acid, the most unsaturated fatty acid. This fatty acid is necessary for cellular oxidation, for metabolizing important sulfur-containing amino acids, and for maintaining a proper balance in prostaglandin production. Deficiencies of omega-3 linoleic acid have been associated with asthma, heart disease and learning disabilities.[66]

Most commercial vegetable oils contain large amounts of omega-6 linoleic acid and very little omega-3 linoleic acid. In addition, modern agricultural and industrial practices have reduced the amount of omega-3.

Commercial fatty acids are available in vegetables, eggs, fish, and meat. For example, organic eggs from hens allowed to feed on insects and green plants may contain omega-6 and omega-3 fatty

---

[65] David F. Horrobin (1983): "*The Regulation of Prostaglandin Biosynthesis by the Manipulation of Essential Fatty Acid Metabolism*". *Reviews in Pure and Applied Pharmacological Sciences*, 4 (4), 339-383. Thomas M. Devlin (ed.) (1983): *Textbook of Biochemistry: with Clinical Correlations*, 429-430. 2nd ed., New York: Wiley Medical. Sally Fallon & Mary G. Enig (1996): Tripping Lightly Down the Prostaglandin Pathways. *Price-Pottenger Nutrition Foundation Health Journal*, 20 (3), 5-8. http://www.westonaprice.org/know-your-fats/tripping-lightly-down-the-prostaglandin-pathways/. http://www.westonaprice.org/know-your-fats/tripping-lightly-down-the-prostaglandin-pathways/

[66] Harumi Okuyama, Tetsuyuki Kobayashi & Shiro Watanabe (1997): "*Dietary Fatty Acids — The N-6/N-3 Balance and Chronic Elderly Diseases. Excess Linoleic Acid and Relative n-3 Deficiency Syndrome Seen in Japan*". *Progress in Lipid Research*, 35 (4), 409-457.

acids at an approximate one-to-one benefit ratio; but commercial eggs purchased at the supermarket may contain up to nineteen times more omega-6 than omega-3![67]

The benefit of saturated fats

The much-maligned saturated fats — which Americans try to avoid — are not the cause of our modern diseases. In fact, they play a very important role in body chemistry:

Saturated fatty acids make up at least 50% of cell membranes. They are what give our cells the necessary rigidity and integrity.

They play a vital role in the health of our bones. For calcium to be effectively incorporated into our bone structure, at least 50% of our dietary fats should be saturated.[68]

They lower lipoprotein(a) [Lp(a)], a substance in the blood that indicates a propensity for heart disease.[69] And

---

[67]   Artemis P. Simopoulos & Norman Salem (1992): *"Egg Yolk as a Source of Long-Chain Polyunsaturated Fatty Acids in Infant Feeding"*. *American Journal of Clinical Nutrition*, 55 (2), 411-414.

[68]   Bruce A. Watkins, John J. Turek, Mark F. Seifert & Hui Xu (1996): *"Importance of Vitamin E in Bone Formation and in Chondrocyte Function"*. In Lester Packer & Maret G. Traber, eds. *American Oil Chemists' Society, AOCS Proceedings, 1996, Proceedings of the International Symposium on Natural Antioxidants: Molecular Mechanisms and Health Effects*. Lafayette: Purdue University. Bruce A. Watkins & Mark F. Seifert (1996): *"Food Lipids and Bone Health"*. In Richard E. McDonald & David B. Min (eds.). *Food Lipids and Health*, 71-116. New York, New York: Marcel Dekker, Inc.

[69]   Gösta H. Dahlén, Sathanur R. Srinivasan, Hans Stenlund, Wendy Ann Wattigney, Stig Wall & Gerald S. Berenson (1998): *"The Importance of Serum Lipoprotein (a) as an Independent Risk Factor for Premature Coronary Artery Disease in Middle-Aged Black and White Women from the United States"*. *Journal of Internal Medicine*, 244 (5), 417-424. Pramod Khosla & Kenneth C. Hayes (1996). Dietary Trans-Monounsaturated

they protect the liver from alcohol and other toxins, such as Tylenol.[70]

Saturated fatty acids improve the immune system.[71]

They are necessary for the proper utilization of essential fatty acids. Long-chain omega-3 fatty acids are better retained in the tissues when the diet is rich in saturated fats.[72]

Fatty Acids Negatively Impact Plasma Lipids in Humans: Critical Review of the Evidence. *Journal of the American College of Nutrition*, *15* (4), 325-339. Beverly A. Clevidence, Joseph T. Judd, Ernst J. Schaefer, Jennifer L. Jenner, Alice H. Lichtenstein, Richard A. Muesing, Janet Wittes & Matthew E. Sunkin (1997): *"Plasma Lipoprotein (a) Levels in Men and Women Consuming Diets Enriched in Saturated, Cis-, or Trans-Monounsaturated Fatty Acids."* Arteriosclerosis, Thrombosis, and Vascular Biology, *17*(9), 1657-1661.

[70] Amin A. Nanji, S.M. Hossein Sadrzadeh, Eun K. Yang, Franz Fogt, Mohsen Meydani & Andrew J. Dannenberg (1995): *"Dietary Saturated Fatty Acids: A Novel Treatment for Alcoholic Liver Disease"*. Gastroenterology, *109* (2), 547-554. Youn-Soo Cha & Dileep S. Sachan (1994): *"Opposite Effects of Dietary Saturated and Unsaturated Fatty Acids on Ethanol-Pharmacokinetics, Triglycerides and Carnitines"*. *Journal of the American College of Nutrition*, *13* (4), 338-343. James L. Hargrove, Jinah Hwang, K. Wickwire & J. Liu. Diets with Corn Oil or Soybean Oil Increase Acute Acetaminophen Hepatotoxicity Compared to Diets with Beef Tallow. *FASEB Journal, The Official Journal of Federation of American Societies for Experimental Biology*, Meeting Abstracts, Mar 1999, #204.1, p A222.

[71] Jon J. Kabara (1978): *"Fatty Acids and Derivatives as Antimicrobial Agents — A Review"*. In *The Pharmacological Effects of Lipids*, 1-14. Champaign, Illinois: The American Oil Chemists' Society. Leonard A. Cohen, Diane O. Thompson, Keewhan Choi, Rashida A. Karmali & David P. Rose (1986): *"Dietary Fat and Mammary Cancer. II. Modulation of Serum and Tumor Lipid Composition and Tumor Prostaglandins by different Dietary Fats: Association with Tumor Incidence Patterns"*. Journal of the National Cancer Institute, *77*(1), 43-51.

[72] Manohar L. Garg, Alan B. R. Thomson & Michael T. Clandinin (1988): *"Effect of Dietary Alpha-Linolenic Acid Fed with High-Levels of Either Saturated Fatty-Acids or Linoleic-Acid on Cholesterol and Fatty-Acid Metabolism in Rat Serum and Liver"*. FASEB Journal, The Official Journal of Federation of American Societies for Experimental Biology, 2,

Saturated stearic acid with eighteen carbons and palmitic acid with sixteen carbons are the preferred foods of the heart, which is why the fat around the heart is highly saturated.[73] The heart feeds on this fat reserve in times of stress.

Short and medium chain saturated fatty acids have important antimicrobial properties. They protect us against harmful microorganisms in the digestive tract.

Honestly evaluated, the scientific evidence does not support the claim that saturated fats that cause "arterial clogging" cause heart disease.[74] In fact, evaluation of the fat in arterial clogging reveals that only 26% is saturated. The rest is unsaturated, of which more than half is polyunsaturated.[75]

What about cholesterol?

What about cholesterol? Here, too, the public has been misinformed. Our blood vessels can also be damaged in various ways — by irritations caused by free radicals and viruses or

---

A852-A852. Rosa María Oliart-Ros *et al.* (1998): *"Meeting Abstracts"*, *American Oil Chemists' Society, AOCS Proceedings*, May 1998, 7, Chicago, IL.

[73] Larry D. Lawson & Fred A. Kummerow (1979): "ß-oxidation *of the Coenzyme A Esters of Elaidic, Oleic, and Stearic Acids and their Full-Cycle Intermediates Rat Heart Mitochondria"*. *Lipids*, *14* (5), 501-503. Manohar L. Garg, Antoni A. Wierzbicki, Alan B. R. Thomson & Michael T. Clandinin (1989), *"Dietary Saturated Fat Level Alters the Competition between Alpha-Linolenic and Linoleic-Acid." Lipids*, *24* (4), 334-339.

[74] Uffe Ravnskov (1998): *"The Questionable Role of Saturated and Polyunsaturated Fatty Acids in Cardiovascular Disease"*. *Journal of Clinical Epidemiology*, *51* (6), 443-460.

[75] Carl V. Felton, David Crook, M. J. Davies & M. F. Oliver (1994): *"Dietary Polyunsaturated Fatty Acids and Composition of Human Aortic Plaques"*. *The Lancet*, *344* (8931), 1195-1196.

because they are structurally weak — and when this happens, the body's natural healing substance steps in to repair the damage. This substance is cholesterol. Cholesterol is a high molecular weight alcohol that the liver and most human cells produce. Like saturated fats, the cholesterol we produce and consume plays many vital roles:

Together with saturated fats, cholesterol present in cell membranes gives our cells the necessary rigidity and stability. When the diet contains an excess of polyunsaturated fatty acids, they replace the saturated fatty acids within the cell membrane, causing the cell walls to become flaccid. When this occurs, cholesterol is "carried" by the blood to the tissues and gives them structural integrity. This is why serum cholesterol levels can be temporarily lowered when we replace saturated fats with polyunsaturated oils in the diet.[76]

Cholesterol acts as a precursor for vital corticosteroids, hormones that help us manage stress and protect our bodies against heart disease and cancer; and for sex hormones, such as androgen, testosterone, estrogen, and progesterone.

Cholesterol is a precursor of vitamin D, a fat-soluble vitamin necessary for healthy bones and a healthy nervous system, proper growth, mineral metabolism, muscle tone, insulin production, reproduction, and immune system function.

Bile salts are made of cholesterol. Bile is vital for digestion and assimilation of dietary fats.

---

[76] Peter J. Jones (1997): "*Regulation of Cholesterol Biosynthesis by Diet in Humans*". *American Journal of Clinical Nutrition, 66* (2), 438-446. A. D. Julius, Kenneth D. Wiggers & Marlene J. Richard (1982): "*Effect of Infant Formulas on Blood and Tissue Cholesterol, Bone Calcium, and Body Composition in Weanling Pigs*". *Journal of Nutrition, 112* (12), 2240-2249.

Recent research shows that cholesterol acts as an antioxidant.[77] This is the possible explanation for the fact that cholesterol levels increase with age. As an antioxidant, cholesterol protects us against free radical damage that causes heart disease and cancer.

Cholesterol is necessary for the proper functioning of serotonin receptors in the brain.[78] Serotonin is the body's natural "feel good" chemical. Low cholesterol levels have been linked to aggressive and violent behavior, depression, and suicidal tendencies.

Breast milk is especially rich in cholesterol and contains a special enzyme that helps the baby use this nutrient. Infants and children need cholesterol-rich foods during their growing years to ensure proper development of their brain and nervous system.

Dietary cholesterol plays an important role in maintaining the health of the intestinal walls.[79] Because of this, vegetarian diets with low cholesterol can lead to gingival bowel syndrome [leaky gut] and other intestinal disorders.

Cholesterol is not the cause of heart disease, but a powerful antioxidant weapon against free radicals in the blood and a repair

---

[77] Elmer M. Cranton & James P. Frackelton, MD (1984): "*Free Radical Pathology in Age-Associated Diseases: Treatment with EDTA Chelation, Nutrition and Antioxidants*". *Journal of Holistic Medicine*, Spring/Summer 1984, 6-37.

[78] Hyman Engelberg (1992): "*Low Serum Cholesterol and Suicide*". *Lancet*, *339* (8795), 727-729. W. Gibson Wood, Friedhelm Schroeder, Nicolai A. Avdulov, Svetlana V. Chochina & Urule Igbavboa (1999). Recent Advances in Brain Cholesterol Dynamics: Transport, Domains, and Alzheimer's Disease. *Lipids, 34* (3), 225-234.

[79] Roslyn B. Alfin-Slater & Lilla Aftergood (1980): "*Lipids.*" In Robert S. Goodhart & Maurice E. Shils (eds.). *Modern Nutrition in Health and Disease; Dietotherapy*, 134. 6th ed. Philadelphia: Lea and Febiger.

substance that helps heal arterial damage — although the plaques that clog arteries contain very little cholesterol themselves. However, like fats, cholesterol can be damaged by exposure to heat and oxygen. This damaged or oxidized cholesterol appears to cause both injury to arterial cells and the pathological buildup of plaques in the arteries.[80] Oxidized or damaged cholesterol is found in powdered eggs, powdered milk — added to low-fat milks to give them consistency — and in meats and fats that have been fried at high temperatures in oil or other high-temperature processes.

High blood cholesterol levels often indicate that the body needs cholesterol to protect itself from high levels of altered fats containing free radicals. Just as a large police force is needed in a place where many crimes occur, so cholesterol is needed in a poorly nourished body to protect the person from the tendency to heart disease and cancer. Blaming cholesterol for coronary heart disease is like blaming the police for murder and robbery in a place with a high crime rate.

Poor thyroid gland function-hypothyroidism-often results in high cholesterol levels. When thyroid function is poor, usually because of a diet high in sugar and low in usable iodine, fat-soluble vitamins and other nutrients, the body floods the blood with cholesterol as an adaptive and protective mechanism to provide an overabundance of materials needed to heal tissues and produce protective steroids. People with hypothyroidism are especially susceptible to infections, heart disease and cancer.[81]

---

[80] Paul Addis (1990): *"Coronary Heart Disease"*. *Food and Nutrition News*, *62* (2), 7-10.

[81] Broda Otto Barnes & Lawrence Galton (1976): *Hypothyroidism, The Unsuspected Illness*. New York, NY: Thomas Y. Crowell.

The cause and treatment of heart disease

The cause of heart disease is not animal fat or cholesterol, but rather a number of factors inherent in modern diets, including excessive consumption of vegetable oils and hydrogenated fats; excessive consumption of refined carbohydrates in the form of sugar and white flour; mineral deficiencies, especially low levels of the very protective magnesium and iodine; deficiencies of vitamins, especially vitamin C, necessary for the integrity of blood vessel walls, and of antioxidants such as selenium and vitamin E, which protect us from free radicals; and finally, the disappearance of antimicrobial fats provided by the diet, mainly from animal fats and tropical oils.[82] These once protected us against the types of viruses and bacteria that have been associated with the appearance of the pathogenic plaque that leads to heart disease.

While blood cholesterol levels provide an incorrect indication of impending heart disease, a high blood level of a substance called homocysteine has been positively correlated with pathological plaque buildup in the arteries and the tendency to form clots, a deadly combination. Folic acid, vitamin B6, vitamin B12 and choline are nutrients that lower homocysteine levels in the blood.[83] These nutrients are found mainly in foods of animal origin.

Therefore, the best way to treat heart disease is not to focus on lowering cholesterol — either with medication or diet — but to consume a diet that provides animal food rich in vitamins B6 and B12; strengthen the functioning of the thyroid gland by using natural sea salt, a good source of usable iodine, on a daily basis; avoid vitamin and mineral deficiencies that make artery walls more susceptible to rupture and plaque buildup; include antimicrobial

---

[82]   Sally Fallon & Mary G. Enig (1996): *"Diet and Heart Disease — Not What You Think"*. *Consumers' Research*, *79* (7), 15-19.

[83]   Johan B. Ubbink (1994): *"Vitamin Nutrition Status and Homocysteine: an Atherogenic Risk Factor"*. *Nutrition Review*, *52* (11), 383-393.

fats in the diet and eliminate processed foods containing refined carbohydrates, oxidized cholesterol and vegetable oils with free radicals that cause the body to be in constant need of repair.

Modern fat processing methods

It is important to understand that of all the substances the body ingests, polyunsaturated oils are the most dangerous in industrially processed foods, especially the unstable omega-3 linoleic acid [subjected to heat]. Consider the following processes inflicted on natural fatty acids before they appear on our tables:

Extraction: Natural oils from fruits, nuts and seeds first have to be extracted. In the old days, this extraction was done with slowly rotating stone presses. But the oils processed in large factories are obtained by grinding the oilseeds and heating them to 230 °C. This oil is then extracted at pressures of ten to twenty tons per square inch, which generates even more heat. During this process, the oils are exposed to harmful light and oxygen. In order to extract the remaining 10% or more oil from the ground seeds, processors treat the pulp with one of several solvents, usually hexane, a petroleum derivative. This solvent evaporates, although up to 100 parts per million remain in the oil. These solvents, themselves toxic, also retain toxic pesticides that adhere to the seeds and kernels before processing begins.

High-temperature processing causes the weak carbon chains in unsaturated fatty acids, especially triple unsaturated linoleic acid, to separate and create dangerous free radicals in the process. In addition, antioxidants, such as fat-soluble vitamin E, which protects the body against the ravages of free radicals, are neutralized or destroyed by the high temperatures and pressures. BHT (*butylated hydroxytoluene*) and BHA (*butylated hydroxyanisole*), both suspected of causing cancer and brain damage, are often added to these oils to replace the vitamin E and other natural preservatives that such heat destroys.

There is a modern extraction technique that pierces the seeds and extracts the oil and its valuable cargo of antioxidants at low temperatures, with minimal exposure to light and oxygen. These unrefined oils, extracted by mechanical pressure (Expeller®), will remain fresh for a long period if stored in dark bottles in the refrigerator. Extra virgin olive oil is produced by grinding the olives between mortar stones or steel rollers. This process is gentle in that it preserves the fatty acids and the many natural preservatives in olive oil. If olive oil is packaged in opaque containers, it will retain its freshness and valuable antioxidant content for many years.

Hydrogenation: This is the process that converts polyunsaturates, normally liquid at room temperature, into solid fats at room temperature: margarine and shortening. To produce them, manufacturers start with the cheapest oils — soybean, corn, cottonseed, or canola, already rancid from the extraction process — and mix them with tiny particles of metal, usually nickel oxide. The oil, with its nickel catalyst, is then subjected to hydrogen gas in a high-pressure, high-temperature reactor. Emulsifiers and soap-like starches are then squeezed out of this mixture to give it a better consistency; and again, the oil is subjected to high temperatures when it is steam-cleaned. This eliminates the unpleasant odor. The margarine's natural color, an unappetizing gray, is removed with bleach [chlorine]. Next, strong coloring and flavoring must be added to make it look like butter. Finally, the mixture is compressed and packaged into blocks or tubes that are sold as health foods.

Partially hydrogenated margarines and shortenings are even worse for you than the highly refined vegetable oils from which they are made because of the chemical changes that occur during the hydrogenation process. At high temperatures, the nickel catalyst causes hydrogen atoms to change position within the fatty acid chain. Prior to hydrogenation, the pairs of hydrogen atoms are together in the chain, which causes the chain to bend slightly and form a concentration of electrons at the site of the double bond. This is called cis-formation, the most common configuration in nature. With hydrogenation, a hydrogen atom is moved to the opposite side so that the molecule straightens. This is called trans formation, which is rare in nature. Most man-made trans fats are a toxin to the body, but unfortunately, your digestive system does not recognize them as such. Instead of eliminating them, trans fats are incorporated into cell membranes as if they were cis fats: your cells actually become partially hydrogenated! Once in place, trans fatty acids, with their missing hydrogen atom, wreak havoc on cellular metabolism because chemical reactions can only take place when the electrons within cell membranes are in a certain order or pattern, which has been disrupted by the hydrogenation process.

In the 1940s, several researchers found a strong correlation between cancer and fat consumption — the fats used were hydrogenated fats, although the results were presented as if saturated fats were the culprit.[84] In fact, until recently, saturated fats were lumped together with trans fats in the various U.S. databases used by researchers to correlate dietary trends with disease.[85] Thus, naturally occurring saturated fats were tarred with the black brush of artificially hydrogenated vegetable oils.

---

[84] Mary G. Enig (1993): *"Trans Fatty Acids: An Update"*. *Nutrition Quarterly*, *17* (4), 79-95.

[85] Mary G. Enig (1995). *Trans Fatty Acids in the Food Supply: A Comprehensive Report Covering 60 Years of Research*, 148-154. 2nd ed., Silver Spring, Maryland: Enig Associates, Inc. Mary G. Enig, Subodh Atal, Mark Keeney & Joseph Sampugna (1990): *"Isomeric Trans Fatty Acids in the U. S. Diet"*. *Journal of the American College of Nutrition*, *9*, 471-486.

Partially altered hydrogenated fats made from vegetable oils actually block the utilization of essential fatty acids and cause many detrimental effects, including sexual dysfunction, elevated blood cholesterol and paralysis of the immune system.[86] Consumption of hydrogenated fats is associated with harboring a host of other diseases, not only cancer, but also arteriosclerosis, diabetes, obesity, immune system disruption, low birth weight babies, birth defects, impaired visual acuity, difficulty breastfeeding, and bone and tendon problems.[87] And yet they continue to promote hydrogenated fats as health foods. The increased popularity of partially hydrogenated margarine compared to butter represents a triumph of advertising duplicity over common sense. Your best defense is to avoid it like the plague.

Homogenization: This is the process by which fat particles in the cream are strained through small pores under great pressure. The resulting fat particles are so small that they remain in suspension rather than rising to the top of the milk. This makes the fat and cholesterol more susceptible to oxidation and

---

[86] Ralph T. Holman (1979): "*The Importance of Double Bond Position in the Metabolism of Unsaturated Fatty Acids*". In Edward A. Emken & Herbert J. Dutton (eds.). *Geometrical and Positional Fatty Acid Isomers*, 283-302. Champaign, Illinois: American Oil Chemists' Society. *Science Newsletter*, Feb 1956. Edward J. Schantz, Conrad A. Elvehjem & Edwin Bret Hart (1940): "*The Comparative Nutritive Value of Butter Fat and Certain Vegetable Oils*". *Journal of Dairy Science, 23* (2), 181-189.

[87] Mary G. Enig (1995): *Trans Fatty Acids in the Food Supply: A Comprehensive Report Covering 60 Years of Research,* 4-8. 2nd ed. Silver Spring, Maryland: Enig Associates, Inc. Bruce A. Watkins, Colin C. Whitehead & S. R. I. Duff (1991). Watkins, Colin C. Whitehead & S. R. I. Duff (1991). Hydrogenated Oil Decreases Tissue Concentrations of n-6 Polyunsaturated Fatty Acids and May Contribute to Dyschondroplasia in Broilers. *British Poultry Science, 32* (5), 1109-1119.

rancidity; some researchers indicate that homogenized fats may contribute to heart disease.[88]

The constant media attack on saturated fats is extremely suspicious. Claims that butter causes chronically high cholesterol have not been substantiated by research — although some studies show that butter consumption causes a small temporary increase — while other studies have shown that stearic acid, the main component of meat fat, actually lowers cholesterol.[89] Margarine, on the other hand, causes chronically high cholesterol levels and has been linked to both heart disease and cancer.[90] The new soft or spreadable margarines, although lower in hydrogenated fats, are still produced from rancid vegetable oils and contain many additives.

Nutrients in butter

Diet dictators have been successful in convincing Americans that butter is dangerous, when in fact it is a valuable element of many traditional diets and a source of the following nutrients:

Fat-soluble vitamins: These include true vitamin A or retinol, vitamin D, vitamin K and vitamin E, as well as all of their naturally occurring cofactors necessary for maximum effect. For Americans, butter is the best source of these important nutrients.

---

[88] John P. Zikakis, Stanley J. Rzucidlo & Nicholas Oliver Biasotto (1977): "*Persistence of Bovine Milk Xanthine Oxidase Activity after Gastric Digestion in Vivo and in Vitro*". *Journal of Dairy Science, 60* (4), 533-541. Kurt A. Oster (1971), "*Plasmalogen Diseases: A New Concept of the Etiology of the Atherosclerotic Process*". *American Journal of Clinical Research, 2* (1), 30-35.

[89] Andrea Bonanome & Scott M. Grundy (1988): "*Effect of Dietary Stearic Acid on Plasma Cholesterol and Lipoprotein Levels*". *The New England Journal of Medicine, 318* (19), 1244-1248.

[90] Gary Farr (1991): "*What are Fats?*". *Nutrition Week, 21* (12), 2-3.

In fact, vitamin A is more readily absorbed and utilized when it comes from butter than from other sources.[91] Fortunately, these fat-soluble vitamins are relatively stable and survive the pasteurization process.

When Dr. Weston Price studied isolated traditional populations around the world, he found that butter was the basis of many native diets — he found no isolated populations consuming polyunsaturated oils. The groups he studied especially valued the deep yellow butter produced by cows fed on fast-growing green grass. Their natural intuition told them that the life-giving qualities were especially beneficial to children and expectant mothers. When Dr. Price analyzed this deep yellow butter, he found that it was exceptionally rich in fat-soluble vitamins, especially vitamin A. He called these vitamins "catalytic" or "activating" vitamins. According to Dr. Price, without them we are not able to utilize the minerals we consume, no matter how abundant they are in our diets. He also believed that fat-soluble vitamins were necessary for the absorption of water-soluble vitamins. Vitamins A and D are essential for growth, healthy bones, proper brain and nervous system development, and normal sexual development. Many studies have demonstrated the importance of milk fat in reproduction; its deficiency results in "nutritional castration," the failure to manifest male and female sexual characteristics. As butter consumption in the United States has declined, sterility rates and sexual development problems have increased.

---

[91] George Stronach Fraps & Arthur Russell Kemmerer (1938): "*The Relation of the Spectro Vitamin A and Carotene Content of Butter to its Vitamin A Potency Measured by Biological Methods*". *Texas Agricultural Bulletin*, 560, 5-21. https://oaktrust.library.tamu.edu/bitstream/handle/1969.1/4517/Bull0560.pdf?sequence=22&isAllowed=y

In calves, butter substitutes have not been able to stimulate growth or maintain reproduction.[92]

Not all the societies Dr. Price studied consumed butter; but all the groups he observed strove to obtain foods rich in fat-soluble vitamins — fish, shellfish, fish eggs, offal, fat from marine animals, and insects. Without knowing the names of the vitamins in these foods, isolated traditional societies recognized their importance in the diet and ate copious amounts of animal products containing them. They correctly believed that these foods were necessary for fertility and optimal child development. Dr. Price analyzed the nutritional content of native diets and found that they consistently offered nearly ten times as many fat-soluble vitamins as the American diet of the 1930s. This ratio is perhaps more extreme today, as Americans have intentionally reduced animal fat consumption. Dr. Price realized that these fat-soluble vitamins promoted faces with the beautiful bone structure, broad palate, flawless teeth without crowding, good looks, and well-proportioned features that characterized members of these isolated traditional groups. Generally speaking, American children do not eat fish and offal, at least not to any great extent, and fats and insects are not part of the Western diet; many do not want to eat eggs. The only good source of fat-soluble vitamins in the American diet, one that they are sure to eat, is dairy fat. Butter added to vegetables and spread on bread and cream added to soups and sauces ensure adequate assimilation of minerals and water-soluble vitamins from vegetables, grains, and meat.

The Wulzen factor: The compound stigmasterol, called anti-stiffness factor, is present in raw animal fat. Researcher Rosalind Wulzen discovered that this substance protects humans

---

[92] Edward J. Schantz, Conrad A. Elvehjem & Edwin Bret Hart (1940): "*The Comparative Nutritive Value of Butter Fat and Certain Vegetable Oils*". *Journal of Dairy Science, 23* (2), 181-189.

and animals from joint calcification — degenerative arthritis. It also protects against hardening of the arteries, cataracts, and calcification of the pineal gland.[93] Calves fed pasteurized milk or skim milk develop joint stiffness and do not thrive. Their symptoms are reversed when raw milk fat is added to their diet. Pasteurization destroys the Wulzen factor, which is only present in raw butter, cream, and whole milk.

Price Factor or Activator X: Discovered by Dr. Price, Activator X is a powerful catalyst that, like vitamins A and D, helps the body absorb and utilize minerals. It is found in the offal of grazing animals and in some seafood. Butter can be an especially rich source of Activator X when it comes from cows that eat fast-growing grass in the spring and fall seasons. It disappears in cows eating cottonseed-based feeds or high-protein soybean-based feeds.[94] Fortunately, Activator X — a scientific mystery for years, finally discovered to be the fat-soluble vitamin K2, menaquinone — [95] is not destroyed during pasteurization.

Arachidonic acid: This twenty-carbon polyunsaturated acid contains four double bonds and is present in small amounts only in animal fat. Arachidonic acid (AA) plays a role in brain function and is a vital component of cell membranes and a precursor to the important prostaglandins. Some diet gurus warn us against consuming foods rich in AA on the grounds that they contribute to the production of "bad" prostaglandins, which cause inflammation. But the prostaglandins that fight inflammation also come from AA.

---

[93]   Willem J. van Wagtendonk & Rosalind Wulzen (1942-1943): *"A Dietary Factor Essential for Guinea Pigs I. Isolation from Raw Cream"*. Archives of Biochemistry, 1, 373-377.

[94]   Personal communication with Pat Connolly, executive director, Price Pottenger Nutrition Foundation.

[95]   www.westonaprice.org/health-topics/abcs-of-nutrition/on-the-trail-of-the-elusive-x-factor-a-sixty-two-year-old-mystery-finally-solved/

Short — and medium-chain fatty acids: Butter contains 12-15 % short — and medium-chain fatty acids. This type of saturated fat does not need to be emulsified by bile salts, but is absorbed directly from the small intestine to the liver, where it is converted into quick energy. These fatty acids have antimicrobial, antitumor and immune-supporting properties, especially lauric acid with twelve carbons, a medium-chain fatty acid not found in any other animal fat. The highly protective lauric acid should be called conditionally essential fatty acid, because it is only produced by the mammary gland and not by the liver like other saturated fats.[96] We must obtain it from one or two food sources — small amounts in dairy fats or large amounts in coconut oil. Butyric acid with four carbons is completely unique to butter. It has antifungal properties, as well as anti-tumor effects.[97]

Omega-6 and omega-3 essential fatty acids: These are found in butter in small, almost identical amounts. This excellent balance between linoleic and linoleic acid prevents the kind of problems associated with over-consumption of omega-6 acids.

Conjugated Linoleic Acid, CLA: Butter from grazing cows also contains a form of conjugated or rearranged linoleic acids (CLA, Conjugated Linoleic Acid), which has strong anti-cancer properties. It also stimulates muscle strengthening and prevents

[96]   Mary G. Enig (1998): "*Health and Nutritional Benefits from Coconut Oil*". *Price-Pottenger Nutrition Foundation Health Journal, 20* (1), 1-6.

[97]   Kailash N. Prasad (1980): "*Minireview: Butyric Acid: A Small Fatty Acid with Diverse Biological Functions*". *Life Science, 27* (15), 1351-1358. Herman Gershon & Larry Shanks (1978): "*Antifungal Activity of Fatty Acids and Derivatives: Structure Activity Relationship*". Jon J. Kabara, ed. *Symposium on the Pharmacological Effect of Lipids*, American Oil Chemists Society 69th Annual Meeting, May 14-18, 1978, 51-62. Champaign, Illinois: American Oil Chemists Society.

weight gain. CLA disappears when cows are fed dry hay or processed feed.[98]

Lecithin: Lecithin is a natural component of butter that aids in the proper assimilation and metabolization of cholesterol and other fatty components.

Cholesterol: Breast milk is high in cholesterol because it is essential for growth and development. Cholesterol is also needed to produce a variety of steroids that protect against cancer, heart disease and mental illness.

Glycosphingolipids: This type of fat protects us against gastrointestinal infections, especially in children and older adults. For this reason, children who drink skim milk have diarrhea at a rate three to five times higher than children who drink whole milk.[99]

Trace minerals: Many trace or trace minerals are incorporated into the fat globule membrane in butterfat, including manganese, zinc, chromium, and iodine. In mountainous areas far from the sea, iodine in butter protects against goiter. Butter is extremely rich in selenium, a trace element with antioxidant properties, and contains more per gram than herring or wheat germ.

One of the most frequent objections against the consumption of butter and other animal fats is that they tend to accumulate poisons from the environment. Fat-soluble poisons such as DDT (dichloro diphenyl trichloroethane) do accumulate in fats; but

---

[98] Martha Ann Belury (1995): "*Conjugated Dienoic Linoleate: A Polyunsaturated Fatty Acid with Unique Chemoprotective Properties*". *Nutrition Reviews*, 53 (4), 83-89. Miriam L. Kelly, Eric S. Kolver, Dale E. Bauman, Michael E. van Amburgh & Larry D. Muller (1998): "*Effect of Intake of Pasture on Concentrations of Conjugated Linoleic Acid in Milk of Lactating Cows*". *Journal of Dairy Science*, 81 (6), 1630-1636.

[99] James S. Koopman, Verna Jean Turkish, Arnold S. Monto, Frances E. Thompson & Richard E. Isaacson (1984): "*Milk Fat and Gastrointestinal Illness*". *American Journal of Public Health*, 74 (12), 1371-1373.

water-soluble poisons, such as antibiotics and growth hormones, accumulate in the aqueous portion of milk and meats. Vegetables and grains also accumulate poisons. An average crop receives ten pesticide applications — from planting to storage — while cows graze in unsprayed pastures. Aflatoxin, a fungus that grows on grains, is one of the most potent known carcinogens. It is correct to assume that all our food, whether of animal or plant origin, can be contaminated. The solution to environmental poisons is not to eliminate animal fats — so essential for growth, reproduction, and overall health — but to look for organic meats and butter from grass-fed cows, as well as organic vegetables and grains. These are increasingly available in health food stores and supermarkets, by mail order and in co-ops.

The composition of the different fats

Before leaving this complex but vital subject of fats, it is worthwhile to examine the composition of vegetable oils and other animal fats in order to determine their usefulness and suitability in food preparation.

Duck and goose fat are semi-solid at room temperature, containing approximately 35 % saturated fat, 52 % monounsaturated fat — with small amounts of antimicrobial palmitic acid — and about 13 % polyunsaturated fat. The ratio of omega 6 to omega 3 fatty acids depends on what the birds have eaten. Duck and goose fat are quite stable and highly prized in Europe for frying potatoes.

Chicken fat is about 31% saturated, 49% monounsaturated — with moderate amounts of antimicrobial palmitic acid- and 20% polyunsaturated, most of which is omega-6 linoleic acid, although the amount of omega-3 can be raised by feeding chickens flaxseed or fish or allowing them to peck freely and eat insects. Although widely used for frying in *kosher* cooking, it is inferior to duck and goose fat, which were traditionally preferred to chicken fat in that Jewish cuisine.

Lard or pork fat is approximately 40% saturated, 48% monounsaturated — with small amounts of antimicrobial palmitic acid — and 12% polyunsaturated. Like poultry fat, the amount of omega-6 and omega-3 fatty acids will vary in lard, depending on the pigs' diet. In the tropics, lard can also be a source of lauric acid if the pigs have eaten coconut. Like duck and goose fat, lard is stable and is the preferred fat for frying. It was widely used in the United States during the change from the 19TH to the 20TH century. It is a good source of vitamin D, especially in third world countries where other animal foods tend to be expensive. Some researchers believe that pork products should be avoided because they may contribute to cancer. Others suggest that only pork presents problems and that fat in the form of lard is safe and healthy.

Lamb meat and tallow are 50-55 % saturated fat, 40 % monounsaturated and contain small amounts of polyunsaturated fat, usually less than 3 %. Tallow, which is the fat in the animal's cavity, is 70-80 % saturated. Lard and tallow are very stable fats and can be used for frying. Traditional cultures value these fats for their health benefits. They are a good source of antimicrobial palmitic acid.

Olive oil contains 75% oleic acid, a stable monounsaturated fat, along with 13% saturated fat, 10% omega-6 linoleic acid and 2% omega-3 linoleic acid. The high percentage of oleic acid makes olive oil ideal for salads and for cooking at moderate temperatures. Extra virgin olive oil is also rich in antioxidants. It should be cloudy, indicating that it has not been filtered, and have a golden yellow color, indicating that it is made from fully ripe olives. Olive oil has stood the test of time; it is the safest vegetable oil you can use, but don't overdo it. The longer the fatty acid chains in olive oil, the more likely they are to contribute to body fat accumulation than the short — and medium-chain fatty acids found in butter, coconut oil or palm kernel oil.

Peanut oil contains 48% oleic acid, 18% saturated fat and 34% omega-6 linoleic acid. Like olive oil, peanut oil is relatively stable and therefore suitable for occasional stir-fry dishes. But the high percentage of omega-6 presents a potential hazard, so the use of this oil should be strictly limited.

Sesame oil contains 42% oleic acid, 15% saturated fat and 43% omega 6 linoleic acid. Sesame oil has a composition similar to that of peanut oil. It can be used for frying because it contains unique antioxidants that are not destroyed by heat. However, the high percentage of omega-6 militates against exclusive use.

Safflower, corn, sunflower, soybean, and cottonseed oils contain more than 50 % omega-6 and, with the exception of soybean oil, only minimal amounts of omega-3. Safflower oil contains almost 80% omega-6. Researchers are just beginning to discover the danger of excess omega-6 oil in the diet, whether rancid or not. The use of these oils should be strictly limited. They should never be consumed after they have been heated, as in cooking, frying, or baking. High oleic oils such as safflower and sunflower, produced by hybrid plants, have a similar composition to olive oil, mainly large amounts of oleic acid and only a small amount of polyunsaturated fatty acids, and are therefore more stable than traditional varieties. However, it is difficult to find truly cold-pressed versions of these oils.

Canola oil contains 5 % saturated fat, 57 % oleic acid, 23 % omega-6 and 10-15 % omega-3. Canola oil, the newest oil on the market, was developed from rapeseed, a member of the mustard family. Canola seed is not suitable for human consumption because it contains a very long-chain fatty acid, called erucic acid, which is associated with fibrotic lesions of the heart in certain circumstances. Canola oil was produced to contain little or no erucic acid and has attracted the attention of nutritionists because of its high oleic acid content. But there are indications that canola oil presents dangers of its own. It has a high sulfur content and goes rancid easily. Products baked with canola oil quickly develop mold. During the deodorization process, the omega-3 fatty acids in processed canola oil are transformed into trans fatty acids, similar to those in margarine and possibly more dangerous.[100] A recent study indicates that "heart-healthy" canola oil actually creates a deficiency of vitamin E, a vitamin necessary for a healthy cardiovascular system.[101] Other studies indicate that even canola oils low in erucic acid cause heart damage, especially when the diet is low in saturated fat.[102]

Flaxseed oil contains 9% saturated fatty acids, 18% oleic acid, 16% omega-6 and 57% omega-3. With its extremely high omega-3 content, flaxseed oil offers a remedy for the omega-6/omega-3 imbalance so prevalent in the United States today. Not surprisingly, Scandinavian popular culture values flaxseed oil as a health food. New extraction and bottling methods have minimized rancidity problems. It should always be kept

---

[100] Personal communication, Mary G. Enig.

[101] Frank D. Sauer, Edward R. Farnworth, Jacqueline M.R. Bélanger, John K.G. Kramer, Ric B. Miller & Shigeto Yamashiro (1997): *"Additional Vitamin E Required in Milk Replacer Diets that Contain Canola Oil"*. *Nutrition Research, 17* (2), 259-269.

[102] John K. G. Kramer, Edward R. Farnworth, B. Kathleen Thompson, A. H. Corner & H. L. Trenholm (1982): *"Reduction of Myocardial Necrosis in Male Albino Rats by Manipulation of Dietary Fatty Acid Levels"*. *Lipids, 17* (5), 372-382. H. L. Trenholm, John K. G. Kramer & B. Kathleen Thompson (1979), *"An Evaluation of the Relationship of Dietary Fatty Acids to Incidence of Myocardial Lesions in Male Rats"*. *Canadian Institute of Food Science and Technology Journal, 12*, 189-193.

refrigerated, never heated, and consumed in small amounts in salad dressings and spreadable sauces.

Tropical oils are more saturated than other vegetable oils.

Palm oil is about 50% saturated fat, with 41% oleic acid and about 9% linoleic acid.

Coconut oil is 92% saturated fat with more than two-thirds of saturated fat in the form of medium-chain fatty acids — often called medium-chain triglycerides. Of particular interest is lauric acid found in large amounts in both coconut oil and breast milk. This fatty acid has strong antifungal and antimicrobial properties. Coconut oil protects tropical populations against bacteria and fungi so prevalent in their food supply; as third world countries in tropical areas have switched to polyunsaturated vegetable oils, the incidence of intestinal disorders and immunodeficiency diseases has increased dramatically. Since coconut oil contains lauric acid, it is often used in infant milk formulas.

Palm kernel oil, used mainly in confectionery coatings, also contains high levels of lauric acid. These oils are extremely stable and can be kept at room temperature for many months without going rancid. Highly saturated tropical oils do not contribute to heart disease, but have nourished healthy populations for millennia.[103] It is a shame that we do not use these oils for cooking and baking — the bad reputation they have received is the result of intense lobbying by the U.S. vegetable oil industry.[104]

Red palm oil has a strong taste that most find unpalatable — although it is widely used throughout Africa — but **clarified palm oil**, which is tasteless and white in color, was formerly used

---

[103] Ian A. Prior, Flora Davidson, Clare Salmond & Z. Czochanska (1981), "Cholesterol, Coconuts, and Diet on Polynesian Atolls: A Natural Experiment: the Pukapuka and Tokelau Island Studies." *American Journal of Clinical Nutrition, 34* (8), 1552-1561.

[104] Personal communication, Mary G. Enig. The Institute for Shortening and Edible Oils, ISEO, has filed this lobby against tropical oils.

as shortening and in the production of commercial potato chips, while coconut oil was used in cookies and cakes.

Fear of saturated fats has forced producers to abandon these safe and healthy oils in favor of hydrogenated soybean, corn, canola, and cottonseed oils.

Summary

In summary, our choice of fats and oils is important. Most people, especially infants and growing children, benefit from more fat in their diet than less. But the fats we eat should be chosen carefully. Avoid all processed foods containing modern hydrogenated fats and polyunsaturated oils. Instead, use traditional vegetable oils such as extra virgin olive oil and small amounts of unrefined flaxseed oil. Familiarize yourself with the merits of coconut oil for baking and animal fats for occasional frying. Consume egg yolks and other animal fats with the proteins to which they are [naturally] bound. Finally, use as much good quality butter as you like, in the happy knowledge that it is a health food, in fact, essential for you and your entire family.

Organic butter, extra virgin olive oil and flaxseed oil extracted by mechanical pressing in opaque containers are available in health food stores and *gourmet* markets. Edible coconut oil can be found in markets in India or the Caribbean.

Mike Geary and the 21ST Century Nutritionists describe the above article as an important document for understanding real nutrition. They invite sharing it on social media. Geary refers to the authors as follows:

Mary G. Enig, PhD, an internationally renowned expert in the field of lipid biochemistry, led a series of studies in the United States and Israel on the content and effects of trans fatty acids and successfully challenged government claims that the animal fat diet causes cancer and heart disease. Recent scientific and media attention on the possible adverse effects of trans fatty acids brought increased attention to her work. She was also a licensed nutritionist with the Board of Certification of Nutrition Specialists, a qualified expert witness, a nutrition consultant to individuals, industry, and state and federal governments, an editor and contributor to several scientific publications, a fellow of the American College of Nutrition, and president of the Maryland Association of Nutritionists.

She is the author of more than sixty technical papers and presentations and a renowned lecturer. Dr. Enig worked until her death on the exploratory development of an adjunct therapy for AIDS from whole food saturated fatty acids.

Sally Fallon, co-author with Mary G. Enig, PhD of *The Nourishing Traditions*, has published numerous articles on diet and health. She is president of the Weston Foundation and a promoter of the Campaign for Real Milk.

Chapter V

Learning to Eat

The second lane argues that, due to lack of knowledge, high rates of poverty and illiteracy, and poor access to information, no one has received, as a minimum, even two hours of food and nutrition education during the educational process by the age of twelve. As ridiculous as it sounds, we all have to learn how to eat. This is achieved through the knowledge of how foods and the combination of foods can affect the body. That is: knowing how nutrients work when ingested. However, when we wake up, we have the habit of eating a piece of toast, a fritter, a donut, an arepa — anything that contains flour —, while we turn on the TV, the radio, or the computer to find out the news while we prepare breakfast. This is how we almost always do it.

But it turns out that changing habits and waking up are not easy. Knowing trophology — the science of combining foods — is a different way of looking at things and explaining them to broaden your perspective and grasp the encompassing enlightenment that starts right when you ask yourself, "What's in what I'm putting in my mouth?"; and later, in the bath or shower, "What's absorbed into my skin; what am I nourishing myself with?"

Breakfast is important

Breakfast is the first full meal of the day. Some people believe that not eating breakfast is a good habit and that it helps to lose weight. But the opposite is true. You are probably thinking: "There is no time!" Well, it turns out that there is. I already hinted at it: it is in the meagre limits and depends on making certain simple changes in your mind: that time that we believe goes so fast and that we are used to measuring in hours, minutes and seconds is malleable and is not an absolute, a theme that Deepak Chopra explains in his book *Ageless Bodies, Timeless Minds* (2008).

The night before you can make these preparations: as the natural need to wake up is to quench thirst, leave ready an infusion with pineapple peels, a natural diuretic that helps you lose weight. The next morning, just heat it, before boiling, add the tea of your choice or aromatic herbs. Pineapple has a high fructose content, so there is no need to add any sweetener to the infusion. *Kombucha* tea, for example, is a natural ferment with a delicious flavor and, if you squeeze half a lemon, you guarantee alkalinity. Above all, you will provide the intestinal flora with a lot of beneficial bacteria that serve to strengthen the immune system. Complementary to this cleansing, eat fruit without added sugar, with all its fiber — that processed orange juice loaded with sugar is not the best option —, so that after twenty to thirty minutes, during which time you will surely have had your first bowel movement of the day, you can proceed to eat your breakfast.

Drinking tea and eating fruit upon waking up provides the body and its metabolism with a complete package of vitamins, minerals, antioxidants, water, and something else extraordinary: on an empty stomach, the fruits pass through the intestine and cleanse it. This habit of coming out of fasting with a warm or hot liquid and whole fruits considerably reduces the risk of colon cancer. If fruits remain in the stomach because of the presence of another solid, their alkalinity potential is spoiled; the gastric juices that try to break down the other solid foods reverse their pH towards acidity. Therefore, do not eat fruit on a full stomach. That "orange gives me acidity" is a mistake that can be corrected by respecting the golden rule: "eat them only on an empty stomach". Fruits are the healthiest and most wholesome because of their alkaline benefits. During the day, you have several options to eat them on an empty stomach: first thing or mid-morning, late afternoon, before bedtime or all of the above. A red apple relieves heartburn and gastric reflux. There is an old English saying: *An apple a day keeps the doctor away*.

What happens when you skip breakfast? Venezuelan endocrinologist Daniela Jakubowicz, in her book *¡Ni una dieta más!* (No more diets) explains this issue in a clear, simple, and didactic way. From a scientific point of view, she confirms what I have maintained: the body and the being are two different entities that affect each other.

Riiinng!

The alarm clock rings, and the brain starts to worry: *"We have to get up already; we used all the fuel"*.

It calls the first neuron at hand and sends a message to see what glucose is available in the blood. The blood replies: "There is enough sugar here for fifteen to twenty minutes, nothing more".

The brain makes a grimace of anxiety and tells the messenger neuron: "Okay, go talk to the liver, see what it has in reserve". The liver consults the savings account and replies that "at most the funds are enough for about twenty to twenty-five minutes". In total there is only about 290 grams of glucose, that is, enough for forty-five minutes, time in which the brain has been praying to all the saints to see if it occurs to us to have breakfast.

If we are in a hurry or find it unbearable to eat in the morning, the poor organ will have to go into emergency mode: "Maximum alert: they are throwing an economic package at us. Cortisone, child, get what you can out of the muscle cells, bone ligaments and skin collagen."

The cortisone will set in motion the mechanisms for the cells to open up like a mother's purse buying supplies and let their proteins out. These will pass to the liver to be converted into blood glucose. The process will continue until we eat again.

As can be seen, those who believe that not eating breakfast is good are deluding themselves: they are eating their own muscles, they are self-devouring! The consequence is the loss of muscle tone and a brain that, instead of taking care of its intellectual functions, spends the morning activating the emergency system to obtain fuel and food.

How does this affect our weight? When we start the day by fasting, an energy saving strategy is put in place, so the metabolism decreases. The brain does not know if the fast will be for a few hours or for a few days, so it takes the most severe restrictive measures. Therefore, if the person then decides to have lunch, the food will be accepted as surplus, it will be diverted to the "reserve fat" store and the person will put on weight.

The reason why muscles are the first to be used as reserve fuel in the morning fast is due to the fact that the morning hours are dominated by the hormone cortisol, which stimulates the destruction of muscle proteins and their conversion into glucose.

Now you know, never again go out without breakfast, your body will thank you and will compensate with better health.

Dr Daniela Jakubowicz, PhD. (Endocrinologist)

Effective nutrition is a matter of greater concern when it involves children. Influenced perhaps by industry, or to maintain the bad eating habits of the last century, in some countries junk food and drink are still served in schools. Historical data suggest: "The harm of these denatured diets can be passed on to succeeding generations". Community pressure on the state is required to implement breakfast education as an effective health and nutrition policy.

However, at very low costs, we can establish serious food policies and start giving children real fruit in schools; in the countryside they are at cost price. For example, panela water — the result of diluting panela (an unrefined whole cane sugar) in hot water — is an ideal low-cost caloric and nutritional accompaniment to nourish brains that need to learn and recharge energy; we can also use the healing power of infusions for study or work.

Then it wouldn't take more than a piece of avocado or lightly sautéed vegetables, such as carrots, broccoli, celery, bell pepper, curly lettuce, endive, Brussels sprouts, and some seeds to accompany the least caloric and cheapest complete source of essential proteins: a boiled egg. A slice of whole wheat artisan bread with butter; potatoes cooked with salt; half a glass of homemade yogurt that preserves the bacilli and probiotics alive and active, mixed with dried fruits; nuts and seeds or a glass of whole milk, which in the countryside is a complete nutrition option, are some alternatives for mid-morning. At lunchtime, a good portion of a different animal protein every day or tofu with salad or fresh vegetables. And in the middle of the week, the alternative can be *pizza*, hamburger, lasagna, stew, goulash, paella, rice with tuna, roast suckling pig. Dessert should be served at mid-afternoon, and each region has many that define them. In schools and educational centers, drinking water is a priority and coastal cities have a great advantage: the mixture of one-part clean sea water to five parts fresh water with lemon is an extraordinary cold drink that lowers body temperature, tastes good, is catalytic, alkaline and an inexpensive way to quench thirst and fortify the immune system.

The above menu may not sound appetizing to many. But hunger is so great in some so-called poor countries that people are sometimes forced to eat cooked dirt. For the sake of the future of these countries, it would be easy and also advantageous to apply and implement this educational-food model based on assertive nutrition. With an extremely cheap breakfast that includes alkaline liquid, vitamins, minerals, healthy fats, fiber, and protein to guarantee the basic nutritional qualities of an arduous day of study, in a few years, a little less than a quarter of a century, impoverished countries would cease to be "poor".

Trophology

In modern times, trophology teaches us how to cultivate or restore health through a diet suited to the body's needs. This nutritional theory, initially followed by few, is attributed to William Howard Hay (1866-1940), an American physician born in Pennsylvania. Then came works such as *Medicina natural al alcance de todos* (Natural medicine within everyone's reach), by the Chilean lawyer and naturopath Manuel Lezaeta Acharán (1881-1959). And *Food combining made easy*, in which the therapist and naturopath Herbert M. Shelton (1895-1985) lists the correct food combinations, and *Fit for Life*, by Harvey and Marilyn Diamond (1945) in the United States.

Man feeds on what he digests, not on what he eats.

Manuel Lezaeta

The theory holds that compatible foods should be combined in the same meal to facilitate digestion. The teaching of medicine in the West has gaps in nutrition and today few scientists in America and Europe make extraordinary contributions to this science.

Trophology, an irrefutable fact, is also wisdom. Almost 2500 years ago, in China, the *Tao te King* (*King*: 'the book'; *Tao:* 'of the way'; *te*: 'its power'), by the philosopher, Lao-Tse, made its principle concerns clear in his approach. In the West, trophology is the scientific concept equivalent to the balance between the yin and yang of the East. It is elementary chemistry: the balance between acid and base. If we add a measure of acid to an equal measure of alkali, the resulting solution is as neutral as fresh water; hence the old idea of drinking it with bicarbonate — an alkaline substance — to relieve heartburn.

The science of combining foods

When we chew a piece of bread, potato, or any other carbohydrate — starches such as rice or pasta — the ptyalin in the saliva coats these starches, because to digest them and optimally complete their digestion, the environment must be **alkaline.** To initiate the digestion of any concentrated animal protein, the stomach secretes pepsin to completely digest the proteins and must act for several hours, but only if the environment remains highly **acidic**.

If at the same time in the same dish we eat proteins — meat- and carbohydrates, starches — rice, potatoes, cassava, banana, pasta, or bread basically —, the acid and alkaline juices are secreted simultaneously and neutralize each other. The body is able to correctly digest one or the other, not the mixture; therefore, it cannot complete an optimal digestion. The issue boils down to the following: when the stomach is immobilized and its digestive functions are disturbed by the consumption of indiscriminately combined foods, the bacteria in the digestive canal have a field day. They take advantage of the nutrients and multiply, and while the body is left with the waste, you suffer the consequences. Gas, heartburn, bloating, constipation, foul-smelling stools or, worse, medium, and long-term digestive problems such as colitis, diverticulitis, hemorrhoids, and the various types of cancer that are often very aggressive and only become noticeable when it is too late for the patient.

Uniqueness makes us uncommon, and commonness is a power that invalidates differences and their coexistence: I differ from totalitarian thinking that ignores uniqueness. What matters here is that there is no 100% protein or 100% carbohydrate food; whether the main nutritional element of a particular food is protein or carbohydrate: if a food contains 15% more protein, it is categorized as protein, while 20% or more carbohydrate makes it a carbohydrate. When combining different types of foods in a single meal, it does not matter much whether a little protein is added to a complex carbohydrate meal or vice versa, especially if raw vegetables are included to provide active enzymes and fiber.

Without a proper combination of foods in the same intake, the body is not able to digest the nutrients. This would not occur if at least half of the daily supply is eaten raw, no matter how many calories or cholesterol it contains. Properly combined foods do not make the body fat and do not slow down the metabolism.

For trophology, the ideal is to consume one food at a time or to combine them well. A glance at nature shows that carnivorous animals do not mix the meat they eat with starches, but they do supplement digestion occasionally and purge their guts by chewing wild herbs with medicinal properties. For centuries, birders have seen birds eat insects and worms at one time of day and seeds and berries at another, but never both at the same time. Among humans, a look at the eating habits of the Chinese shows that, at home, they had been eating rice alone or combined with plenty of fresh vegetables, soy products and very few meats. And, usually, when they give a banquet, rice is not served — it is not on the table — so that it does not interfere with the enjoyment of the meat, fish and poultry that always appear on those menus. Since the MID-20TH century, especially in urban areas, modern lifestyles have been eroding these healthy eating habits, with detrimental effects on health and longevity; and not only among the Chinese.

In the 1920s, before the impact of the West on Chinese customs, expert nutritionists compared the eating habits of the Chinese and Americans: the study revealed that the average Chinese obtained more than 90% of their energy from grains and grain products, fresh vegetables and fruits, and only 1% came from animal products; the data for Americans showed that 39% of their energy came from grains, 38% from animal products and most of the remaining 23% was from refined sugars. Of course, vegetables and fruits accounted for a miniscule portion of their diet. You can hardly have a more unbalanced diet without fiber-rich, whole, unprocessed, complex carbohydrates.

In July 1986, a study carried out in the United States, reported by the Associated Press, revealed that 49% of the population complained daily of stomach pains, chronic gastrointestinal discomfort, constipation, and other disturbances of the digestive system. And another more recent study among men — also in the United States — concluded that they carry an average of more than four and a half pounds of putrefying and undigested meat in their intestines.

What happens when we leave a four and a half pounds of meat in a dark, humid, and warm place for several days? The severely septic state of the human intestinal tract is unique in nature. Yet Western doctors insist that it is normal and harmless to the rest of the body.

The reality is different. To protect itself from chronic toxic irritation caused by poorly combined foods, the colon secretes large amounts of mucus to envelop toxic particles before they damage its sensitive mucosa. When this happens at every meal, every day, every week of the year — as is common in the Western diet — the colon ends up with a constant flow of mucus that accumulates and becomes embedded in its folds. This results in a narrowing of the colon lumen and a constant leaking of toxins into the bloodstream by osmosis. When the encrustation of toxic mucus in the colon reaches a critical pressure, it produces a pouch that swells outward like a balloon, leading to diverticulosis. Colitis and cancer are the subsequent stages of colon deterioration.

From the point of view of **trophology,** the direct consequences of poorly combined foods are putrefaction and fermentation, which also cause many allergies: the bloodstream absorbs toxins from the fermented and putrefied mass that fills the intestines and these toxins in turn cause rashes, hives, headaches, nausea, and other symptoms that are usually categorized as allergies. The same foods capable of triggering an allergic reaction when improperly combined often do not produce a harmful effect when consumed according to the standards suggested by **trophology.**

When you change your habits, digestive problems — gastritis, indigestion and flatulence — decrease and a host of improvements are triggered: your metabolism speeds up; detoxification strengthens your immune system; episodes of colds and allergies become fewer and fewer; your energy gradually increases; your physical appearance improves and your empathy with others increases; your smile and self-esteem increase; and the challenge of losing weight and fighting obesity ceases to be an impossibility.

Protein and tuber starch
— cereal starch —.

This is the worst combination that can be made in the same meal, but it constitutes the main course of modern Western diets: meat with mashed potatoes, hamburgers with French fries, eggs with bread. The alkaline enzyme ptyalin, present in saliva, when starches are ingested, mixes with proteins; when that chewed food reaches the stomach for digestion, those alkaline enzymes that coat the starch neutralize the action of pepsin and the other acidic juices that digest the protein. This mixture causes the bacteria present in the stomach to go into action to trigger fermentation of the starches and putrefaction of the proteins. As a result, toxic wastes and fetid gases are produced in which there are poisons such as indole, skatole, phenol, hydrogen sulfide, phenyl propionic acid and others.

Why does the stomach have no trouble digesting foods such as whole grains, which by nature contain protein and starch? Shelton said: "There is a great difference between the digestion of one food, however complex its composition, and the digestion of a mixture of different foods". Faced with a simple food combining protein and starch, the body can easily regulate its secretions, both in potency and timing, according to the digestive demands of that food. But when two foods with different, even antagonistic, digestive requirements are consumed, this precise dosage of secretions becomes impossible.

The norm is: eat concentrated proteins, such as meat, fish, eggs, or cheese, separate from concentrated starches, such as bread, potatoes, and rice. For example, eat toast or eggs for breakfast, NOT both; hamburger meat or the bread roll that goes well with butter for lunch, NOT both; chicken, fish, or potatoes for dinner and, in all cases, accompany them with the neutral group of fresh vegetables and greens.

Protein and protein

Different proteins have different digestive requirements. For example, the greatest enzymatic action on milk occurs during the last hour of digestion, while in meat it occurs during the first hour and in eggs towards the middle of digestion.

Thus, two similar meats, such as beef and lamb, or two kinds of fish, or fish and shellfish, such as cod and shrimp — shrimp, crayfish, prawns, king prawns — are not sufficiently different in nature to cause digestive conflict in the stomach and can therefore be eaten at the same time.

The norm is: consume only one main type of protein at each meal. Avoid combinations such as meat and eggs, meat and milk, fish, and cheese. Make sure you assimilate all the essential amino acids by varying the type of protein concentrate you consume at each meal.

Starch — starches — and acid

Any acidic food consumed at the same time with a starch interrupts the secretion of ptyalin, a biochemical fact on which all physicians agree. Therefore, if you eat oranges, lemons, or other acidic fruits — or acids such as vinegar — together with a starch, you will not have ptyalin in your mouth to initiate the first phase of starch digestion. Consequently, the starch reaches the stomach without the alkaline juices essential for proper digestion and bacterial fermentation occurs. A single teaspoon of vinegar — or its equivalent in other acids — completely inhibits the salivary digestion of starch in the mouth.

The norm is: consume acids and starches in separate meals. For example, if you eat toast or cereal for breakfast, skip the orange juice and eggs. If you are going to have a meal composed basically of starches — rice or any kind of pasta —, do without vinegar and all concentrated proteins.

Protein and acid

Since the proper digestion of proteins requires an acidic environment, it would be logical to assume that acidic foods facilitate the digestion of proteins; however, this is not the case. When they reach the stomach, acidic foods inhibit the secretion of hydrochloric acid and pepsin — the enzyme that digests proteins — can only act in the presence of hydrochloric acid, not any acid. Therefore, orange juice inhibits the proper digestion of eggs and strong vinegar in salad inhibits the digestion of steak.

The norm is: avoid combining acids and concentrated proteins in the same meal. This leads to choosing a salad dressing without citrus or heavily laden with vinegar when eating meat, and at the table, if an accompanying liquid is required, water is ideal.

Protein and fat

In John James Rickard Macleod's *Physiology in Modern Medicine,* we find a statement shared by physicians: "Fat has been shown to exert a distinct inhibitory influence on the secretion of gastric juices". During the two to three hours following the ingestion of fat, the concentration of pepsin and hydrochloric acid in the stomach is considerably reduced. This delays the digestion of any protein that has been ingested along with the fat, allowing bacteria to initiate putrefaction of the protein. This is why fatty meats such as bacon, fatty steaks or lean meats fried in oil are heavy on the stomach for several hours after eating them.

The normal thing is to consume fats and concentrated proteins in different meals. When you can't avoid mixing them — for example, that steak with that golden fat that many of us like —, accompany them with plenty of raw vegetables to facilitate their digestion and their passage through the intestine.

Protein and sugar

All sugars without exception inhibit the secretion of gastric juices in the stomach. This is because sugars are not digested in the mouth or in the stomach but pass directly to the small intestine for digestion and assimilation. When consumed in combination with some protein, such as a cake after a steak, not only do they inhibit protein digestion by inhibiting the secretion of gastric juices, but the sugars themselves become trapped in the stomach instead of passing quickly to the small intestine, and this delay allows bacteria to ferment the sugar, which releases toxins and harmful gases that further impair digestion.

The norm is to avoid consuming sugars and proteins at the same meal. That dessert immediately after lunch can wait until mid-afternoon.

Starch and sugar

It has been established that when sugar arrives in the mouth accompanied by a starch, the saliva secreted during chewing does not contain ptyalin, which sabotages the digestion of the starch, even before it reaches the stomach. In addition, this combination prevents the sugar from passing beyond the stomach until after starch digestion is complete, resulting in fermentation. The by-products of sugar fermentation are acidic, which further inhibits the digestion of starches, which need an alkaline medium. Bread — starch — with butter — fat — is a perfectly compatible combination, but when a spoonful of honey or jam is added, sugars are introduced into the mixture, and this impairs the digestion of the starchy bread. The same principle applies to sugar-sweetened breakfast cereals, highly sweetened gateaux, sweet cakes and so on.

The norm is: consume starches and sugars separately.

Melon

Melon is a food so suitable for human consumption that it does not require any digestion in the stomach, but passes quickly into the small intestine, where it is digested and assimilated. This can only happen when the stomach is empty, and melon is consumed alone or accompanied exclusively by other raw fruits.

When consumed with or after other foods that require complex stomach digestion, cantaloupe cannot pass into the small intestine until after digestion of the other foods is complete. This causes the melon to be retained, ferment rapidly and produce all kinds of gastric discomfort.

The rule of thumb is as with all fruits, eat melon only on an empty stomach or don't eat it at all.

Desserts

Avoid all kinds of sweet desserts after a large meal, as this kind of food combines poorly with everything. Even fresh fruits should be avoided after a big meal, as they accumulate in the stomach and ferment instead of being digested. If you are tempted by sweets and feel like eating cakes, sweets, and pastries, you can indulge in them from time to time. They are not going to do you much good, but at least if you consume them alone, they will not cause as much gastric discomfort or produce as many toxic by-products as if you consume them after a meal.

The standard is: avoid fruits and starchy sweet desserts after a large protein — or carbohydrate — based meal.

Source: adapted from Daniel Reid (2014): *The Tao of Health, Sex, and Long Life*. Barcelona: Urano, Vintage.

Where there is a will, there is a way, and now that you know the way, it all depends on your willingness to practice it.

DANIEL REID (2014, p. 116).

There is no doubt that the above is normal; as long as it corresponds to the following definition of normal: "according with, constituting, or not deviating from a norm, rule, procedure, or principle", and "occurring naturally...within a range considered safe, healthy, or optimal", instead of "conforming to a type, standard, or regular pattern: characterized by that which is considered usual, typical, or routine" (Merriam Webster), which is also a definition of normal. It is ironic that in this text you'll find relatively frequently the words "normal" or "normally", which contain the valid and precise meanings that reflect polarity and antagonism between the lanes in which we drive. I insist, learn to navigate them; it's your choice!

What an outburst!

"So, everything was wrong! And now they're telling us that we even have to learn to eat? Oh, no! Not that! A *pizza* without Coca-Cola® is unimaginable. My body needs that dessert after lunch; do you really think I'm going to give that up too?"

I know it sounds like an outburst, but it's not. None of this matters... for now. Don't worry. I agree with you. It takes time to accept that many of our previous habits were wrong and to assimilate these concepts that pull the rug out from under us; it produced an enormous resistance in me, and I guess in you too.

True, thought-provoking, educational processes are not imposed and do not happen overnight. Step by step, the brain processes the information as soon as it gets it, which is why I advise reading and consulting frequently. "This is not for me", we may think, but without us noticing it, the brain will be removing the locks to make those changes we need, which are confirmed by our welfare. Calm down! The behavioral patterns, established by inherited bad eating habits, can also be broken. At the table, only answer if you are asked about those changes that go hand in hand with your acquired knowledge. But to avoid entering conflicts, there will always be the friendly: "over tastes there is no dispute".

Let's carry on with the change of habits. I ask you to keep some of your resistance though, because it will be your main weapon to lose weight by using a sensational scientific discovery of the 21ST CENTURY that works in practice.

A fair trial for the four white murderers

Milk, sugar, salt, and white flours have been accused of being "the four white killers" and known as "the white poisons: foods that have very little nutritional value and in excess can damage your health to the point of killing you". They have in common that they are industrially processed. In the case of milk and its derivatives, by pasteurization and homogenization; sugar, salt and flours by another industrial process, refining. Let's review each case.

In contrast to alkaline superfoods, animal milk, sugar and refined flours generate acidic metabolic reactions. To counteract the acidity, the body resorts to its own base substances or alkaline components: the mineral salts of teeth and bones. The possible results are osteoporosis, kidney stones, arthritis, fluid retention, atherosclerosis, inflammation, coronary heart disease and the appearance of cancer cells: in short, aging prematurely. Fresh water and common salt in their natural state are neutral with pH 7. Seawater, loaded with more than eighty minerals in perfect molecular balance, is alkaline with pH 8. Carbon, high fructose corn syrup or substitutes such as aspartame, coloring chemicals and preservatives are added to fresh water and packaged for sale as a soft drink. Salt loses many of its minerals in the refining process, which alters its qualities; the addition of artificial sodium turns it into the alkaline food of choice for cancer cells and thus they survive the acidic environment that surrounds them.

Generic, non-industrial milk, flours, sugar, and salt are healthy alternatives that deserve to be studied individually.

Milk

Milk, one of the many sources of calcium, appeared on the menu, at the same time as sedentism and agriculture, more than 10,000 years ago. In that last gastronomic second of mankind, animal grazing made milk from cows, goats, sheep, and other mammals the new food. Cereals, which were cultivated as fodder, were exclusively food for farm animals and, only after a long period, also became for human consumption.

In the NINETEENTH CENTURY, Louis Pasteur discovered and developed a process that consists of subjecting a food, usually liquid, to a temperature of approximately eighty degrees for a short time and then cooling it rapidly. This process eliminates toxic bacteria and minimizes the probability of people getting sick from drinking milk. For mankind, pasteurization was a great advance because it allowed the commercialization of this product on a massive scale.

Although pasteurization allowed the population access to this food, this process, when evaluated with the technological advances of 21ST century microbiology, is also establishing another great difference that trophology clearly explains.

Calves only feed on cow's milk from birth to weaning and, even if they try, they never go back to it for the rest of their lives. They are mammals like us and once they start consuming pasture and forage, they never go back to milk. Breast milk, as a raw and natural food for the newborn, is fundamental and irreplaceable.

After weaning, stopping milk does not make any difference to the normal growth and development of mammals. Calcium, essential for bones and teeth, body tissue, neurons, blood, and other fluids, can be obtained from various sources, such as shellfish, clams, mussels, cod, tuna, salmon, fruits, nuts, legumes, cabbage, broccoli, carrots, and spinach. However, those who believe that by drinking a lot of milk they will never have calcium deficiencies do not realize that the opposite is true. Milk of animal origin is an acidifying food; with this excess, if the balance of daily intake tends to acid, the body eventually appropriates calcium from bones and teeth to balance the pH.

Pasteurized milk according to trophology

We come to one of the most controversial and poorly understood issues of the Western diet. Orientals and Africans avoid the consumption of milk, except as a purgative. In nature, mammalian animals feed exclusively on milk until they are weaned. Humans, by taste or whim, drink milk daily throughout their lives.

The natural decrease of lactase, the enzyme that allows digesting milk, in the organism of any mammal shows that, as it grows, a human being has no more need of milk than a tiger or an adult chimpanzee. Although milk is a complete protein food, it contains fat which slows digestion and should not be combined with any other food except itself; nevertheless, many adults accompany their meals with cold milk. Milk curdles (from the Latin, *coagulāre*) as soon as it reaches the stomach, so that, if other food is present, the milk forms lumps around the food particles and insulates them from the action of the gastric juices, which delays their digestion long enough for putrefaction to begin. Therefore, the first and most important rule about milk consumption is: "Drink it alone or don't drink it at all". Today, milk is made even more indigestible by pasteurization, which destroys the natural enzymes and alters its proteins. Natural milk contains the active enzymes lactase and lipase, which make its digestion possible. Pasteurized milk, devoid of lactase and other active enzymes, cannot be properly digested, even by infants, as evidenced by colic, rashes, respiratory problems, gas, and other ailments so common in bottle-fed babies. In addition, the absence of enzymes and the alteration of vital proteins mean that the calcium and other minerals contained in milk are not well assimilated.

Calcium deficiency has become so widespread that more than 90% of American children suffer from chronic dental conditions. Europeans and Americans have been fed pasteurized milk for three generations; to make matters worse, the custom of "homogenizing" milk to prevent the cream from separating has taken hold. Homogenization, which consists of fragmenting and pulverizing the fat molecules to the point where they cannot separate from the rest of the milk, leaves tiny fragments of fat that are easily filtered through the walls of the small intestine and greatly increase the amount of cholesterol and denatured fats absorbed by the body; in fact, more milk fat is absorbed by drinking homogenized milk than by consuming pure cream.

Milk denatured by homogenization and pasteurization does not provide sufficient calcium to combat osteoporosis. Recent studies at the Human Research Center in Grand Forks, North Dakota (USA), indicate that the element boron is also essential for the absorption of calcium from food and bone formation. The estrogen level in the blood of women receiving adequate amounts of boron more than doubled and eliminated the need for hormone replacement therapy, which is a common "patch" against osteoporosis in Western countries. And where is boron found? In fresh fruits and vegetables, especially apples, pears, grapes, and all nuts, cabbage, and other leafy greens. There we also find calcium. Nature provides us with abundant sources of all the nutrients we need, but humans insist on cooking and processing them until they are all removed and then wonder why their diet does not work.

The standard is to eliminate homogenized and pasteurized milk completely from your diet. If you can get natural milk, consume it as a complete meal by itself, never combined with other foods.

Source: adapted from Daniel Reid (2014): *The Tao of health, sex and long life*, pp. 95-98. Barcelona: Urano, Vintage.

In conclusion, breast milk of any species is not as bad as it is portrayed. In its natural state it retains intact its unique vitamin nutrients, fats, minerals, and enzymes, which indicates that real milk is a complete and irreplaceable food for the newborn. Of course, milks other than breast milk provide a beneficial alkaline balance and are healthy, but not indispensable in post-breastfeeding feeding. These are almond, rice, coconut, birdseed, soy, nut, and seed milks (*organic & non-GMO*), other than those just mentioned.

The COVID-19 pandemic forced the development of methods to transport vaccines at very low temperatures. These advances and modern packaging and milking hygiene techniques may make it easier to get real fresh milk into supermarkets. In Spain and countries in the rest of Europe, cold "real whole milk" is sold in local stores and comes from nearby.

Refined flours

Colombia, Mexico, and El Salvador, for example, have traditional flours for their dough and their arepas, tortillas or pupusas contain slow absorption complex carbohydrates. They are healthier roasted than fried, and it is better to get used to whole wheat flours that provide fiber. Not so refined flours which, due to refining and the addition of chemicals that remove the lipids that degrade over time, are simple carbohydrates that are rapidly absorbed. Most refined flours, ready for the preparation of biscuits, tortillas, arepas and cakes, or that white bread whose aroma makes us close our eyes and sigh with pleasure, have hidden sugar added to them and, when the preparations are ready, they are also sprinkled with powdered sugar devoid of nutrients. The effect of this easy absorption on the metabolism is that blood sugar levels rise and the pancreas releases insulin to promptly stabilize this excess. After enjoying a delicious dessert, in less than two hours, the craving and desire for more of the same is confused with increased appetite and hunger. By misinterpreting this message of anxiety, we do not realize that we are falling into dependence on flour and sugar, a vice that makes us sick.

In this resplendent universe of delicious multicolored preparations in the form of cakes, pastries, breads, cookies, candies, and biscuits that bend the strongest will, at some point came donuts and churros fried in refined oils that generate trans fats, the result of bathing refined flour with lots of sugar. This is, without a doubt, one of the worst trophological combinations. Donuts and coffee are, according to Hollywood, the favorite combination in police stations in the United States. Donuts and churros are delicious, of course, but you can only very occasionally give in to their charms. As for coffee, in Colombia — not Columbia, as some believe — we learned to cultivate and prepare a very exclusive, smooth, and very aromatic variety, because only the ripe bean is harvested. The baristas recommend only drinking it in a small cup and without sugar, or latte in a medium cup to enjoy its aroma, because the rest... it is also an excess to drink it watered down in a huge mug. Coffee is stimulating: one or two cups a day does not unbalance the body towards acidity. With coffee — as with bread, cookies, cereals, potatoes, snacks, and other foods, regardless of whether they are fried, baked, roasted, or toasted —, due to industrial processes and the high temperatures to which it has been subjected, acrylamide, a neurotoxicant that increases the probability of suffering from cancer, is produced naturally. Although it is lower in coffee, the study[105] carried out by the biologist Amaya M. Ortiz-Barredo, in collaboration with the Neiker Institute in the Basque Country, shows that the levels of acrylamide increase according to the exposure to heat and the different roasting or burning processes; this level is higher in espresso; among the soluble coffees, the level is higher in decaffeinated ones.

Refined flours do not provide fiber; moreover, consuming them in excess causes a rapid rise and fall of sugar in the blood, with long-term consequences. For now, the serious thing is the glycemic effect; it consists of the metabolic action of converting starches into sugars: fast-absorbing carbohydrates. It is as simple as that. We have not considered being overweight and obesity, two diseases that translate into hypertension and other diseases with worse risks; the body's capacity to process so many things is overwhelmed that it cannot evacuate them and, instead of providing us with energy we do not need, it converts the resulting

---

[105] Amaya M. Ortiz-Barredo (2004): *Determination of acrylamide levels in coffee*. Vitoria, Basque Country, Spain: NEIKER-Tecnalia (Basque Institute for Agricultural Research and Development). http://www.izenpe.eus/s15-4812/es/contenidos/informacion/resultados_investigacion/es_9873/adjuntos/acrilamida.pdf

excess glucose into fat and accumulates it. Let's no longer blame premature aging, alopecia, moles, varicose veins, freckles, gray hair and wrinkles on age or genes; let's call it what it is: the path of acidification. I learned this years ago, in the worst way, when I met with a prestigious neurologist at Celebration Hospital in Central Florida to present a special case to him and I'll never forget his words: "Neurology, as a strictly academic science, is still in its infancy". His diagnosis, without being able to state it, was that it was a rare form of multiple sclerosis; four years later, despite all medical care, my brother passed away at the age of forty-two. This was the main reason why I became fully involved in these issues and I was able to conclude that my brother was killed by too much sugar and refined flour, long before diabetes occurred. His daily exaggerated taste for desserts that he accompanied with Coca-Cola®, without fiber and full of preservatives, toxic dyes, sugar, and more sugar exacerbated the underlying disease that led to his death.

I mentioned that the +SUGAR = ACID path leads to cancer and every other rare disease there is. If you do well, it will only lead to type 2 diabetes or, if you carry on, to type 1. And that body, which tries to get you to listen to it and heed its messages because you constantly poison it and deprive it of its normal supply of oxygen, will condemn you to death, but not without first allowing you to suffer from Parkinson's, Alzheimer's, or senile dementia. The alarming thing is that it now happens to middle-aged people. Sclerosis begins with excess acid that drips directly onto the body of the axons — transmitters of electrical signals in the cells of the nervous system — burns and melts the myelin sheath covering the axons which, when exposed, creates a short circuit that produces the imminent failure of the individual's muscular response; progressively, the vital organs degenerate, collapse and you die. How I wish — pardon me for using useless words — that

I had become involved in these issues earlier. But as the quantum universe, which obviates space-time, connects everything and in its tendency to balance uses unforeseen forces, both from us and towards us, to make everything happen, I was able to understand the value of sacrifice: "it corresponds to the extraordinary effort to achieve a greater benefit by overcoming interests, tastes and comfort" — not to mention, naked selfishness — ; I have been able to concentrate, to write, and to share my experience.

Let us return to the subject of starch. Here I must mention three foods — rice, pasta, and potatoes — with which something important is happening. According to a report by the Environmental Working Group, rice contains traces of arsenic, due to the abuse of farmland that is not allowed to rest. Instead of white rice without fiber and devoid of nutrients, brown rice, wild rice of different colors — organic —, parboiled rice, quinoa, or quinoa or both mixed together is to be preferred. In pasta, Italy has achieved a magisterial magic: noodles from China and tomatoes from America. Integral or not, choose well what goes with the pasta, what you add to it. A pasta primavera, pesto or *puttanesca* is not the same as a pasta carbonara, al burro or marinara; the latter are a complete dish with a higher caloric contribution that considerably reduces your caloric budget. Finally, potatoes. Let's face it: with these three white foods we have problems. They are not complements; we turn rice, pasta, and potatoes into indispensable accessories without their being so. In trophology, white foods that accompany proteins are cauliflower, mushrooms, eggplant, cucumber, garlic, radishes, various onions, zucchini, bamboo, or alfalfa sprouts among others, either alone or in addition to the salad.

Now, if you want to put the starches to work to lose weight, first analyze the list of carbohydrates you consume in a typical day. These are cereals, starches, and sugars: corn tortilla at breakfast, Danish pastry, donuts, pancakes, cereal, slice of bread, cheesy rolls, arepa, empanadas, pasta, potatoes (cooked, fried or packaged), candy, banana slices, cassava, puff pastry, rice. And what you eat in the afternoon or at night: other tortillas or arepas, chips, corn cakes, chocolate cake, cookies, cheesecake, ice cream. In short, a long list, because in the same dish you eat two, three, or more different starches. With pasta, many people also eat rice, a piece of bread or even potatoes. Consume one starchy food per day: maximum two from the whole list. At times of high anxiety, mid-morning, afternoon, or evening or before bedtime, look for convenient snacks: fruit, nuts, seeds, or probiotic yogurt and, to accompany the protein at meals, vegetables and salads are ideal replacements for your usual ones. Sweetness is in a prune or two with no added sugar. If you can't avoid it, eat just one square from the whole chocolate bar. Prefer dark chocolate containing 70% cocoa (or more), without milk. After three days, as a bonus and reward, a couple of times a week, on spaced days, for example, Wednesday and Saturday or Sunday, do a "cheat day", because you're in for a treat, and choose from the list whatever you wish: on Wednesday, pasta with the sauce of your choice; cream of broccoli with cheddar cheese; or, eating out, that dream burger with fries? It's OK. For breakfast on Sunday, have pancakes with honey and butter or that bowl of cereal you top with sugar. The other day you choose in your plan, how about pizza? Or dare with a feijoada or *frijolada* and in the afternoon, for dessert, a coconut and caramel flan. Counterproductive? Maybe, but for the sake of well-being and self-esteem, what was everyday will now be only occasionally, part of the chapter of cravings.

"What's the point of that if you were doing so well on the diet!", some will ask. Over the next three days, promise yourself that on the first day you will not eat any starchy foods and only one or two on the following days, until the next cheat day. This is to balance out the excess you just enjoyed the day before. As you will see, your diet consists of eliminating the habit of consuming six to twelve starches per day. The amazing thing about this technique is that, though you don't forbid yourself anything, you gradually change your habits without starving yourself, and you gradually lose weight. It works very well.

The preamble to our next theme is a dramatic story, in which one who loves with passion dies, but not before revealing his desire for revenge. It is also sweet, very sweet. This love story is literally killing us.

There once was a charming and long-lived character of whom it is said:

Originally from New Guinea, this flirtatious character was born about five thousand years ago, slender, tall and with a fine figure. Natural charms that allowed him to first seduce the mysterious India. Not content with that, five hundred years later, though today it is not known whose attraction came first, China for him or he for China, it is said of his boldness that after traveling all over the country for millennia, leaving a hint of his desire to travel, he escaped at night to visit elegant Persia, by jumping over walls and mountains. The records indicate a date of 510 B.C. And, not tired of seducing such beautiful ladies, much more than a century later, in the company of his friend Alexander the Great, he set out on the silk road to drive the beautiful Eastern Europe crazy. His sweetness echoed in the Mediterranean. So much so that Greeks, Arabs, and others of the Middle East, jealous of his charm, knelt before the powerful and dominant Rome, begging on their knees, to try to catch him and subdue him. Overflowing with strength and energy, a proof of love was enough for Rome to persist. He did not think of fleeing and for some time our wily knight, unbeknownst to her, preferred to enjoy Rome and her dominions. It was after so many breakfasts with Europe, but not the same, it was another the one from the west, you know of his irremediable infidelity, and perhaps tired of the glare and the cloying that produced his last conquest, the demure Spain, he decided to escape. One dark night, after 1492, slipping away in one of the many ships, he crossed the Atlantic and, not knowing what fate had in store for him, imagine his surprise upon arriving in new lands: what an appearance and nothing like it! Cuba, tropical and dancing, smiled flirtatiously at him and welcomed him with a sense of wonder; he did not realize that there, amid a great gala, he would be introduced to the young lady who would change his life: the tender, restless and crazy America. Splendid amidst the honeys of her charm, vulnerable and with nowhere else to go, our original lover succumbed. He plotted silently. He had not been himself since the first day America possessed him. Subdued, in cruel revenge for losing his precious integrity, almost five centuries later, our sad and famous character became mass consumption: he was so desired that he became degraded, and he let himself be groped to such an extent that substitutes were created for him. Stripped of his charms and in honor of what was once vigorous, latent, and healthy, our character, the cane sugar, refined, of white appearance and brown heart, and his cronies — created in the laboratory, full of empty calories — do not provide anything other than a high degree of acidity and generate addiction. Refined white sugar and its artificial substitutes, nutrient free, have become a public health hazard.

For more than a century, advertising has used terms, slogans, and catchy phrases that over time and for the benefit of the industry keep us in the inertia of paradigms. "Substitute: a person or thing that takes the place or function of another." (Merriam Webster). The definition is not value-laden and so could be good, bad, or mediocre. But when it comes to health, the word "substitute" suggests that something is an equal, good, or better replacement. Sugar substitutes were a great contribution at the time; the word "substitute" is a message that circulates in our minds, and we assimilate it without questioning it because it is another established paradigm.

Sugar

Fertile valleys bathed by rivers form the geography of my warm and tropical hometown, Cali, which is in the valley of the Cauca River. It was once a multicolored landscape, but over time, the wheat, cotton, soybeans, sorghum, rice, millet, avocado, mango, barley, beans, peanuts, peas, sunflower, soursop, strawberries, and other crops lost the fight against sugar cane, and it became a boring monoculture. In the economy of scale, supply and demand favored the sugar industry, which managed to displace them. Its enormous boom allowed it to become the first mass-consumption sweetener. But certainly, the underlying reason has always been our exaggerated taste for sweet, sugary things. On the other hand, salt, smoke, freezing and dry shady places are the natural preservatives par excellence, which have served to preserve fish, meat, vegetables, fruits, and grains. Something extraordinary was discovered about sugar in the 20TH century that made it remarkable, and it was not exactly its property as a food preservative. With industrialization, stored foods required greater preservation, and sugar increased at the same rate as our love for sweet things.

The proliferation of refrigerators in the middle of the century had little influence on the avoidance of excess sugar, which was no longer required as a preservative, but as an addition to foods that already have natural sugars. We may wonder why a packaged fruit juice, in addition to the natural sweetness of the fruit, contains up to two outrageous ounces of sugars, or why sodas and juices come in personal containers of sixteen or more ounces, which is another exaggeration. Surprisingly, the sugar industry, pleased with the profits, managed to expand its supply due to the demand from other sectors of the food industry that were also favored by the excessive consumption of sugar. But it is only now, in our day, that studies linking the empty calories of refined white sugar and artificial sweeteners with anxiety and addiction have emerged; others even claim that it produces cancer. It is implicit that empty calories only provide energy; food does not retain its original flavor and, without the contribution of nutrients, the taste that persists alters the psyche and addiction to sweeteners. This is reason enough for an industry under fire to have marketed new products of natural origin, and others that are mixtures of artificial, either with natural or other artificial.

A sweetener is any substance that communicates a sweet taste and, when added to foods, changes their original flavor; this concept is common to all of them. Common sugar is sucrose, a disaccharide compound made up of two molecules: fructose and glucose, and its low price makes it palatable to the masses who, without hesitation, prefer it and tend not to include sweeteners with strange names in their purchases. The choices are confusing. The point is that without sufficient information we cannot establish a clear criterion about what we can or cannot consume without risking our health; for our wellbeing, we do not know what to include to relish sweetness. My criteria, based as always on the natural, is focused on maintaining alkalinity in the body.

At first, humans used ripe fruit or honey to sweeten, then sugar cane, then sugar from white beets and, to reinforce the sweet taste, we used cinnamon, vanilla, cloves, and nutmeg as flavorings.

Human health should not be a commercial issue. Today, in a table of sweeteners, those with the lowest recall and consumption — the most alkaline and beneficial — are relegated to the bottom of the table. I will start with those at the top of the list, which have the lowest pH, corresponding to the most acidic, and imply the greatest health risk; on the other hand, those with high pH, the nutritive sweeteners, have the greatest alkaline effect.

First, most industrially processed foods contain high levels of fructose corn syrup — transgenic — which is not suitable for diabetics. *High fructose corn syrup* is the result of biochemically converting corn starch — glucose — into concentrated fructose. This is achieved by means of genetically modified living microorganisms, i.e., transgenic.

In second place on this scale, *light* products contain artificial substitutes that are supposedly non-caloric and others of natural origin. Ever since the creation of the first synthetic sugar, the industries goal in the 20TH CENTURY has been to limit the energy in food for dieters, reduce the formation of dental plaque, and regulate blood sugar levels in diabetics. Let's analyze what these sweeteners are and what happens with these sugars.[106]

In the 1960s, the sodium or calcium salt of cyclamic acid — cyclohexylsulfamic acid — came on the market as cyclamate. Sucaryl and Sugar Twin became popular. But in 1969, the FDA banned its use in the United States because experiments with mice showed that in large quantities it could cause bladder cancer. It is still approved in more than fifty-five other countries. On November 21, 2017, the scientific journal *PLOS Biology*

---

[106] http://www.scientificpsychic.com/fitness/edulcorantes-artificiales.html.

brought the issue back to life and rescued the history, precedents, and commentary on the controversial 1965 Project 259.[107]

Approved by the FDA and promoted as NON-caloric sweeteners are:

Saccharin — Sweet'N Low — : basically dextrose, it contains 3.6% soluble saccharin and anti-caking agents. Out of 0.35 oz. of the product, almost 0.32 oz. are dextrose and provide 36 kilocalories; if they were refined sugar, they would provide 39. Invented in 1879, saccharin is the oldest artificial sweetener used in beverages, candies, medicines, and toothpaste.

Glucose for doctors; and dextrose for the food industry are the same as sugar: caloric carbohydrates!

Sucralose — Splenda — : is a chlorinated sugar. 0.35oz. of Splenda provide 33 kilocalories and contain 0.28 oz. of dextrose — sugar — and 0.03 oz. of maltodextrin — starch —. The rest, 0.4 oz., corresponds to sucralose, a non-caloric chlorinated organic compound. The same 0.35 oz. of sugar would provide 39 kilocalories.

Aspartame — Equal and NutraSweet — : is a sweet salt from the condensation of alcohols and acids. Aspartame is the product of methyl alcohol and two amino acids: phenylalanine and aspartic acid — aspartyl phenylalanine-1-methyl ester.

Neotame — also from NutraSweet — : similar to aspartame, but sweeter and more stable, was approved for general use in July 2002.

Acesulfame potassium — Ace-k — : two hundred times sweeter than table sugar, it is the potassium salt of 6-methyl-1,2,3-oxathiazin-4(3H)-one-2,2-dioxide.

---

[107] Cristin E. Kearns, Dorie Apollonio & Stanton A. Glantz (2017). *"Sugar industry sponsorship of germ-free rodent studies linking sucrose to hyperlipidemia and cancer: An historical analysis of internal documents."* PLOS Biology, 15 (11), 1-9. http://journals.plos.org/plosbiology/article?id=10.1371/journal.pbio.2003460.

As the fundamental objective is to lower the glycemic index when absorbed by the body, other FDA-approved sweeteners are either not digested or are absorbed as fiber and not as glucose. This happens with polydextrose — soluble fiber — and with non-caloric sweeteners that are mixed with dextrose or maltodextrin to increase the volume of the product and allow them to be compared and measured as if they were refined sugar. The problem is that dextrose and maltodextrin are caloric sweet carbohydrates.

Sugar alcohols: these are polyols or polyols of sugar and are found naturally in fruits and vegetables. They are produced in two basic ways: by exudation of some trees, mushrooms and seaweeds, mannitol; or by catalytic hydrogenation of the sugar to which they correspond: from xylose, xylitol; from glucose, sorbitol (also called glucitol), and from maltose starch, maltitol. Also from glucose, lactitol is obtained by reduction in the disaccharide lactose, and by fermentation with the yeast *Moniliella pollinis*, erythritol.

Sugar alcohols are not well absorbed in the intestines. Xylitol, for example, is partially digested and provides 40% fewer calories than sugar — one ounce of refined sugar provides 113 kilocalories — which means about 68 kilocalories per ounce ingested. Sorbitol and xylitol are common ingredients in "sugar-free" candies and chewing gums; when fermented in the intestine, they produce gas, colic and diarrhea, common symptoms in those who overindulge in treats. In a study with dogs, xylitol, which seems harmless to humans, caused convulsions and liver failure. Not even in exaggerated amounts: just 0.35 oz. of sorbitol can cause gastrointestinal problems. However, erythritol, with only 60 to 70% of the sweetness of sugar, provides 6.80 kilocalories per oz., does not promote dental caries, and does not cause gastric side effects.

Isomaltitol, which is known as Isomalt, is obtained from hydrogenated isomaltose, which in turn is obtained from sucrose, the sugar of the white or sugar beet; it is preferred by modern confectioners. It provides two kilocalories per gram, half that of refined sugar. With a pH higher than 5.5, it is considered non-cariogenic: it does not produce cavities. However, there are no guarantees because the industry generally mixes sweeteners: erythritol and aspartame, or Splenda and stevia, for example. Let us not forget that excessive consumption of sugars leads to metabolic syndrome.

The issue with non-caloric artificial sweeteners is this: as noted above, 0.35 oz. of Sweet'N Low, Equal and Splenda provide 33 to 36 kilocalories compared to 39 kilocalories for sugar. By weight, these sweeteners can reduce calories by only 10 to 15% compared to sugar. However, these sugar substitutes can reduce sweet-tasting calories by 80%. For example, a packet of Splenda containing 0.035 ounce (1g) of the product with 3 to 4 kilocalories, has the equivalent sweetness of one teaspoon of sugar — 0.15 ounces and 16.3 kilocalories. Food rules allow the numbers to be rounded down to zero when small packages contain fewer than five calories per serving; in this way, brands can advertise themselves as "zero-calorie" products. However, animal experiments show that "non-caloric" artificial sweeteners — ironically, the most widely consumed — have the most drawbacks.

Completing this group, in third place, are two fully caloric sugars: refined white sugar and brown sugar. Although the original pH of sugar cane — 6.8 — or beet — 5.6 — is almost neutral, the different clarification processes to which they are subjected to obtain refined sugar cause the resulting pH in foods to remain acidic. What a great surprise I had when I researched brown *sugar*. I thought it was the best, least harmful option in the carousel of multicolored sachets offered by restaurants, roadside rest areas and gas stations; that brown sachet is just refined white sugar with a molasses coating: what a disappointment! I accepted it based on its caramelized, supposedly natural taste.

A study conducted by dentists on twenty-three different beverages evinces the pH lowering effect of liquids when mixed with sweeteners:[108] with pH 2.30, regular Coca-Cola is the most acidic. Gatorade: 2.71; Fuze Tea-lemon tea: 2.96; Red Bull: 2.98. The best scored, so to speak, is Sprite Zero with pH 3.40, still far from the 5.5 factor. In the same study, distilled water and still Dasani water with 6.54 and 6.23 do not reach 7 of neutral pH. From natural lemonade, citric acid with pH 2.3 sounds strange, but its magic lies in the fact that lemon contains ascorbic acid essential for oxygenation and cell regeneration and decreases acidity in the blood; lemon is absorbed by the body as an alkaline element.

Dentists have established the critical point of acidity at 5.5 on the scale of hydrogen potential between 1 and 14. Below this pH, the most acidic liquid solutions are conducive to the appearance of caries due to demineralization of tooth enamel. This limit is used to measure *biocorrosity* in the mouth — the body — which increases when we ingest substances with pH below 5.5. Therefore, the excessive addition of sugar to food damages the human body.

Adding sugar to food is NOT essential. And it is, like drugs, alcohol, or cigarettes: more than a taste: sugar is a vice. The difference is that most of us acquire the sweet habit with breast milk replacement formulas. Sugar-laden bottles have perpetuated this vice and we haven't even noticed. Like other vices, if we take

---

[108] Hwadam Suh & Estefania Rodriguez (2017). "Determination of pH and total sugars content of various soft drinks: their relationship with erosion and dental caries." *OdontoInvestigacion*, *3* (1). https://www.usfq.edu.ec/publicaciones/odontoinvestigacion/Documents/odontoinvestigacion_n005/oi_005_002.pdf

on the sugar vice as such, we can deal with it. You too can kick the sweet habit.

Of the average calorie intake — 1800 men and 1400 women —, leave only 10% for added sugars. The remaining 90% corresponds to the foods you eat that already contain natural sugars. Increase the consumption of fruit, because there is an added value in the connection between mouth, tongue, and brain to recover the ability to capture the taste as it is. This correction occurs gradually with the frequent consumption of fruit, which is the ideal way to become fond of vegetables and salads that are part of that 90%. Between unripe, green, and ripe, eating fruits allows us to adjust to the real healthy sweetness. By amplifying the sense of taste, you capture the sweetness in everything that, in excess, had been doing you a lot of harm.

I repeat: +SUGAR = +ACID, which means that *biocorrosity*, cancer's best friend, can appear at any moment. The changes you require to recover your health bring unsuspected benefits; for example, if you reduce your consumption, sugar is no longer a priority part of the family shopping basket; its price would not matter and you could choose a better sweetener; and if you limit the consumption of red meat to only one day a week and buy the finest, the budget will even have enough left to enjoy a bottle of wine.

With a pH around the 5.5 limit of *non-biocorrosity*, we have:

Rebiana: The nutrient-free extract rebiana, the sweetest compound of the plant, is synthesized from the South American plant stevia. Experiments with rodents showed that, with high doses of this extract, males produced fewer sperm and females fewer offspring. The stevioside known as *rebaudioside A* or Reb-A, a purified version, was approved in December 2008 by the FDA for general use. Reb-A is used mixed with erythritol or dextrose, as in the Truvia and PureVia brands. One packet of

Truvia — 0.12 oz. — in addition to Reb-A, contains undisclosed "natural flavors" and 0.11 oz. of the "filler" erythritol.

Agave, used for thousands of years by the Aztecs and Mayas, is presented as a diabetic-friendly and a vegan substitute for honey. Its basic compound is fructose with little glucose; fructose, a fruit sugar, does not raise insulin levels in the blood in the short term. However, the concentrated fructose in agave syrup is metabolized exclusively in the liver and is easily transformed into fat. This is why it is advisable to be careful with the consumption of agave, because it compromises liver function and contributes to excessive weight gain.

Brazzein: this sweet-tasting protein is extracted from the fruit of a West African vine (*Pentadiplandra brazzeana baillon*), and tastes similar to sucrose — common sugar — but with a very wide pH range — between 2.5 and 8 — depending on its origin. As commercial quantities cannot be extracted from its natural source, it has been produced from genetically modified corn varieties and industrially distributed under the name Cweet since 2009.

Stevia and monk fruit — raw and pulverized — are not new. Both were rediscovered in response to synthetic sweeteners and were finally allowed to come on to the market by the FDA. They are offered as zero-calorie and suitable for diabetics. Being the leaves and fruit of these plants, respectively, with minimal processing they are almost raw, and even when pulverized, they retain most of their nutrients. However, it is necessary for them to be mixed, for example with maltodextrin, so that they acquire volume and weight. A little less than half a teaspoon of stevia — stevia in the raw — supplements three or four teaspoons of refined sugar. On top of this, many complain of its bitter taste and, therefore, it should not be used in a 1:1 ratio as if it were sugar. With refined white sugar, the price ratio is four times higher, but in practice, stevia, or monk fruit in the raw yields four times as much, i.e., they cost the same. The monk fruit is the small *Luo han guo* melon (*Siraitia grosvenorii/Momordicae grosvenori*), which is three hundred times sweeter than sugar and has been used as a natural sweetener for centuries in China.

Though we have not yet reached the top of the chart, the choices for diabetics seem to be over: the remainder, all natural sweeteners that are full of nutrients and caloric content, are not recommended for diabetics.

In the first lane, nobody ever says, "Hey, why don't you cure yourself of that diabetes!" as it would immediately draw the response, "Don't you know it's incurable? It can only be controlled with medication". Therein lies the misconception that minimizes a serious problem by reducing it to a "controllable medical condition" so that we remain fixated on bad habits and pay for expensive medications that alleviate and sustain life, but do not cure. Accepting the indoctrination of modern medicine and the pharmaceutical industry is a personal decision; things change when we educate ourselves to break out of the inertia.

Bee honey is a special case: with a pH between 4 and 7, it is a complex mixture of water, sucrose, fructose, glucose, maltose, proteins, minerals, and other substances with acid pH that prevent and inhibit the proliferation of microorganisms; this animal secretion resulting from the processing of flower pollen is a natural medicine.

In Canada, between February and April, sap is collected from the trunk of the sugar maple, which is then boiled and results in maple syrup (or maple honey). Imitated for decades, it has been confused with *pancake syrup*, which is a mixture of high fructose corn syrup (HFCS) with artificial colors and flavors. The genuine maple syrup is of course pricey, but economics in health is in avoiding the consumption of waffles and pancakes on a daily basis. The link between this healthy sweetener and "maple syrup disease", a rare hereditary condition in which the odor of the urine of patients — usually children — is similar to that of maple syrup, is in name only.

Molasses is obtained by industrial processes of diffusion or extrusion. Fermentation is the natural method. Unlike the extraction of sugar — 18% — from white sugar beet, which is by diffusion, i.e., by running warm water in a countercurrent, the processes to obtain refined sucrose from sugar cane begin with simple steps that go from milling, in which the cane pieces begin to release juices and molasses by extrusion and cooking, to the processes of evaporation, crystallization, centrifugation and cooling, which change the characteristics of the product, and give rise to the sugar crystals that are later refined.

The centrifugal action, which cleans the impurities and dries the molasses inside a turbine, releases a natural product for sweetening. In the United States it is called *sugar in the raw*, and it comes from Hawaii. Similar products are in England, *Demerara* sugar, named after the province of Guyana, where it is produced; in France, *cassonade* or tertiary sugar, the product of a second crystallization of molasses. There is also *Sucanat* (SUgar CAne NATural), with a similar level of crystallization.

When the juice that results from crushing the sugar canes is cooked, but not centrifuged, a dry and compact honey called panela is obtained, which is very common in Colombia and the Caribbean. It is known by a variety of other names: *chamgay* in Peru and Chile; *raspadura* in Brazil and Ecuador; *gur* in India and Pakistan; *chancaca* or *piloncillo* in Mexico, Guatemala, and Central America; *papelón* in Venezuela. With a pH close to 7, with a very pleasant taste, it contains nutrients with some "impurities", pulp granules — fiber —, antioxidants, B complex vitamins, and minerals such as potassium, magnesium, iron, and calcium. It is natural, vital, and nutritious energy. Ground panela is similar to Barbados *mascabado.*

Panela: panela water is obtained by dissolving a piece of panela in water; sometimes, lemon and cinnamon are added. This is the perfect energy drink at breakfast for children and young people, who go to school, because they require a high energy charge and the battery, an alkaline energy source that avoids oxidation, must be well chosen.

In the fully alkaline spectrum, molasses is the product of the controlled fermentation of some fruits, berries, and cereals. Examples of these molasses are barley molasses, with a slightly bitter taste; rice syrup, especially suitable for celiacs because it does not contain gluten; or coconut sugar extracted from the flower of this palm tree.

The most complete sweetener with extraordinary medicinal properties is at the top of the table. It is the leaves of the stevia plant, the free sale of which is prohibited in the USA, where it has been monopolized by the food industry. Stevia owes its name to the Spanish botanist and physician Pedro Jaime Esteve (1500-1556), who first investigated it. Described in 1887 by the naturalist Moisés Bertoni, *Stevia rebaudiana bertoni* is a magnolia of the asteraceae family that has always been part of traditional Guarani healing practices in Paraguay and parts of Brazil: totally alkaline with pH 9, it prevents tooth decay, is diuretic, non-caloric, helps to lose weight and fights constipation. When consumed alone or as an ingredient in salads, the sweet leaves of the stevia plant contain the active nutrients, vitamins and minerals that reduce cravings and sweet addiction. Because it regulates blood sugar, stevia neutralizes hypertension and poor blood circulation; all these qualities make it a cure for hypoglycemia and facilitate the reversal of type two diabetes.[109]

For years, the interests created by the large corporations that own the sweetener multinationals and pharmaceutical laboratories have not allowed the dissemination, distribution, and free sale of stevia leaves. The great crusade against it has caused a disadvantage for naturalists, and the antecedents confirm it. It was already banned in Europe and the USA when the application to authorize its use was submitted to the European Union on September 26, 2007; and it was only on December 2, 2011, that the World Health Organization, WHO, declared that stevia leaves as a food and natural sweetener that are beneficial and safe for human health. In the United States, for example, the FDA banned its consumption in a resolution that favored NutraSweet in 1991, which was later reversed in 1995. The multinationals Coca-Cola® and Cargill, owner, and producer of Truvia, registered since 2007, hold at least twenty different patents related to the use of stevia extract, but it was only in December 2008 that the FDA authorized the specific use of stevia extracts as natural sweeteners in food and beverages. In 2018 and 2020, the FDA declared, "The use of stevia leaves and crude extracts is not *generally recognized as safe* (GRAS) in the United States, and their importation is not permitted for use as a

---

[109] Rachel J. Perry, Liang Peng, Gary W. Cline, Yongliang Wang, Aviva Rabin-Court, Joongyu D. Song, Dongyan Zhang, Xian-Man Zhang, Yuichi Nozaki, Sylvie Dufour, Kitt Falk Petersen & Gerald I. Shulman (2018), *"Mechanisms by which a very-low-calorie diet reverses hyperglycemia in a rat model of type 2 diabetes."* Cell Metabolism, 27 (1), 210-217. https://www.cell.com/cell-metabolism/fulltext/S1550-4131(17)30616-2?_returnURL=https%3A%2F%2Flinkinghub.elsevier.com%2Fretrieve%2Fpii%2FS1550413117306162%3Fshowall%3Dtrue

sweetener."[110][111] With this attitude, and that of other countries, it seems that stevia leaves are banned practically worldwide.

It is time to clarify that treating the alkaline concept as a law and sticking to trophology is impossible: they are NOT diets; but by putting them into practice you will be avoiding the inflammatory and acidifying processes that cause all kinds of diseases.

Conveniently related to the candy vice, I want to include a topic that may help others. Addictive substances are the most acidifying and there is no doubt that they become vices that dominate us. Though I always knew it, I only admitted it when I understood that addictions lead to suicide and, with acceptance, will and determination, I managed to quit the vice of cigarettes.

The first thing to overcome — even with physical pain — is the withdrawal syndrome. And that's how it was. I set myself a threshold of four days to quit smoking, because I sensed that something important would happen after those ninety-six hours: I felt that between the brain and the mind a fine thread of mastery and control was reconnected that corresponded to the lost will. Don't fool yourself. Nothing works better than self-will to not break your resolve and relapse. The withdrawal syndrome must be overcome without aids such as nicotine patches and gums. Only after overcoming the ninety-six hours, with better judgment and without irritation, is reason heeded; the comments of friends and loved ones, who tried to encourage me, now do work and the products offered by the market to alleviate the process of detoxification of this, and other vices, do inhibit anxiety, which results in a strengthening of the will. Those who have never been addicted do not understand that to an addict

---

[110] https://www.fda.gov/food/food-additives-petitions/additional-information-about-high-intensity-sweeteners-permitted-use-food-united-states.

[111] https://www.accessdata.fda.gov/cms_ia/importalert_119.html.

— especially during detox — comments such as "you're almost there" or "have you seen the picture on the cigarette box?" hurt and are counterproductive. It is understandable: real changes do not come from outside, from external influence; in humans, real changes are gestated and only occur within the being.

Think you're ready? Just think, no one is going to help you. On the contrary, more problems will appear, and they'll be the perfect excuses for you to give up. Dare, and from that last cigarette remember the unhealthy pleasure that makes us fools: 7500 toxins — many of those radioactive — have to do a lot of damage. You hated that last puff, and you are ready: then, the night before, next to the coffee pot and the oatmeal — it tasted good with my coffee —, leave a spoon ready for you to use both hands and avoid that first fateful moment of the cigarette that you have always "married" with the coffee when you wake up. Think that you have already spent six, seven, even eight of the ninety-six hours asleep and lean on this, because this is what you are going to do: add hours. As soon as the day starts and you begin to work, concentrate and during the break try to find an immediate distraction, count the hours, and go on. You cannot smoke in public transportation, and even less in the car; it is two or three hours that you add to your will. At home, surround yourself with your loved ones and don't tell anyone about your challenge; talk to yourself or your pet and, if you watch TV after dinner, kill anxiety with nuts and fall asleep early. That extra time gets you closer to forty-eight hours. Whether you exercise or not, if you walk, you break the routine; it is the ideal way to face the difficult third day. It usually happens that, when you breathe, you feel pain in your chest; a direct message from lungs and bronchial tubes grateful that they finally started to heal. And that phlegm, don't worry, will increase for a while as the tissue repairs itself. After seventy-two hours, you are already one day away from achieving your goal. Do you notice that everything smells like cigarettes? Your sense of smell also recovers. And, above all, you will realize that it is a matter of the body and also of the soul; faith arises without warning at the right time, and you manage to overcome the goal of ninety-six hours. From now on, you can keep in your pocket the list that you yourself made of all the evil that this vice, whatever it is, has been doing to you. This memorial of grievances is very useful in sustaining you when you feel the desire to relapse; after the abstinence syndrome; if you keep the faith, it will be enough to overcome the vices. Do not stop and, with a firm step, do not try them again, because total detoxification is achieved over the years, keep going. Good luck!

Salt

When we discovered its virtue to naturally preserve fish and game, salt became a currency and appreciated like gold. In ancient Rome, a *salaried* worker was the person who received a bag of salt, *salarium argentum,* for participating in the construction of the Via Salaria between the military and commercial port of Ostia Antica, where the salt quarries were located near the Tyrrhenian Sea, and the capital, Rome. Salt and other indispensable items for the economy have been the source of many schemes and intrigues. A clear and transcendental example in the 20TH CENTURY was the electric light bulb, which Edison patented in 1880. From the moment of its invention, so that it would last a lifetime,[112] the industrialists, including Edison, signed the first global pact of programmed obsolescence[113] for a product: to limit the electric light bulb to a maximum duration of 1500

---

[112] http://centennialbulb.org/cam.htm. This prototype has been on since 1901.

[113] https://es.wikipedia.org/wiki/C%C3%A1rtel_Phoebus.

hours. These pacts consolidated the great monopolies and, in the end, inspired consumerism. I mentioned Edison. You will be surprised by the corroded relationship he had with the American Serbian immigrant Nikola Tesla (1856-1943), whose discoveries and pioneering inventions —

like those of Leonardo da Vinci (1452-1519) and Albert Einstein (1879-1955) — which were ahead of their time, and which we have only just begun to enjoy. His prodigy will gain validity in the 21ST century.

This policy of selling a non-perishable product with an expiration date has become the paradigm of the industry, which believes that when consumption is full, production will cease, and the direct and indirect jobs generated by the industry will be lost; programmed obsolescence is the subliminal tool that perpetuates the idea that consumerism is the only way to sustain and expand jobs. How ironic: in counter-politics, monopolies reduce jobs to increase profitability, net profit, and rivers of money. In relation to human achievement, planned obsolescence is a twisted, retrograde, and irrational idea that has led to the depredation of the planet. Today, innovative, resource-conscious companies that take advantage of the dynamism of global communication to interconnect regions are successful. With more jobs, people do not have to leave their homes, their farms, their environs to acquire products and services of the highest quality, or to promote their own to the world. This satellite business model focuses on promoting and commercializing local products and consumption; and rescues the identity of the locality and the pride of its inhabitants.

In the salt industry, an intriguing phrase is obligatory on the front labels of salts other than common refined table salt: *THIS SALT DOES NOT CONTAIN IODIDE, A NECESSARY NUTRIENT.* More than simple information, it is a warning that generates confusion in the uninformed consumer to abstain from acquiring 100% natural salt and buy the usual refined salt.

Salt began to be refined in the early 1930s to facilitate its solubility and to give it a better presentation, but with the need to combat thyroid problems — both goiter and hyperthyroidism —, in the 1920s and 1930s, it was considered appropriate to include a strong dose of iodine. Also, from 1980, fluoride was added to prevent tooth decay. The daily dose of iodine should be 150 micrograms for adults and up to 290 in pregnant women, because iodine deficiency is the main cause of brain damage in the fetus during pregnancy. Iodized salt contains between 30 and 100 micrograms of iodine per gram of salt and, if you consume five grams of iodized salt — one teaspoon contains up to seven grams —, you would be ingesting between 150 and 500 micrograms of iodine in addition to that naturally contained in food: undoubtedly, a toxic excess. For example, a portion of one hundred grams of codfish contains 170 micrograms of iodine, or *kelp* has four times more than we need daily, two servings a week are enough.

With the practice becoming the norm, a genius idea led to the paradigm and the clever phrase *THIS SALT DOES NOT CONTAIN IODIDE, A NECESSARY NUTRIENT*, which tends to misinform by not saying on the labels of sea salt and other 100% natural salts what would be true: "This salt does NOT contain the amount of industrial iodine that is usually added to table salt to combat thyroid problems". If by medical recommendation you need iodine, include in your weekly diet, seaweed; fish; seafood; blueberries and cranberries; yogurt with probiotics; and increase the consumption of white beans; strawberries; dairy products; eggs; lentils; spinach; watercress; garlic, beets; caviar, and drink plenty of tea, which contains it. Among other things, fish, nuts, and seeds provide us with fluoride. If you want to limit salt intake, you can season with pepper, bay leaf, turmeric, rosemary, basil, garlic, onion.

We can look for healthy alternatives to enhance the flavor of foods. There are others: natural salts contain trace minerals and essential trace elements that, although they seem insignificant, are in perfect balance and proportion, and are precisely amount of each element needed for the metabolism and to establish the connections in the biological function of any living organism on Earth. When buying sea salt, for example, check the ingredients on the label and make sure that it only reads "*sea salt*" and that it does not contain anything additional. Food provides the amount of essential trace elements and minerals that the human body requires on a daily basis; otherwise, or to supplement it, additional 100% natural salt to meals should not exceed 0.1 oz. in a single day. Promoting and protecting food diversity on the planet is a matter of urgency, as today, the food supply comes from many different places: the well-intentioned argument that made iodized table salt an indispensable product can be ignored.

In its pure state, salt has a perfect balance: one tenth is composed of the 84 stable elements of the periodic table — including iodine and fluorine — minerals essential for life. The rest is chlorine and sodium — in a ratio of approximately 40-60 % — in percentages that vary due to the physical and environmental characteristics at the extraction points. Hence, in urine tests, sodium is the element that determines the patient's salt intake. The problem with what is added to this basic compound is not only quantitative. In addition to iodine and synthetic fluoride, the refined compound includes bleaching agents, anti-caking agents such as sodium ferrocyanide, ammonium citrate, aluminum silicate and artificial sodium in greater quantities and proportions. What is serious is the qualitative aspect: due to the effect of the heat to which the substance is subjected to disaggregate and refine it, the resulting sodium chloride is not pure in nature — the same happens with sucrose and white sugar — and nitrates resulting from the introduction of iodides and fluorides, probably carcinogenic substances that the body does not metabolize, the organism does not recognize them and biologically rejects them.

Natural salts come from the sea or from deposits on land and not all natural salts are sodium chloride. Indian black salt, of volcanic origin, is odorless and has a sulfurous taste due to its sulfur content, an element different from the sodium characteristic of rock salts. It is recommended for people suffering from high blood pressure and is preferred by vegans. There are at least two salts of vegetable origin: the South American Indians obtain it from the ashes — by combustion — of the *Holmbergia tweedii* shrub, and the South Africans — by concentration — by boiling a grass plant endemic to the Kalahari Desert.

Rock salt for refining is extracted from halite. The mines of Zipaquirá - Colombia, Cardona Salt Mountain - Spain, Kansas Salt Museum -USA, and the Wieliczka mine in Krakow -Poland, which was declared a World Heritage Site by Unesco in 1978, among others, have become world-famous tourist landmarks. It is worth mentioning that there is another refined salt other than common iodized salt: *kosher* salt, which does not contain additives, although some brands include anti-caking agents.

Ninety-three percent of refined salt is used for industrial purposes. In the food industry, 4 % is used as a preservative and only 3 % is marketed as common table salt. Sodium is a necessary mineral; however, the salt used by the food industry contains more than 90% sodium in order to make processed foods such as baked goods, canned goods, pickles, dehydrated foods, sauces, dressings and chips last. In sausages and processed meats, nitrosamines prevail, preservative salts with high carcinogenic potential: nitrites and nitrates. Brands that avoid them are on the rise. Even dressings that claim to be salt-free contain monosodium glutamate, MSG, to enhance flavor, another salt discussed for its neurotoxic effects and for causing addiction. Those that advertise themselves as NO MSG do not contain it.

In relation to cancer and the accumulation of sodium, Dr. Otto Heinrich Warburg, winner of the Nobel Prize for Medicine in 1931, said: "Tumor cells thrive in an acidic environment without oxygen, they are anaerobic; an external acidic environment, rather than attacking them, sponsors their existence, but to continue living healthily, to begin to mutate, cancer cells need their interior to be very alkaline in order to reproduce". In other words: to bypass the acidic environment and get the sodium — alkaline — that the tumor needs to survive; cancer cells use dextrorotatory proteins — turned to the right — in a process called the "acid fermentation pathway".

Salt as a seasoning is additional and requires caution to get the full benefit of its use, and not only for its alkaline contribution. For example, use coarse-grained sea salt to enhance the flavor of the meat on the grill, just before putting it on the griddle or grill; with the first temperatures, the grains of salt retain the juices that come out of the meat. They are not lost, the coarse-grained salt contains them so that the heat dilutes them, reverses them, and exalts their flavor. Turning the meat only once is a doctrine rigorously taught by the gauchos of Argentina, Brazil, Chile, Uruguay, and other experts in the art of grilling. At home, we use natural salts: sea salt for cooking and for the saltshaker; in the mortar, we prepare *gomasio* salt with toasted sesame and Himalayan salt in equal proportions. In all these years, my family's thyroid stimulating hormone (TSH) and blood sodium reading have always been in the normal range.

Seawater cures all the ills of man.

The seawater molecule contains in balance towards alkalinity the acid minerals: sulfur, iodine, phosphorus, chlorine and fluorine, and the alkaline minerals: calcium, sodium, cesium, magnesium, zinc, potassium, iron among others. When we consume unrefined salt or seawater, the body we inhabit recovers the natural patent of trace minerals. Seawater is extraordinary because of its pH 8. Curiously, however, the planet Earth is composed of 71% water: this percentage varies in the human body between 65 and 75%, an interesting aqueous correlation. Frequently drinking a solution of one part seawater to four — or five-parts fresh water and, for each 4 cups of this mixture, the juice of a lemon restores the body quickly and naturally. The French physiologist and naturalist René Quinton (1867-1925) observed that cancer cells in an oxygenated, alkaline environment died instead of thriving. Of course, you know that the same thing happened to him as to others: his voice was not echoed in the media because his time coincided with the first steps of industrialization. Quinton's plasma cured diseases that had been thought to be untreatable. Considered as a great benefactor of humanity, at his death, he was honored by the scientific community.

The production of sea salt has not only increased. On the Brittany coast, in France, a traditional technique has been revived and has spread to other countries to harvest the *fleur de sel*, rich in minerals, and salt flakes, the result of controlled crystallization of seawater. These *gourmet* salts are highly appreciated for their flavor. Also traditional, gray (or Celtic) salt, which has a slight water content and is grayish, that comes from the Celtic Sea. When I referred to rock salts, I was alluding to some that require special attention.

Originally from the Epsom region in England, where it was produced, Epsom salts today comes from the extraction of the mineral called epsomite — different from halite. Its main component is magnesium, and it is called magnesium sulfate. This hydrated salt, known as English salt, does not absorb moisture. This characteristic makes it special for flotation therapy and salt baths, because in high concentrations and dissolved in water, the density of the solution increases. Also unrefined, with a characteristic pink color, Himalayan salt and its Andean counterpart have something that makes them extraordinary. The molecules of these salts, fossilized residue from the evaporation of ancient seas more than 250 million years ago, a product of the extremely high pressures of rock folding, retain a trapped beam of light that makes them different. There are only four deposits in Bolivia, Peru, Poland and, of course, the ancient Khewra mine in Pakistan, the second largest salt mine in the world, near the Himalayas.

Suzanne Powell, an Irish writer based in Spain, tells us about *gomasio* in her book *We Are What We Eat*. After World War II, scientists focused their research on the very particular almost daily diet of a group of children from an orphanage in Hiroshima who were not affected by the radiation of the atomic bombs. It is called *gomasio* and consists of a plate of red rice one half, and in equal proportions roasted sesame and Himalayan salt the other half. We know that salt, in general, absorbs moisture and excess heavy metals are trapped in its molecules for the body to eventually evacuate. In later studies it was discovered that, due to the pressures, biotectonic transformations gave the molecular structure of Himalayan salt a unique energetic pattern: a light particle capable of trapping the surrounding radioactive residues.

Himalayan salt should not be cooked, because from one hundred — and four-degrees Fahrenheit it dilutes quickly. Use it directly or as a condiment in the dish to release the light beam that traps radioactive waste. To ingest with prudence any natural salt helps us to clean and to eliminate the heavy metals and the free radicals that intoxicate the body.

Is it really harmful and dangerous to consume salt? No. But everything in excess is bad. You will have already concluded that you should eat natural, unrefined products. I would be wrong to pretend to write a medical treatise, but I will try to explain what among other things could happen in the body when you do not consume the basic supply of minerals present in unrefined salt.

When practicing some exercise such as walking, swimming, dancing, you may have a muscle spasm with which the body sends you a message: "I need salt". Minerals maintain the electrical conductivity that is momentarily lost in a more aqueous plasma. The neuromuscular system fails, loses control and the muscle involuntarily retracts; it causes pain, and we call it a cramp. By eating salt or drinking mineralized water, preferably alkaline — without sugar —, the electrolytic conductivity improves, the neurotransmitter system instantly comes back to normal, and the brain resumes the voluntary control of the muscles.

What happens if you consume more salt than necessary for an indefinite period of time?

Minerals heavier than water retain in their molecules more liquid than normal, which makes you constantly thirsty not because of the absence of liquid, but because the excess salt retains it and makes room for more water and food to accumulate; the volume expands, and the less dense mass becomes flabby. In terms of automotive mechanics: blood overloaded with heavy minerals in relation to the liquid to be displaced and dense as oil increases the pressure in the hoses and walls of the pump. The heart, which moves all that non-oil fluid and is designed to pump blood, could fail at any time due to internal inflammation from this excess salt.

Not to mention possible kidney failure. Arterial hypertension is among the diseases related to the heart, veins, and arteries, and is directly linked to high triglycerides in people with enlarged hearts. In response to constant hypertension, which involves extra strain, the heart muscle grows, softens, and loses tone over time. Cholesterol and hypertension result in aneurysms, strokes, or heart attacks. If people changed their habits, they would not depend on drugs that barely control the symptoms, but do not cure the diseases.

The fact that salt retains fluid can be harnessed in an almost "miraculous" way. Instead of further damaging the body's plasma by adding excess salt to this internal liquid environment, you can add lots of salt to a bathtub or hot tub and soak in it for twenty to thirty minutes to create a very dense liquid external environment surrounding the entire body.

Remember that I mentioned a person who the doctors had been given up on, who made a different decision from the conventional one and who has already managed to outlive his life expectancy. My recommendation was that, for some time, he should take daily baths in a hot tub or bathtub with lots of salt. After several months with the disease, his prognosis was reversed, and he was cured of leukemia.

Chapter VI

Why People Get Sick

From Hierapolis and Troy in ancient Greece, Ulysses in Homer's *Odyssey* already spoke of the delight and pleasure of a thermal bath. In Rome they became popular, but over time they ceased to be free and were exclusive to the aristocracy. Today, thermal baths are charged at a not so healthy price. They are medicinal. Their millenary fame is due to the deep cleansing of the skin. On contact with hot water, the pores open and the specific saline concentration of minerals such as potassium or magnesium allows the thermal function to cleanse the lungs, kidneys, and liver, which are the body's filters. Through the skin, the thermal function involving sweating throughout the body, which is uniquely human, removes from these organs the carbonic and uric acids and fats that accumulate and prevent them from functioning properly. It is as simple as that. If we replace the old, dirty filters in our vehicles with new ones every few miles, it is ironic that we do not adopt this habit with the body. When the machine fails, we complicate things and find different, complex, and useless explanations and solutions.

Do you remember what I said: "As long as I can walk, breathe, have no pain and go to work..."? It seems natural for us to think like that. The first thing we do today — with respect to the car — is to protect a patrimony, because money is what matters. The second thing is to protect life. Given the current inhumanity and selfishness of some, who do not pay attention to elementary scientific recommendations, such as wearing face masks in public places while the COVID-19 crisis is happening all over the world, it is evident that even life itself is at the bottom of the list of values.

The Greek physician Galen of Pergamon (130-200 A.D.), father of pharmacology and tablets, warned: "In the face of obesity, we must unblock the sewer and start with the thermal function of water". The thermal function of water not only takes care of obesity, but also of the disease that surrounds the body's universe. Nowadays, we forget to include the thermal bath as a method of detoxification in the chapter of hydrotherapy in the book on the human health.

The thermal bath is a percutaneous dialysis, it is a kidney, it is a lung, it is a high performance and low-cost artificial liver.

DR. ALBERTO MARTÍ BOSCH

Dr. Martí Bosch asks: "How many times have you heard the word "bath salts"? But how many times have you asked yourself why you have to put salt in the bath?".

"Human plasma has a concentration of 9.4 grams of salt per liter and hot springs twenty grams of salt per liter of water. With more than twice the salt concentration, this osmotic gradient causes the extraction of the acids retained inside the body through the skin, a permeable organ". Replicating a thermal bath is easy if you have a bathtub or hot tub at home. Regardless of the type of salt, when you soak in the hot tub, the real benefit is in the environment created by the different densities between the plasma and the salty water surrounding the body.

How much water and how much salt in the tub? A standard bathtub filled halfway — more than that would overflow —, averages one hundred liters (i.e., 26 gallons). If we multiply one hundred liters of water by twenty grams of salt — the required density per liter — we need two thousand grams of salt (i.e, 70 oz.). Then, to the half-filled bathtub, we add 70 ounces of salt. They say that bathtubs are no longer used, but as an architect, I worry that we are removing the bathtub from houses in remodeling. Bathtubs differ according to the model; for example, one that is filled halfway with 150 liters (39 gallons) of water should have three kilos (105 oz.) of salt added.

Must it be hot water? If so, at what temperature? Not necessarily, but we know that the skin pores open faster in hot water. The temperature: whatever temperature you can stand, without exceeding 98.6 degrees Fahrenheit. Above that limit, the tissue shows some degree of scalding, it burns. Those who indulge in extremely hot foods or drinks unknowingly provoke additional internal inflammation that is debilitating because it directly compromises the immune system. The idea is to try to match the external aqueous environment to the normal internal body temperature — 98.6 °F — so water at ninety to ninety-three degrees would be fine; the blood vessels expand and facilitate osmotic exchange. After the bath, the feeling of weakness is similar to when you come out of a sauna. Nothing to worry about.

How long and how often should we take this bath? As in the hydromassage, it should not exceed thirty minutes. The frequency could be weekly: each person can acquire the healthy habit of cleaning the filters of the body. And to educate the children, once a month, share the bath as a family. To this pleasant plan you can add aromatherapy and music therapy. How about Yanni, Enya, Kitaro; or the classics, Beethoven, Chopin; perhaps a modern and inspiring pianist like George Winston; or the radio station of your choice with music for meditation.

Treating a disease requires a different frequency. Dr. Marti speaks of having had success after thirty or forty consecutive sessions, in the most severe cases, which include different types of cancer. Of course, not all patients survive, and let it be clear: mental attitude, faith and perseverance come from within yourself.

Well, in the previous chapters we have focused on explaining how what we ingest could be affecting our health. The second pillar of my work is Dr. Martí's scientific explanation of what happens in the body. In his experience, one word enshrines the concept that holds the "secret" to recovering and maintaining good health: alkalinity.

"Doctor, I'm here to be cured," he is told by many people who knock on his door. Patients with rare, complicated diseases and different types of cancer. So much so that other colleagues ask him: "Do you cure cancers, Alberto?" And his blunt answer: "No, I don't cure cancers, but we do give a manual with instructions that allow the body to be placed in such conditions that it can then cure itself".

By describing physiological processes, I intend to generate concern and curiosity. The scientific explanation of why people get sick makes things clear: where and how diseases are born and develop. The lecture by Dr. Alberto Martí Bosch, an endorsed member of the WACR (World Association for Cancer Research), on how to deal with cancer holistically is a good start in the educational process on health and nutrition.[114]

Alberto Martí Bosch, who was born in Pamplona, Spain, has a doctorate in oncology and specialist in homeopathy, orthomolecular nutrition, and biological medicine. His foundation is the thesis of Dr. Alfred Pischinger (1899-1982), who discovered that the most elementary basic functions of

---

[114] https://www.youtube.com/watch?v=26n11gv5Z1w.

life — which include the defense systems and the acid-alkaline regulation of free radicals, water, oxygen, and electrolyte exchange — do not occur inside the cell, but in the connective tissue of the extracellular matrix that surrounds it. In this respect, Dr. Martí comments: "Dr. Pischinger was a genius because he made us understand diseases; the disease is not generated inside the cell and then spreads to the outside: it is its environment that causes it". And I understand it like this: the cell even defends itself against itself, in spite of the environment that surrounds it. Doing whatever is necessary to continue to live and to be able to reproduce is equivalent to having found in the cell the biological instinct of survival. Disease is generated in the periphery of the cell: if the environment is alkaline, the cell will have enough oxygen and will not require excess sodium to live normally: everything will be fine. But if we start to retain acids and free radicals between the cell and the venous capillary, when the cell cannot get rid of its excrement, it accumulates it in the interstitial space. If the stagnation of metabolic waste persists, problems begin.

Dr. Martí explains that endotoxins — when they surround the cell — burn like acid and begin to cause cellular nutritional distress; accumulated free radicals destroy nutrients and impede the passage of oxygen; caustic aggression occurs, and the cell will eventually drown in its own excrement. Faced with negative circumstances, cells have two options:

Option 1: die chemically burned by the action of free radicals accumulated around them or through lack of oxygen. What happens if the brain cells die? Alzheimer's disease occurs. And the cells at the base of the brain? Parkinson's. Those of the nervous system, those of the myelin covering the axons of neurons? Sclerosis. If the cells in the fibers die? Pulmonary fibrosis, muscular fibrosis, hepatic fibrosis, etc. Except those of viral or bacterial origin, which are acquired by contagion, this is how diseases are generated inside the body.

Option II: in order to survive, cells defend themselves. And they do so in a way that will make us suffer because of their ability to react. In the meantime, with manifest diseases that are not very serious, we persist in responding: "I'm fine!", and others, the silent ones, get worse with time.

How do they defend themselves?

They retain fluids in the interstitial space — the external space between them — in order to dilute acids and thus allow the passage of nutrients from the capillary to the cell. Hydrocephalus and acute renal failure are good examples.

They sequester calcium, sodium, and potassium; the alkaline trace elements in bones and teeth form salts to precipitate acids in soft tissues and lead to decalcification, which causes, for example, osteoporosis or dental caries.

They drain acids through skin and mucous membranes: yellow and excessive sweating; oily and yellowish urine; or sores and ulcers; these are important warnings just before cell death. For example, some skin diseases, although not very serious, indicate premature aging.

Finally, they defend themselves by mutating: cancer.

What does mutation consist of? A cell that is attacked by the external acidic environment can defend itself from dying by mutating into a tumor cell. To live without oxygen, it becomes anaerobic; in this acidic environment, it manages to live with a lot of sodium — salt — and instead of levorotatory proteins — molecules that react to light with a left-handed twist — it uses dextrorotatory proteins — molecules that react to light with a right-handed twist — to feed itself. Eventually metastasis occurs, which is the uncontrolled reproduction of these tumor cells.

So much for the explanation of what happens when what we ingest keeps the body acidic, not alkaline. Dr. Marti makes a brilliant historical analogy to support his methodology to combat this dreaded enemy. In examining the subject of cancer in conventional medicine, he takes us back to the Middle Ages, to the 12TH century, to expose its limits and underlines what we are missing by treating cancer in the same way that an enemy was attacked and liquidated in the Middle Ages.

Let us continue. In Medieval Europe, engrossed in the struggle for power and submerged in obscurantism, the exploited, fearful, and ignorant common people served their fief and were guided by the interests of a great lord, who in return protected them, from his walled castle; and nobles in dispute, or their followers, were often branded as heretics by the Church or turned into enemies of the kingdom who had to be eliminated.

How was an enemy annihilated in the Middle Ages?

The first would be to "cut off the head" of the tumor — if possible — with surgery. Secondly, we have the option of "burning" and, if possible, scorching the tumor with radiotherapy. And the third option commonly offered by conventional medicine consists of "poisoning" the enemy. Tumor cells are poisoned with chemotherapy. We are stuck in the 12TH century.

Only those who investigate the past have a future, because by investigating the past, the future can be rediscovered.

JULIUS ROBERT OPPENHEIMER (1904-1967)

Dr Alberto Martí Bosch, a specialist in oncology and orthomolecular nutrition, noted that we missed the most successful outpatient strategy, which is simple, categorical, definitive, and more successful than single combat; it required a lull and perseverance. At the end of the day, "the siege" consisted of cornering the enemy in his castle and leaving him without supplies, without water and without food until he "starved to death".

And how do we corral the tumor?

We alkalinize the patient.

We hyperoxygenate the system: tumor cells — anaerobic — find an oxygenated environment toxic.

We opt for a low sodium hyposodium diet: on the contrary, the tumor cell needs a lot of sodium to alkalinize its cytoplasm and thus be able to live and counteract the external acid attack.

To starve it and eventually starve the tumor to death, the patient also receives selective proteolytic enzymes. This means that they destroy certain proteins, but not all of them; only the dextrorotatory ones, which are those that the tumor uses to feed itself.

How do we alkalinize the patient?

Unlike traditional medicine, based on surgery, radiotherapy, and chemotherapy, which acidifies, invades, and destroys the immune system of patients, Dr. Martí Bosch's holistic therapy is based on common sense and history; a whole in which neither order nor priority matter. The treatment is based on four pillars:

With hydrotherapy, we recover the function of the liver, kidneys, and lungs. The need for filters in the body is evident: one liver, two kidneys, two lungs, five filters equivalent in size to eight fists. The heart under normal conditions pumps 170 fl oz. of blood per minute, 10,200 fl oz. per hour and 244,800 fl oz. in 24 hours, which is equivalent to the weight of a truck weighing more than seven tons. The blood continuously irrigates the lungs, liver, and kidneys to filter from the cells the toxins accumulated in the interstitial space, the garbage and metabolic waste, the cellular excrement. If a car's filters are clogged, they are changed. And in hydrotherapy, thermal baths — with lots of salt — perform the function of cleaning the body's filters. The next time you enjoy your salt bath, watch your arms: the arteries carry oxygen to the tissues and back through the veins; again, and again the blood plasma passes through the filters and carries away cellular debris. Then, with confidence, step up to the whirlpool jet if the tub has one. Your salt bath is a percutaneous dialyzer. Additionally, to reinforce alkalinization, Dr. Javier López Garcés, a colleague of Dr. Martí Bosch, has successfully used peroxidase enzyme delivery, ozone therapy and hyperoxygenation, which enhance oxygenating function in patients.

Aimed at restoring energy mechanisms and vital cellular functions — nutrition, relationship, and reproduction — physical treatments — acupuncture, chiropractic, physiotherapy, radiofrequency, magnetotherapy, music therapy, osteopathy, deep massage, photonic laser therapy and color therapy, among others — activate the healing process.

Orthomolecular nutrition takes into account the principle of the uniqueness of the individual. Usually, the patient receives a personalized food plan with nutritional supplements such as vitamins and trace minerals, substances that occur naturally in food and are directly involved in metabolism. Oligotherapy allows the constant monitoring of the reinforcement minerals so that their presence does not vary, and the catalytic functions are reactivated and improve the activity of the lungs, liver, and kidneys of the patients. Phytotherapy, the use of products of plant origin for the prevention, cure, or relief of a wide variety of symptoms and diseases, consists of ingesting teas, infusions, or aromatic water of medicinal herbs — the healthy habit of accompanying a solid food with warm or hot liquids — and goes beyond the simple supply of minerals. Thus, for example, the infusion of horsetail, a powerful diuretic, improves renal function. Chamomile, boldo, artichoke, dandelion and *oolong* tea, or blue tea — great for encapsulating fats — cleanse the liver and regulate the choleretic function: the production of bile. Thyme and mullein improve the elimination of carbon dioxide; ginseng and cat's claw are immunostimulants. With these two simultaneous treatments, we make sure to supplement the minerals required by the body.

The fourth pillar of this holistic treatment that makes the necessary adjustments in the body and restores the conditions that fully stimulate the immune system is alkalizing nutrition. Healing depends on the patient and is not a miracle, because at some point, body, mind, and soul conspire: the "siege" is forceful, and the body heals itself.

On the vegetarian issue, Dr. Alberto Martí Bosch says: "A meat diet acidifies the urine, and a vegetarian diet alkalizes the urine. A dirty filter is not a broken filter; it can be washed with water. 95% of fruit and vegetables are water and with the vegetarian diet the filters are washed: lung, liver, and kidney". To the question of whether one should be a vegetarian, Dr. Martí answers:

No, not at all. It is one thing that a vegetarian diet is good and another thing that we have to be vegetarians. Cows eat vegetables because they can: they have four stomachs designed by evolution to digest a diet consisting of fiber and forage; we can't because we only have one stomach. No, we can't be cows, we lack digestive mechanism. One can survive being vegetarian, but not live; we are purely omnivores, neither carnivores nor herbivores; we are, I repeat, omnivores. It is extremely prudent to have moderation with red meat. Not for nothing is it said that "not eating meat on Fridays is for priests". And yes, the word "cure" comes from cure. "Prevention is better than cure", the famous phrase of the physician Galen, consequently, gave rise to this relationship with the priests: *Mens sana in corpore sano*, because the priests after Galen cured. However, the kings and the aristocracy that followed them, due to the Protestant theology of five centuries ago, exaggerated gluttony so they could eat meat on Fridays in protest. They did not wash their filters and what did the kings die of? Of gout, of excess uric acid; acids are what kill if you block the kidney; just as, if you block the liver, you will not be able to eliminate cholesterol and, if you block the lung, you will not be able to eliminate CO_2: acids kill us.

"The cells must swim in a clean pool of transparent water that is the body, but no one has made us understand the importance of eating vegetarian one day a week, of bathing one day a week with hot water with salt and of taking depurative plants that help us to keep our filters clean". This siege to the tumor and to any disease proposed by Dr. Alberto Martí Bosch results in apoptosis — programmed cell death to control cell growth and development — of the tumor cells and the remission of the disease. With this holistic approach, the body will be fully functioning, and the cells will be clean and healthy for a lifetime.

Finally, Dr. Alberto addresses a message to the United States:

How is it that, as successful and original as they have always been — congratulations to them in advance for their ability to teach with cartoons, and even more so with their theme parks — nobody has ever thought of drawing or creating characters explaining that cells are the citizens of the body, organs are the buildings where citizens live, arteries and veins are streets and avenues where we transport drinks, food and collect garbage. The nerves are both the telephone lines and the electrical wiring. The lungs, liver and kidneys, the purification plants; the recycling centers and the central nervous system is the City Hall, the mayor's office.

Preventive health can be taught to solve — once and for all — the serious problems that burden humanity: obesity and diabetes, among many others. The solution is different: to provide the education that is needed to correct the mistakes that we made in the past due to simple ignorance and that only now the second lane highlights. In the first lane of the predominant reality, this and many other truths fully exonerate all those in the second lane, who were pointed out as naive and innocent, who — ironically — can toss back this accusation at the mainstream.

I have never understood why we only focus on what doctors say about what pills to take or what procedure to follow; and depending on the outcome, we praise them, criticize them, or take them to court. What we don't do is research to understand the problem in its full context. Much of the information is already available for educated common sense to constitute itself in sound criticism; with solid bases, reason rejects or accepts the logical procedures to follow. But we insist on rushing to the pharmacy to buy the magic pills; the ones the doctor ordered — or worse, blindly, those the propaganda says we should — without even trying to know what is going on because presumably we would not understand it. In other words, we get sick and don't recognize that we are our nearest and dearest get sick and die. Aside from ranting, the usual explanation is that their demise was due to a "very rare" illness or complication. I recognize that researching, experimenting, and writing is a sacrifice, for which I will be rewarded, if my text helps someone or, at least, I manage to save another life.

Metabolism, the body, and the human self

The metabolism is the set of chemical reactions — among exergonic, i.e., spontaneous, occurring without additional energy, with the capacity to release heat and emit free energy[115] or not (endergonic) — that occur in the cell, by which it extracts from the food the energy that allows the living being to fulfill its vital functions: nutrition, respiration, interaction, and reproduction. A purely scientific explanation. I intend to show from another perspective, my point of view, what we let pass.

The cycle of life is common to every embryo that manages to gestate and survives the change of environment. With its birth, the spirit is established in the creature: the being exists and the body subsists on what mother earth can offer. From that moment on, in the individual, the internal process of life that provides energy, the metabolism, changes its design and makes things more complex in order to fulfill a single objective: to achieve the full reproductive capacity in the subject and multiply the species.

Having found the "bioinstinct" of conservation in the cell, is proof that the objective is reproduction, because in spite of

---

[115] https://es.khanacademy.org/science/biology/energy-and-enzymes/free-energy-tutorial/a/gibbs-free-energy.

the hostile environment in which it finds itself — in the case of mutations — the cell seeks to survive and reproduce at all costs. From the strict natural sense of conservation, this function corresponds exclusively to metabolism; this is proven by the species that die at the moment of procreation. And others, for example, at the top of the food chain, whose families form clans, evolution has endowed them with reproductive apparatuses with a predetermined period of fecundity so that they can fulfill this reproductive function without rest. And while it may have happened to the chimpanzee — and not to us, humans — in addition to thriving, they were granted the divine privilege of procreating at will. Once the natural objective is fulfilled, the care of the body remains under the entire responsibility of the "being": the "human self" is the one who decides whether or not to affect the body: the container that identifies the individual. However, contrary to our intellect, we did not realize that growing and feeding by instinct has been the instinctual alternative common to all species.

When we feed instinctively, we underestimate the brain; the superego governs our will and, for example, by overeating, the "diet of the eye" leads to gluttony. At the beginning of obscurantism, in the 6TH CENTURY, Pope Gregory the Great pointed it out as one of the seven deadly sins. In the midst of so much fear and ignorance, at the beginning of the 14TH century, between 1304 and 1321, in addition to the seven deadly sins, Dante Alighieri immortalized what awaits the sinner after death, their supposed suffering, by the staging of the *Divine Comedy*. Of great help to the clergy, this poem sings of monotheism and evokes ideas of hell, purgatory and paradise, places we believe to be true. I firmly believe that sin has always been an easy way to manipulate the fearful and ignorant, because not knowing how to act comes mainly from not knowing things. Then in the human being with full capacity to think, but dominated by the superego, the being is not so wonderful.

Fears, phobias, lack of self-esteem or excessive desire for control can have unusual and difficult to diagnose physical repercussions that can only be resolved by learning to stay in touch with our deepest self.

CAROLINE MYSS, PhD, *Anatomy of the Spirit*

All this makes me think that the fundamental problem of humanity lies in the "human self". Through evolution, the brain tends to develop greater aptitudes. And we are surprised, for example, that children are born with an almost immediate ability to make friends with a computer, a tablet or a smart phone, devices that took us adults a long time to master. We evolved and, even so, we have not understood that in the absence of supervision and strict control, they are ultimately educating our children with harmful messages and twisted information that definitely alters their moral and social behavior. In schools, the classroom had not changed in the last two hundred years until the pandemic forced us to design more effective architectural configurations that take advantage of connectivity and distance education. However, to do so, with an educational system set up to teach groups, it is difficult — almost impossible — to train individuals.

Stuck between fear and ignorance, the human self is the threat that puts our species at direct risk of extinction. It is not enough to fill young people with information in schools; an educational concept, which involves guiding them in the search for balance between body, mind and soul is the appropriate one to bring out in individuals their specific potential and train them to quickly solve the most complex problems posed by coexistence. Educators understand that learning is mutual and young people are born fit to pay attention to the subjects that are needed: health and nutrition; emotional intelligence; creativity and innovation; civics;

social intelligence; positivism and happiness; and an introduction to quantum physics; all of which are as high priority subjects as mathematics, history of civilizations, language, or biology.

Let's tell it like it is today's average educational scheme is obsolete and a waste of time. According to UNESCO in 2018,[116] 750 million people — 10% of the world's population, two thirds of whom are women — do not know how to read and write; and of those, 260 million are children and adolescents who do not attend school. In 2020,[117] illiteracy in the world reached 773 million people: the pandemic worsened the figures. The serious thing is that these statistics show carelessness and confirm another abstract truth that worked very well in the Middle Ages: all uneducated people are manipulable for the convenience of politicians, the State, the clergy, and individuals who have governed the economy, the system of the day. This is how we all live; our children only begin to use their brains to think about all these issues when they enter school or university. And only 2% of the world's population has access to higher education.

The self and my body: two distinct entities?

When we depart, the body decomposes and, if we all departed, the planet would be completely regenerated. We say "me and my body" or "me and my planet"; this egocentric position is wrong because, if we believe that they belong to us, we can dispose of them until they are destroyed! It is said that "ignorance justifies

---

[116] https://www.aa.com.tr/es/mundo/en-el-mundo-750-millones-de-personas-son-analfabetas/1250093#:~:text=The%20Unesco%20indicates%20that%20the%20International%20D%3%ADa%20of%20literacy%20.

[117] https://unesdoc.unesco.org/ark:/48223/pf0000374187_spa.

and knowledge condemns", because if we do not have the prior knowledge of how they work, insisting on saying "my body" and "my planet" is harmful and suicidal for the individual, the collective and the planet. But if you learn how they work and what happens, you can become aware and confirm that "your being" is only an integral part of them as long as it is present. It is urgent that we change our beliefs and habits; we are going to irremediably destroy the planet unless our ideas evolve soon. Then, if with individual attitude, we take care of the body and, with collective attitude, we take care of the planet, then body and planet will allow us to inhabit them, to live and enjoy them longer than we thought, and perhaps transcend eternally.

The body reflects our imbalances and, moreover, makes itself felt so that we listen to it. But in order to feel healthy, we prefer to silence its messages with antacids, anti-allergic and anti-flu drugs. We think it sufficient, and then the muzzled body becomes a comfortable, pleasant, and silent entity, it stops bothering us and simply transmits the message that we are alive and relieved: we do not listen to it. And both, body, and planet, send us signals to try to communicate to the "I" clear messages with real facts: the winters are getting harsher, the summers hotter, the thaws more profuse, the storms more aggressive and the floods more surprising and unpredictable; not to forgetting the wildfires, which are becoming more and more voracious. The truth is that these are "urgent messages", but we insist on calling them climate change; a subliminal message that de facto excludes human impact. For example, in 2009, the American sailor and captain, Charles Moore, discovered a gigantic island of plastic debris that drifts around the Pacific Ocean. It is not the only case; at least four other garbage islands are known to exist at the confluence of macro-ocean currents. And to counter it, among others, the Dutchman Boyan Slat leads its collection with his Ocean CleanUp project (oceancleanup.com); companies that collect plastic waste from the seas and resort to innovation to generate jobs and, for example, reuse garbage to produce bags, straws, cups and biodegradable tableware from sugarcane bagasse, pineapple[118] or cassava, avocado pits, coffee grounds, with economic benefits, are on the rise. Quite an interesting race to watch. Formula E? Yes, that too. Fast electric car races are gaining fans every day. The funny thing is that most of these inventors are very young people. Although the most closed-minded politicians refuse to accept it, according to Alan Gordon, professor of environmental policy at the University of California and a former deputy treasurer of that state,[119] to stop the economy from emitting carbon and avoid catastrophic effects in the world, 93 billion dollars are needed, less money than the wars in Iraq and Afghanistan cost the people of the United States — who commonly call themselves Americans without realizing that, despite customs that have existed for centuries, we're all Americans from Alaska down to Patagonia. Wherever you live, it is up to all of us to take up the global challenge of rescuing the planet, and it would be unfair to leave the bill to any one nation.

However, the other side of the coin has yet to be resolved.

The main environmental problem of the 21ST century is POVERTY. When you don't know where your next meal will come from, it's hard to think about the environment for the next hundred *years.*

BJØRN LOMBORG

---

[118] https://lifepack.com.co/.

[119] http://www.economiahoy.mx/economia-eAm-mexico/ noticias/8228078/03/17/Se-necesitan-93-billones-de-dolares-para-salvar-al-mundo-del-cambio-climatico-.html.

As you assimilate knowledge, the incomprehensible makes sense and, if you have already accepted that the body — the container — and the being — the occupant — are two different entities, it will be easy for reason to find in the being the probable causes — conscious and unconscious — of our imbalances. They are deep inside, and the worst thing is that the being somatizes them as a scourge that the body almost always ends up paying for. This is why, for example, in response to anxiety we tend to overeat or believe we can assuage it by lighting up a cigarette or, more seriously, by using drugs and drinking alcohol. In any case, we continue to believe that the great loser is the body and we do not realize that, by subtracting time from the existence of the body that welcomes us, the undisputed loser is ourselves. Your "being" is the one which, perhaps before its time, could be decimated or disabled.

We have a tendency to punish ourselves, to self-flagellate when facing difficulties and weaknesses or, worse, in response to our anxieties and passions, we tend to exercise violence against our fellow humans. "Do not do to others what you would not want them to do to you"; and there are those who, with or without a mask, pull the trigger left, right and center, mowing down lives by dogmatically following any idea that, since they were children, other humans have made them believe to be a divine mandate. The naive and ignorant allow themselves to be manipulated without allowing their own spirit to rule and enlighten. They do not realize that, susceptible to misinterpretation, the books produced by the enlightenment and converted into sacred doctrines were also written by men who, without paying attention to reasoning, believed they were in possession of the absolute truth; this question always concerns the imagination and human creativity.

How ironic, suffering for the sake of suffering acquires a level of imbalance, as when we accept to submit ourselves to absurd diets. It is a cultural issue. All this comes from a single place: the mind, where the fears that others make us feel directly or subliminally are hidden in order to manipulate our thinking and, therefore, our actions. These fears are transmitted generationally. It is very difficult for us to accept that we need therapy with a psychologist or psychiatrist, experts in the field of the mind. However, there are other alternative sciences that help to confirm and recognize that our deepest limits are in the mind. Metamedicine and bioenergetic medicine — among others — invite us to explore their discoveries: in a high percentage, the body's illnesses have a specific meaning that relates them directly to the self. Undoubtedly, an important part of the equation "healthy mind in a healthy body" needs to be mentioned:

> The fundamental difference between the person who governs his own life and the one who suffers from it is that the former is in command of his instrument, the brain, while the sufferer follows his orders.

CLAUDIA RAINVILLE

How to proceed with self-healing

Have you ever wondered where that desire to sing, cry, smile or pray under a stream of water comes from? The next time you are taking a shower, think that in this pure act of love the water interacts with your feelings and, reciprocally, blesses you and activates its healing properties to cure you of many ills. Other societies, before the time of Jesus, already performed this communion in a ritual way this connection with the element water.

According to chemistry, water lacks carbon and is considered inorganic. However, it is organic in living things because it acts as a solvent to transport, combine and compose the elements that make up cellular protoplasm: the basic material of life. And since you are more than 75% water, we can start by recognizing that water "feels". The Japanese observer with a doctorate in alternative medicine Masaru Emoto (1943-2014), in his experiments with water, demonstrated that in the face of microwave radiation, strident music and negative emotions such as anger, molecules that were once harmonious appear grotesque and amorphous. Emoto has not been the only one to notice the transcendent power of being, feelings, emotions and thought.

Noesiology studies the effects of thought on human life and activity. Its creator, the Spanish physician and surgeon Angel Escudero Juan, succeeded in developing noesitherapy. *Noesis* in Greek is the action of thinking and therapy means treatment: healing by thought. According to an article on August 4, 2019,[120] the BBC made a three-part documentary with three different cases to show how a surgeon had operated for decades without using chemical anesthesia or antibiotics and without postoperative infections.[121] A unique experience in the world.[122] None of these programs has been broadcasted or recognized in Spain. The success of this Valencian doctor, who recently retired at the age of eighty-six, was such that even the Royal Academy of History requested that his biography in 2004 be included in the Biographical Dictionary of the History of Spain. Dr. Escudero states: "The operations and deliveries with psychological analgesia that I have been practicing for more than forty years, until the

---

[120] https://www.larazon.es/local/comunidad-valenciana/dr-angel-escudero-cuarenta-anos-operando-sin-anestesia-quimica-FE24469297/.

[121] BBC: Your life in their hands (1991). *Noesitherapy:* http://www.bbc.co.uk/dna/h2g2/A27371513.

[122] https://vimeo.com/13416916.

implementation of the natural mechanisms of healing, have their origin in the correct use of the creative power of thought".

Science cannot underestimate that thought, emotional charge and feelings affect in such a way that they are capable of transforming the DNA in living organisms. Not only that, far from recognizing that water lives and feels, Dr. Masaru Emoto concluded: "Water is the universal medium of information transmission". It is logical to suppose that, in order to be able to communicate information between living things, at least some portions of DNA, the codes that store information, must swim freely in water. This is when we must give space to quantum physics; there is much to investigate, and no one could boast of possessing the absolute truth.

It is estimated that about 1.5% of the human genome corresponds to protein-coding DNA — the genes. It was assumed that about 90% was useless and was called junk DNA. Biopolymer DNA constitutes the 3 % capable of capturing, storing, modifying, and transmitting information. Most of it, 87% of the total, is an energetic tangle that it is up to biophysics to solve. We already know that light in DNA or electrical impulses, luminous or not, are the way to spread information. For the rest, we are left with that undecipherable quantum something, which is normal, because therein lies the secret of life.

We are light, spirit and matter that come together so that we can exist. But sometimes, although we do not understand it, we forget that in this constant struggle between good and evil, positive, and negative, healthy, and unhealthy, we belong to that something that creates, transforms, or destroys at the same time to balance everything.

As a preamble to the topic to be discussed, the writer Caroline Myss states in one of her books:

Cure is not the same as healing.

The healing process is passive, that is, the patient is inclined to surrender his or her authority to the physician and the prescribed treatment rather than actively challenging the disease and regaining health. Healing, on the other hand, is an active, internal process that involves investigating attitudes, memories, and beliefs with the desire to free oneself from all negative patterns that prevent full emotional and spiritual recovery.

Is healing the same as self-healing?

We usually take for granted that the term "healing" implies an external intermediation associated with the divine, a power that is specifically granted to "someone" and comes from a "something". It is that powerful spiritual ingredient that enables one to heal, that you can find to heal yourself. Wholeness — as has always been affirmed — is found in the balance between body, mind, and soul; in imbalance, we tend to get sick. It stands to reason that, with a permanent attitude of acquiring knowledge, we are able to lead ourselves in self-healing, an explicit term that associates mind and body. With a knowing attitude, we can find what is necessary to achieve that full state of healing. Let us begin by rescuing common sense.

Of course, you have to acquire knowledge so that you can rely on your own experience. We know that alkalinity leads to recovering the immune system and restoring the DNA. As far as the body is concerned, favoring the alkaline internal environment is the right path to self-healing. Now, as far as the soul is concerned, faith is required not to doubt your reinvention, your acquired knowledge, your re-evaluated principles. Of course, faith is there for you to find or come to you simply and spontaneously. But keep in mind that, regardless of its origin, religious or not, faith without spirituality does not work and spirituality does not require religiosity.

To connect with your spirit, do not be afraid to accept the spiritual path. Motivation is what it is all about and part of it comes from something external, it comes with faith. The other part is drawn from the mind with meditation. Exercise is the easy way and even walking invites meditation. Or if you prefer different disciplines, try yoga, tai chi, *reiki*, Zen, and others — some martial arts, for example — that probe deep, beyond the mind, the inner self. To connect the spirit, both energies are required: they come from faith and meditation. They have the combined purpose of consolidating the spirit that, when you least expect it, empowers you. But right here, because of the fear that subsists in the religious foundations, many are afraid to meditate; they forget the mind and the spirit do not find how to connect. By connecting the outer with the inner, with the precise mix that spirituality provides, the fuel is ignited and what is truly important emerges: the light of truth that invites us to review history. It shines to illuminate the path of awakening.

The constant search for knowledge not only allows us to visualize the goal of healing, which is to reach the right physical and mental state so that the body can heal itself. This search has also always been an infallible remedy to correct fanaticism, the most persistent and dangerous mental deviation used by the ignorant to manipulate the ignorant. History indicates that it has been the perfect fuel to ignite conflicts and wars of all kinds: religious, political, and even sporting. The irony is that fanaticism has always arisen in the midst of peaceful societies which, without knowing why, remain silent. And we believe that a fanatic is a self-absorbed madman who does no apparent harm, and that fanaticism does not affect us; yet millions have died.

> The ultimate tragedy is not the oppression and cruelty by the bad people but the silence over that by the good people.
>
> MARTIN LUTHER KING JR.

When I take the salt bath on weekends, I go inside myself and practice deep abdominal breathing. Also sometimes, in the mornings, I do two exercises, the sun salutation and the *Jin Ji du Li* or golden crane, which consists in keeping the balance alternately on each leg for as long as possible. Both relaxation exercises take no more than ten minutes and train physical and mental balance. And, instead of asking, I thank God.

Even the hopeless find enough reasons — like holding their breath and living — to thank God: the love that connects everything. On the contrary, anchored in supplication, others pray to endure the limits of the sacred and the fear of God does not allow them to act; they prefer not to take the leap into that apparent emptiness that means living the present fully.

What happens and how does gratitude work? Let's imagine a situation of extreme need and, for the practical purpose of understanding — it's easy, because that's how we learned — prohibit yourself from asking. The emptiness is so great that, on the verge of despair, before going mad, the only thing left is to be grateful. And without asking — although quantum physics already offers clues —, things are resolved by your constant gratitude. Try it, because it increases day by day: with faith *in situ*, that emptiness in the soul is filled and, when anxiety and anguish explode, with your spirit burning free of ties you will be strengthened, and you will be able to overcome all your fears.

Then, to follow through with your desire for self-improvement and self-healing, feelings of security and self-esteem will fully emerge that help you achieve the worldly goal of losing weight and body fat.

Even in a vacuum, the *quantum* represents the purest form of energy that connects the energy matrix which is not seen, but that through experiments we can visualize and know it exists. Now, let us remember that we are light and that everything, even matter, functions this way because of some kind of energy.

Perhaps you have heard of the *chakras*. In the human body, the energy that passes, the energy that is concentrated, the energy that is distributed and the **energy that the being creates from his feelings** connect with the whole and cross at least twenty-one times in seven *chakras*, points or centers at different levels or meridians. Bioenergetics says that they are wheels that turn by the flow of energy. Inward to capture, concentrate and distribute it; and outward to emanate it from the being. Depending on whether you are a man or a woman, they turn in opposite directions. Then, from the bioenergetic point of view, the genders are complementary, and the following is confirmed: taking into account that there may be male or female gender identity in a non-corresponding body, neither of the two — male or female — is more than the other, because we could never know what the exact contribution is of each one to the complement.

To connect us with the cosmos — the energetic whole —, the first three *chakras*, located between the anus, the sexual organs, and the lower part of the stomach, handle the energy coming from the Earth — the yin, from below to above — ; and the last three distribute the energy coming from the Sun — the yang, from above to below —.

The first coccygeal *chakra* — between the anus and the sexual organs — is related to survival in general; stress management and the adrenal glands, which are closely related to metabolism. The second is the umbilical, at the level of the sacral vertebra, between the pubis and the navel; the sacral center is related to reproduction and the sexual glands and involves the greatest amount of body energy. The third, the solar center, located below the sternum — in the place where we feel butterflies — operates the *emotions* and desires. At the highest part of the body is the seventh center or crown *chakra*, which also encompasses the brain. The traits of intelligence and the ability to observe are related to the sixth *chakra*, called the third eye; the ability to speak and communicate resides in the fifth *chakra* or neck *chakra*.

In the universe, yin and yang define us and turn us into a tiny dynamo of toroidal energy. Toroids are spherical, doughnut-shaped vortices. As in galaxies, planets or subatomic particles, self-sustaining toroidal energy generates magnetic fields around a center. In us, this personal space extending about three feet around is special. Around the heart is the essential source capable of receiving, **creating,** and emitting infinite energy at the same time. While we are alive, this field is active because it emits the energy that identifies the human being and that, when we die, it releases.

Without jumping to conclusions, what happens during the contact between yin — emotions — in the first three *chakras* and yang — thought — in the last three? This contact manifests around the fourth *chakra*, the heart or cordial center, located in the chest behind the sternum; there is the thymus, a special gland of the adaptive immune system. In the thymus are mixed the unique inclusive ingredients of feeling, which corresponds to saying: "What I feel in the chest I feel in the soul". And the soul would not exist if by nature the breath of life, the potential essence, the animal instinct; by evolution, the intellect; and the spirit by divine gift were missing. The individual, in life, decides the energy and the thought he wishes to emit; the energy capable of changing everything. Still to be mentioned is what the maximum proof of what human identity consists of.

Feelings — the product of emotions and thought — are catharsis equivalent to any point on the spectrum between love and hate. Therefore, the indivisible bond, which consists in the ability we have to turn love into hate and vice versa at will and in an instant, constantly offers the opportunity to resolve everything between us at any time.

The high percentage of studies of women with cancer, who reveal having maintained an unresolved conflict with their parents, are proof that it is not possible to achieve wholeness without first achieving inner peace. By the way, and to dilute this utopia in the equation "healthy mind in a healthy body", surgeon Jorge Iván Carvajal Posada, pioneer of bioenergetic medicine in Latin America and creator of syntergetics with its holistic approach, explains aspects relevant to feelings, disease and bioenergetic medicine:

Interview with Dr. Jorge Carvajal

Surgeon, University of Antioquia,[123] Colombia
Pioneer of bioenergetic medicine

Health and emotions

Which gets sick first, the body or the soul?

The soul cannot get sick because it is what is perfect in you, the soul evolves, learns. In fact, most of the diseases are the opposite: they are the resistance of the emotional and mental body to the soul. When our personality resists the design of the soul is when we get sick.

---

[123] Department of Antioquia in northwestern Colombia.

Are there emotions that are harmful to our health? Which are the ones that are most harmful to us?

Seventy percent of human illnesses come from the emotional field of consciousness. Diseases often come from unprocessed, unexpressed, repressed emotions. Fear, which is the absence of love, is the great disease, the common denominator of most of the diseases we have today. When fear is frozen it affects the kidney, the adrenal glands, the bones, the vital energy, and can turn into panic.

Do we act tough and neglect our health?

Cemeteries are full of heroes. You have to take care of yourself. You have your limits, don't go beyond them. You have to recognize what your limits are and overcome them because, if you don't recognize them, you will destroy your body.

How does anger affect us?

Anger is holy, it is sacred, it is a positive emotion because it leads you to self-assertion, to the search for your territory, to defend what is yours, what is right. But when anger becomes irritability, aggressiveness, resentment, hatred, it turns against you and affects the liver, digestion, the immune system.

Does joy, on the contrary, help us to be healthy?

Joy is the most beautiful of emotions because it is the emotion of innocence, of the heart, and it is the most healing of all because it is not contrary to any other. A little bit of sadness with joy writes poems. Joy with fear leads us to contextualize fear and not to give it so much importance.

Does joy soften mood?

Yes, joy softens all the other emotions because it allows us to process them from innocence. Joy puts the rest of the emotions in contact with the heart and gives them an ascending sense. It channels them into the world of the mind.

What about sadness?

Sadness is a feeling that can lead to depression when you get wrapped up in it and do not express it, but it can also help you. Sadness leads you to get in touch with yourself and restore inner control. All negative emotions have their own positive aspect, we make them negative when we repress them.

Is it better to accept those emotions that we consider negative as part of oneself?

As part of transforming them, that is, when they are accepted, they flow and no longer stagnate and can be transmuted. We have to channel them so that they reach from the heart to the head. So difficult! Yes, it is very difficult. Really the basic emotions are love and fear — which is the absence of love —, so everything that exists is love by excess or defect. Constructive or destructive. Because there is also love that clings, love that overprotects, toxic, destructive love.

How do we prevent disease?

We are creators, so I think the best way is to create health. And if we create health, we will neither have to prevent disease nor attack it because we will be health.

And if disease occurs?

Well, we will have to accept it because we are human. Krishnamurti also got sick with pancreatic cancer, and he was not someone who led a disordered life. Many spiritually valuable people have fallen ill. We must explain this for those who believe that to get sick is to fail. Failure and success are two teachers, but nothing more. And when you are the learner, you have to accept and incorporate the lesson of illness into your life. More and more people suffer from anxiety. Anxiety is a feeling of emptiness that sometimes becomes a pit in the stomach, a feeling of breathlessness. It is an existential emptiness that arises when we look outside instead of looking inside. It arises when we look for external events, when we look for crutches, external supports, when we do not have the solidity of the inner search. If we do not accept loneliness and do not become our own company, we will experience that emptiness and we will try to fill it with things and possessions. But since it cannot be filled with things, the emptiness increases each time.

And what can we do to free ourselves from that anguish?

Distress cannot be overcome by eating chocolate or eating more calories or looking outside for a prince charming. Distress is overcome when you go inside yourself, accept yourself as you are and reconcile with yourself. Distress comes from the fact that we are not what we want to be, but neither what we are, so we are in the "should be" and we are neither one nor the other.

Stress is another of the evils of our time. Stress comes from competitiveness, that I want to be perfect, I want to be better, that I want to submit a grade that is not mine, that I want to imitate. And you can only really compete when you decide to be your own competition, that is, when you want to be unique, original, authentic, not a photocopy of anyone else.

Destructive stress damages the immune system. But good stress is a wonder because it allows you to be alert and awake in crises and to be able to use them as an opportunity to emerge to a new level of consciousness.

What would you recommend to us to feel better about ourselves?

Solitude. To be with oneself every day is wonderful. To be twenty minutes with oneself is the beginning of meditation; it is to build a bridge to true health; it is to access the inner altar, the inner being.

My recommendation is that people set their alarm clock twenty minutes earlier so as not to take time away from their occupations. If you dedicate those first minutes of the morning, when you are fresh and rested, to meditate, not the time you have to spare, that pause will recharge you because, it is in the pause that the potential of the soul dwells.

What is happiness for you?

It is the essence of life. It is the very meaning of life, we incarnate to be happy, not for anything else. But happiness is not pleasure, it is integrity. When all the senses are consecrated to being, we can be happy. We are happy when we believe in ourselves, when we trust in ourselves, when we entrust ourselves transpersonally at a level that transcends the little self or the little ego. We are happy when we have a sense that goes beyond everyday life, when we do not postpone life, when we do not displace ourselves, when we are at peace and safe with life and with our consciousness.

Living in the present.

Is it important to live in the present, but how can we achieve it?

We let go of the past and we do not mortgage our lives to future expectations when we focus on being and not on having. I tell myself that happiness has to do with realization, and this has to do with the capacity to live in reality. And to live in reality is to leave the world of confusion.

Are we that confused, in your opinion?

We have three enormous delusions that confuse us. First, we believe that we are a body and not a soul when the body is the instrument of life and ends with death. Second, we believe that the meaning of life is pleasure; but more pleasure does not mean more happiness, but more dependence. Pleasure and happiness are not the same thing. It is necessary to consecrate pleasure to life and not life to pleasure. The third delusion is power; we believe we have the infinite power to live.

And what do we really need to live - love?

Love, so brought, so carried and so slandered, is a renewing force.

Love is magnificent because it creates cohesion. In love everything is alive, like a river that renews itself. In love one can always renew oneself because it orders everything. In love there is no usurpation, no displacement, no fear, no resentment, because when you order yourself because you live love, each thing occupies its place, and then harmony is restored. Now, from the human perspective, we assimilate it with weakness, but love is not weak. It weakens us when we understand that someone we love does not love us.

There is great confusion in our culture. We believe that we suffer because of love, that our catastrophes are because of love. But it is not because of love, it is because of infatuation, which is a variety of attachment. What we usually call love is a drug. Just as we depend on cocaine, marijuana, or morphine, we also depend on infatuation. It is a crutch to lean on instead of carrying someone in my heart to set them free and set me free. True love has a fundamental essence which is freedom, and it always leads to freedom. But sometimes we feel tied to a love. If love leads to dependence, it is *eros*. *Eros* is a match and, when you light it, it burns quickly, in two minutes you burn your finger. There are many loves that are like that, pure spark. Although that spark can serve to light the log of true love. When the wood is lit, it produces fire. That is the impersonal love, which produces light and heat.

Can you give us some advice on how to achieve true love?

Only the truth. Trust the truth; you don't have to be like the princess of another's dreams, you don't have to be more or less than what you are. You have one sacred right, which is the right to be wrong; you have another, which is the right to forgive, because error is your master. Love yourself, be sincere and consider yourself. If you do not love yourself, you will not find anyone who can love you. Love produces love. If you love yourself, you will find love. If you don't, it will be empty. But never look for a crumb; that is unworthy of you. The key then is to love yourself. And your neighbor as yourself. If you do not love yourself, you do not love God or your child because you are becoming attached, you are conditioning the other. Accept yourself as you are; what we do not accept we cannot transform, and life is a permanent current of transformation.

Blue Consciousness Newsletter, March 10, 2009

After this brief passage through the mind that confirms that fear is the origin of many of our ills, the transcendental thing is that, understood as the absence of love and a common denominator between people and society, fear is the great disease; it is also true that we can change this truth.

To culminate the topic of why people get sick, I thought it pertinent to use the following article by Mike Geary to address fear in a practical way with information and undo another false belief that links illness to weather changes.

Top seven tips to stop you from getting sick

First of all, many people still fall into the huge mistake of thinking that the cold can make them sick. This is false. In fact, there are studies that show that exposure to cold increases immunity; cold therapies, ice water baths or some other type of cold exposure stimulates or enhances the immune system.

Why do more people get sick in the winter? I'll give you a hint: in winter, in the northern hemisphere — Canada, the United States, Europe — diseases skyrocket, but, at the same time, it is summer in the southern hemisphere — South America, Australia, New Zealand — : while diseases strike in the northern hemisphere they are at their lowest in the southern hemisphere. And vice versa.

So, in warm temperatures does the disease decrease? Really this is all about the strength of the sun's UVB rays[124]

---

[124] In general, UVB rays are strongest between 10 a.m. and 3 p.m. to activate vitamin D production. But this depends on the time of year, latitude, and altitude. For example, in New York, although you can produce vitamin D between 9 a.m. and 4 p.m. in June or July, that period — when UVB rays are strong enough-might be reduced from 11 a.m. to 1 p.m. by late September, and according to charts of the sun's height in the sky, by late

and how much vitamin D the body produces due to UVB contact with the skin.

There are two theories as to why more colds, flu and illness occur in the winter.

Theory 1. This may be due to the fact that people spend more time indoors in the winter and are thus exposed to more germs in closed buildings.

Theory 2. People get sicker in the winter because of the drastic reduction in the production of vitamin D, which is responsible for how strong their immune system is.

In the winter, above and below the tropics, the sun's rays are weak, therefore, vitamin D levels in the body drop significantly, which reduces immunity. This vitamin D deficiency triggers a hormonal imbalance. Although many viruses and bacteria reproduce and the environment is conducive in the summer, this lack of vitamin D production and decreased immune strength in the winter months is the real reason why people get sicker in the winter.

So how can you boost your immune system so your body can fight off disease?

1. Focus on vitamin D — but NOT in synthetic forms, pills or "fortified" foods.

Unless medical tests show a catastrophic vitamin D deficiency — in which case and you should immediately see a doctor —, ordered vitamin D3 treatment, for which I advise consuming foods with sufficient vitamin K2 such as *natto* — fermented soybeans — and animal fats such as egg yolk, goose liver, certain cheeses, butter and lard from free-range grazing animals, which are the best **sources** of **K2**, necessary to prevent calcification

---

October in New York you cannot produce vitamin D even at midday, as the sun is too low and UVB rays are too weak.

of soft tissues in the body; although D2 exists naturally in mushrooms and fungi, a small daily dose of cod liver oil ensures that in the winter months vitamin D levels do not drop too low. Cod liver oil is the best natural vitamin D option if you're not getting enough sun. Take cod liver oil only in small doses, half of what the bottle recommends, as it can produce an overdose of vitamin A. The synthetic version of vitamin D is ergocalciferol — vitamin D2 —, while the natural form is cholecalciferol — vitamin D3 —. By the way, pasteurized milk "fortified with vitamin D" usually has synthetic vitamin D2 of vegetable origin added to it, and **NOT** natural vitamin D3 of animal origin, so it is **NOT** a good source.

Garlic strengthens your immune system!

Garlic is one of the most potent superfoods in several forms: garlic powder in fresh foods, minced garlic in meals or in capsules one or two per day.

3. Kombucha tea strengthens your immune system.

The health of your immune system depends on the protection of those microorganisms that reside in your gut flora against disease-causing pathogens. *Kombucha* is a fermented tea — naturally effervescent — that contains billions of probiotic organisms — bacteria and yeasts — that help strengthen the immune system by boosting levels of good organisms in the gut. A good source of probiotics is kefir, a fermented — cultured — milk drink that has been used for thousands of years as a health elixir in many parts of the world. But keep in mind that when it comes to probiotics, the variety of sources offers greater benefits and drinking *kombucha* and kefir or eating foods such as *sauerkraut* — not canned —, yogurt, *kimchi* and other fermented foods is great for your immune and digestive system.

4. Green tea, chamomile tea and other teas

Both are loaded with powerful antioxidants unique to each tea. For that reason, with a couple of cups of green tea with a little raw honey early in the day and in the evening or chamomile or peppermint tea or other teas such as *rooibos* tea, which contains more antioxidants than green tea, you can strengthen your immune system.

5. Antioxidants

We already know the importance of antioxidants. For this reason, be sure to consume antioxidant-rich fruits, berries — blackberries, strawberries, etc. — teas, red wine, organic unsweetened cocoa — in smoothies, etc. — and vegetables to help prevent disease. Sometimes, you can quickly boost the immune system with a "smoothie" of antioxidant-rich berries, some greens, raw cacao, maca, spirulina, chia seeds and any other superfoods like *açaí* or pomegranate that you have on hand.

6. Gentle exercise — yes, low intensity exercise —.

An intense workout is not a good idea when you think a disease is coming, because a hard workout requires a lot of strength and recovery, and the body needs all its strength to fight the disease. This is why gentle exercise is better.

7. Avoid all processed foods, foods with wheat and artificially sweetened beverages.

Except on cheat days to increase leptin levels, if you are committed to your health and want to stay lean and healthy, it should be the rule every day. Processed foods, soybean oils, corn oil, etc., with inflammatory omega 6, fried foods, high fructose corn syrup, refined sugars and chemical additives bombard your body and are the worst choice for when illness strikes. All of this forces the body to work extra hard to get rid of this junk and the inflammation it causes. By the way, grain-based foods — such as bread, cereals, *muffins*, pasta, and *bagels* — cause internal inflammation and disrupt normal bowel function. Avoid grains as much as possible, as recommended by Paleolithic nutrition; humans did not need grains to survive, and they were not part of the ancient human diet until agriculture arrived about ten thousand years ago. At the time of approaching illness, you should give your body only healthy, unprocessed, single-ingredient foods: fruits, berries, vegetables, eggs, nuts, seeds, grass-fed meats, etc.

These seven tips will get you on the right track and help ward off that disease that is trying to enter your system.

Source: adapted from *The Top 7 Tips to Stop Getting Sick,*[125] by Mike Geary, author of the books *The Truth About the Six Pack Abs*; *The Fat Burning Kitchen*; *The Top 101 Foods That Fight Aging.*

---

[125] https://www.truthaboutabs.com/prevent-sickness-increase-immunity.html.

Chapter VII

The Genetic Factor

DNA repair and more

The decoding of the human genome has made it possible to find in the memory chain — of which DNA is a tiny part — the visible genes that constitute the genetic factor transmissible by consanguinity. With this discovery, we can now verify the total percentages of the ethnicities (éthnos in Greek means 'people') included in our genealogical ancestry.

Regarding the origin or lineage perpetuated by inheritance, recent studies and findings have concluded that after the interbreeding of humanoid species — Neanderthals, Denisovans and another to be determined, probably *Homo erectus* — with *Homo sapiens*, in a range from 12,000 to about 126,000 years ago, no pure-blooded humans can have survived in our prevalent species. Another study in 2019[126] states categorically that "all modern humans have been genetically related to each other for at least 300 000 years". With migrations, due to different climates and the incidence of the sun's rays in the places of settlement,

---

[126] Mayukh Mondal, Jaume Bertranpetit & Oscar Lao (2019): "*Approximate Bayesian computation with deep learning supports a third archaic introgression in Asia and Oceania*". *Nature Communications, 246.* https://www.nature.com/articles/s41467-018-08089-7.

evolution took care of shaping the eyes and discoloring the skin in various groups of humans, which because of their cultural, linguistic, and physical affinities we have erroneously typified as distinct races. All current genetic studies[127] have led science to prove that the human race is one; the once dark-skinned race — around Lake Victoria in Africa — gave rise to our species and intellect: *Homo sapiens*. Those with white skin are thought to be more intelligent. And I wonder: what could be expected from children who are constantly physically and morally mistreated, beaten, neglected, sullied, minimized, humiliated? I am sure — and even more so when they surprise us — that none of this has anything to do with their intelligence, but it does have to do with that of the abuser. As it turns out, this abuse is identical to what has happened to every "race" considered inferior by some other at different times, sometimes for centuries. But there is NO scientific reason to justify racism.

The National Geographic Genographic project led by geneticist, researcher and anthropologist Spencer Wells, in association with IBM and the Waitt Family Foundation, which began in April 2005, has been fully demonstrating the above and it is time for history to show how certain things happened: for example, NASA's achievement in putting the first man on the Moon was, in part, thanks to the help of a small group of black women experts in mathematics and physics that the agency dubbed "the human computers". Among them were Dorothy Johnson Vaughan, Mary Winston Jackson and space scientist Katherine Coleman Goble Johnson, leader of the group, in

---

[127] Extracted from Wikipedia.org: After analyzing the DNA of people from all regions of the world, geneticist Spencer Wells argues that all humans living today are descended from a single individual who lived in Africa some 60,000 years ago. From the above, the monogenism of the human species is demonstrated and, consequently, polygenism, which served as an "argument" for racist theories, is discarded.

charge of reporting to the directors of the National Advisory Committee for Aeronautics (NACA), the agency at the time. This story told in the book *Hidden figures: the American dream and the untold story of the black women mathematicians who helped win the space race*, by Margot Lee Shetterly, was brought to the big screen in 2017 in the film *Hidden figures* by Allison Schroeder and Theodore Melfi and directed by Melfi.

Back to DNA, the previous drafts that allowed science to decode the human genome have provided the opportunity to establish which are the diseases that "haunt" us. The bad thing is that we believe that they will be able to harm us at some point and we just hope that it will not happen soon without even thinking about what this discovery means: we can act in time.

Let's move to the future, here is the scenario: you went to your medical check-up appointment and, as part of the protocol, you were given a questionnaire about you and your family's history: has there been anyone with hypertension, diabetes, obesity, overweight, deaths due to heart attack, cancer or any other disease that can be linked to the hereditary factor?

Imagine that your grandchildren, great-grandchildren, or great-great-grandchildren are in the same situation. Just like you, they try to remember and ask their wife or sister or their mothers — who are your daughters or granddaughters — : "Mom, my grandfather — you — was Antonio; my great-grandfather suffered from hypertension, didn't you have that, Mom? It sounds dangerous! Is it true that Nana Betty died of a heart attack, and my other grandma died of cancer? At what age did they die? Did they suffer from heart disease or diabetes? Were they obese? The questions are endless. You may no longer be around, but your offspring, proudly, could be answering as you are now: NO and NO to questions related to Alzheimer's and other diseases that years ago were considered "rare," but there is nothing rare about them now. Don't get your hopes up too high. With the current landscape, unfortunately, many of your answers will still be yes. And they, of course, will continue to answer impertinent questions about ancestors they may have known: "Excuse me, sir, I don't quite understand your handwriting: does it say breast cancer here and does it say colon cancer here as well, did your paternal great-grandfather die of prostate cancer, is that right, Mr. Perez?" "Did I understand correctly, Mr. Johnson?" "Yes, Miss, you did! Forgive me for not writing it clearly". To reflect on the above, we must again appeal to common sense.

The hereditary factor can be repaired, it can be modified. In other words, that gene — the genetic reason — can be frozen before the problem or disease is diagnosed. In short, you could change everything starting with your existence if for the rest of your life you dedicate yourself to avoiding, reversing, or curing the problem or disease. For better or worse, you can affect your genes and make that disease trait that comes from your genealogical past — present in your DNA — remain frozen, or it may even fade over time.

Yes, it is possible that it is in your genes, that you have already acquired or were born with the disease, or — worse — that you are creating it. It is a fact that, with time and education, the risk factor could diminish in the generations to come. Genetics is important, but it is largely not the determining factor in the occurrence of certain diseases. If you have noticed, you are the one who usually decides to activate or freeze the gene that facilitates the emergence of the disease and not to remain immobile, subjected to the error of thinking that other diseases will appear with age because heredity dictates it. Living also means having the attitude to change habits and beliefs; this aspect would be equivalent to transcending.

Well, say that you are the beginning and the end: "I am the beginning and the end". The phrase that a human being, the most wonderful that ever walked this earth, Jesus, in order for us to understand it, pronounced about two thousand years ago. He also taught us to pray the Lord's Prayer; slowly and thinking about the meaning of each word, its lines possess extraordinary powers that, like mantras, connect with the *chakras* of the body. Jesus was a man of few words, but he managed to concentrate multitudes with short phrases that only he pronounced with a clear, simple, and contemporary language. Without the complexity that others later added to his words, he spoke to men without distinction of gender, age or preferences for any particular ethnicity or culture and addressed the world hoping to be understood someday, as in this case applicable to the genetic factor; a clear example of his practical teaching that we understand with hindsight.

Then there is that special gene that science cannot prove and that goes beyond the skin, as Jesus demonstrated on Calvary for all of us long ago. You have it too. For good, if you decide to **unfreeze** the genetic reason for His being, which in Him ascends and from Him descends, it is Love: God, the antidote to fear, a possible act. And alien to any concept of holiness that surrounds your brain; only you could feel it and verify that no scientific proof would be necessary, since it will be evident: it is Jesus who lives in you; the power and the light for you to achieve what you propose on the path of the good that will be born in your heart.

Educating the mind without educating the heart is no education at all.

ARISTOTLE

A bit of history

Human development has been made possible by the intellectual activity of a few hundred geniuses, and we have all contributed to it. But what would humanity achieve if we break the paradigm of fear and ignorance in which we live? In addition to the daily passage in the first lane, we have the three realities that drive in three different lanes which are identified by fear and ignorance, knowledge, and love. However, if we learn to navigate all three at the same time, love and the spiritual reality will transcend the others; the relentless pursuit of knowledge in the second lane will combat the fear and ignorance of the first: the perfect framing, which already sets us back into our ability to discern and reason. But our behavior as a society still leaves much food for thought.

After ancient history, the little we inherited from cultured Greece and further back — what we were able to rescue —, since the rise of the Roman Empire in 27 B.C., two apparently isolated events — the First Council of Nicaea in 325 A.D. in present-day Turkey and the successive plundering until the total destruction in 642 A.D. of the library of Alexandria, in Egypt — ended up plunging humanity into obscurantism: the Middle Ages. The people, generally ignorant and illiterate, without access to knowledge, protected by priests, scribes and nobles in convents and castles, immersed in religious fundamentalism, remained at the mercy of ecclesiastical power and feudal lords for well over a thousand years. History — consistent with the evolution of societies and the evolution of thought, science, and new discoveries — shows that this has resulted in xenophobia, male chauvinism, contempt for women, modern slavery, and racism, among so many other social ills. Fear and ignorance are evident in the fact that, right in the 21st century, a large part of society still conceives the stale idea of building walls to divide regions as the only way to control interference — positive or negative — between peoples.

Jesus is the lantern of the lighthouse of time. Not in vain did ancient history reach him and the new history began to be counted from the time of his birth. From the FIRST century in yesterday's history, in the three centuries following his death, testimonies began to appear — not only from apostles — about the good news of his life, his work and his word: the Gospels, which, before becoming manuscripts, were inevitably affected by the daily life and feelings of the authors.

By the FOURTH century, Rome, with its empire in shambles, was already experiencing a serious social, political, and economic crisis due to divisionism and border wars: the emperor Constantine I, the Great, noticed the growth of its Christian population, which did not follow the Sun god, one of the many gods that the empire allowed to be worshipped, other than Christ. Constantine — from a merely political point of view — solved the problem with skill: instead of continuing with the persecution and sacrifices, through the signature in 313 of the Edict of Milan, he promulgated freedom of religion and tolerance of Christianity: the empire stopped persecuting them and gained followers. The doctrine tells the rest, starting from the account of Eusebius of Caesarea, who influenced Christian historians to attribute Constantine's victory over Emperor Maxentius at the Battle of the Milvian Bridge in 312 to divine intervention, because he supposedly saw a cross in the sky with the legend "by this sign you will conquer" which awakened his tendency to Christianity, and later, on the advice of Bishop Hosius of Cordoba — one of many tormented Christians — who ordered and presided over the convocation of the first council of Nicaea — the present-day city of Iznik in Turkey — in 325 A.D..

The news spread and the pseudo-Christians compiled 270 documents — the basis of their doctrines — to be presented to the council and approved in the synod, which, among bishops, priests, and Constantine himself, had about three hundred participants. The accounts of early Christianity chosen to shape the New Testament and the Bible established the sacred for the majority of Christianity. And Catholicism — which absorbed some currents and rejected others — emerged as the new catholic and apostolic religion. The council condemned as heretical the doctrine of Arius, presbyter, and priest of Alexandria, because he denied the consubstantiality of the Father with the Son, the divinity of Jesus. Although many of his sympathizers tried to defend him, Arius, who escaped capital punishment, was exiled, and took refuge in Palestine, a vast geographical region corresponding to the united provinces of Judea and Galilee that the Roman emperor Hadrian renamed Syria Palestine in 135 A.D. It must be said that the product of that strangulation of destiny, the orthodoxy — strictly in line with the apostolic testimony — created at that time religious heresy in Christianity and any proposal or belief contrary to any established dogma would be paid with death; imposing by terror, the fear already well permeated in ignorance. And, in favor of what is known as the Holy Trinity, the Nicene Creed was written: a dogmatic social contract that until recently was celebrated three or more times a day and that, according to most Christian confessions of the present, must be endorsed at least once a week, preferably on Sunday.

It should be noted that the FOURTH century marked a very important turning point in history. Among the 270 manuscripts collected — thirty or more of them Gospels — there were fanciful documents, of improper content or style, extemporaneous and discordant with the apostolic account and others attributed to the apostles, but which failed to prove their authenticity, loose copies, and confiscated books, branded heretical, which evaded the pyre; the Council called a large majority apocryphal. In Latin, *apocryphos* ('to hide away') derives from the Greek verb *apokrypto*, 'to hide', 'to set apart'. And, of course, with the chosen testaments — forty-six for the Old and twenty-seven for the New — the Holy Bible was made official at the Council of the African Mediterranean port of Hippo in 393, at the end of the FOURTH century.

Reading and collating 270 documents takes time. However, there are those who affirm that after much prayer, by divine intervention, the books that fell off the table were discarded. What we know is that after a month, between May 20 and June 19, 325, when the doors of the Council were opened, the Gospels of Matthew, Mark, Luke, and John were left on the table, not exempt of contradictions — the Nativity in Matthew happens two years before Herod's death and in Luke after nine —. From the intellectual and literary point of view, these discrepancies invite us to read and investigate — without the blindness that produces the fear for the sacred — in the sources of the time that the bias of history "hid far away" and it is already possible to consult the books and apocryphal fragments[128] unearthed or rediscovered in the 20TH CENTURY.

Of more or less complicated reading — according to historians and theologians —, in the first centuries, the Gospels of Thomas and Philip were the most sought after and read, not so those of somewhat childish reading that were chosen for the New Testament almost three hundred years later. To read the apocryphal Gospels — as was feared — did not mean an attack against the faith. On the contrary, in the first centuries, without

---

[128] http://enigmasdelmundo.com/2012/01/descargar-en-pdf-evangelios-apocrifos.html.

the accusation of falsehood, they were highly esteemed and today they are being spread because the complete perspective was needed to broaden the mind and to be able to elaborate one's own judgment of what happened yesterday. And this is the story today:

In April 2006, after many studies and analyses that dated its antiquity to the end of the 3RD century, the National Geographic Society, from its headquarters in Washington, D.C., convened a live international conference on the Internet to announce the discovery of the Gospel of Judas. As expected, it did not have the desired repercussion. What is relevant is that in this codex found in a cave on the banks of the Nile in the seventies, Judas Iscariot acquires a different dimension than it has had until today, because it is Jesus who, after expressing that the time has come to leave the body in which he lives, asks his disciple and best friend — besides John — Judas Iscariot, to hand him over to the authorities[129]. He could not carry so much weight. Recall that a Roman emperor was who ordered the Council, and it is worth saying that for Christian doctrine, during the distancing of its Jewish origins that had been occurring since the FIRST century, the representation of a treacherous Judas was a convenient stereotype and, in the four Gospels, for example, the figure of the Roman procurator Pontius Pilate is contested and opposed to the condemnation of the Jewish people — represented in Judas and the high priests of the temple — for the death of Jesus. Then, was it really Judas as he is painted in the works of art, the

---

[129] There is no hiding the fact that most modern bibles have been using the word betray instead of deliver, which by concept and subject to interpretation could coincide, but they do not mean the same thing. And the parallel study bible English/ Greek analysis shows 'deliver" instead of "betray": https://biblehub.com/interlinear/apostolic/matthew/26.htm https://www.bibliacatolica.com.br/en/la-biblia-de-jerusalen-vs-new-jeru-salem-bible/mateo/26/

avaricious Jew who sold Jesus for a few measly coins? I think the time has come to say that issuing a conviction based on apparent circumstances and without hearing the accused makes the anti-Semitic idea an unfair and null judgment. Not in vain, in order to defend themselves from their own history with outsiders, the Hebrew people — enslaved and persecuted so many times — early on assimilated that "having" is power. And by force and over time, they had to learn to separate their feelings from the monetary aspect stipulated in the contracts.

I can't hide the fact that talking about apostles left me wondering how likely it is that at an official banquet — for the photo — on one side sit your wife and children, if you have them, and on the other your best friends. Mary Magdalene — a woman out of the ordinary for her time — might or might not be the same Mary of Bethany. Little is said about her in the sacred texts, but in the apocryphal Gospels attributed to Mary [¿?] and Mary Magdalene, *roughly speaking*, we read the following: "However, if the Savior made her — has judged her — worthy, who are you to reject — despise — her? It is certain that the Savior — He, seeing her — knows her perfectly; that is why He loved her — He has loved her, no doubt — more than us". Today is the feast day of Saint Mary Magdalene. And there is a reason why Francis — the Pope — elevated her liturgical memorial to the rank of a feast, which was already celebrated on July 22. What we were led to believe about her comes from Letter 33 of Pope St. Gregory the Great — from the VI century, in the year 591 —, in which he presupposes: "She, whom Luke calls the sinful woman, whom John calls Mary [of Bethany], we believe to be Mary, from whom seven demons were expelled — according to Mark — ".

It has been easy for male chauvinism to cast doubt or defame in order to misinform. For example, it is recorded in the Bible, the concept of Mary as a virgin influenced the worldly notion of virginity to gain strength and persisted for millennia the fixed idea that a woman was an object to be used only once, an inferior being to serve and please men. Not to mention what happened three centuries after the consolidation of the biblical texts, when male precepts about women became edicts in the Koran, the Muslim holy book. And machismo — which had been dictating the way they dress, look, express themselves and behave — has gone even further and, even today, the role of women is almost nil in "legal discussions" — with a male majority — on issues such as abortion, contraceptives, or the use of certain vaccines. Machismo, feminism, sexism, racism, fundamentalism, nationalism, hedonism; the "-isms", all of them extreme tendencies that deny, marginalize, or invalidate contrary positions, entail hatred and there is no moral position that justifies them; it is hypocritical, and I would not like to be one of those who throw the first stone, but the worst thing is that it happens.

The effect of this is that fifty-three countries still have laws on the age of marriage for girls one to three years lower than that of boys at sixteen. This tradition persists and violates the rights of girls: families who force them to marry older men see their virginity as a commodity that is a repository of family honor to be traded. "And they do not understand that because they are neither physically nor mentally prepared for a sad and loveless commitment, these babies have to accept a reality that is equivalent to slavery for the rest of their days", as explained and denounced by the non-governmental organization PLAN INTERNATIONAL, which, since its foundation in Spain in 1937, with presence in seventy countries, watches over their protection and aspires to eradicate the horrifying and cruel practice of female genital mutilation: more than sexist, ablation is a huge aberration by ignorant parents who allow it and make it customary.

Let's resume. With the Bible established, the different interpretations of religious fundamentalism eventually caused the schisms of the Christian and Jewish faiths and were a source of inspiration for another exuberant doctrine to emerge more than six centuries after the year 0. In response to the patterns of social behavior among the descendants of Abraham in the Arabian Peninsula, the Muslim religion, which upon the death of Imam Hussein, Muhammad's grandson, in 680, also split into Sunni and Shiite; buoyant in fervor, all of them were widening mental chasms. The dogmatic discrepancy that has caused war and enmity among peoples has marked an aimless course of darkness in the human mind quite evident in those who have based hatred as a synonym of love, so as to impose their religious beliefs through terror. And not only in them, because when exposing and defending the human and the divine, our existence, creation and God, swarm those who, with meager interpretations, say they do not harm anyone. No wonder this is another late sign — like inhumanity — that history is once again beginning to repeat itself. For example, democracy, the gift of Greece, was completely lost with the passing of the republic; that is exactly where we are: despising it and sponsoring dictators who dismantle it in order to perpetuate themselves. In the timeline of history, changes usually take place in moments. A new circumvallation of empires has already begun with the present weapons, if the planet holds out, the regression could be back to the Stone Age for the survivors of the mankind.

At the beginning of the Christian era, there were three hundred million inhabitants. In the face of the theocracy and persecution that persisted in the known world until Constantine, with the debacle of the empire and the barbarism that resurfaced at the end of the FIFTH century and deepened the darkness in what was once the Roman Empire and beyond, a great majority accepted the dogmas of religious fundamentalism and found refuge in Jesus, their redeemer. But what else had been happening in parallel — since the consolidation of the Bible three centuries before and three centuries after — that caused us to fall to such a low point in the culture of fear and ignorance and caused us to remain in the backwardness of such darkness? What else happened to make this the whole that caused civilization to regress?

The destruction of the library of Alexandria sealed a process in which — without books at its disposal — the world went backwards in its ideas, and many do not remember or do not know that with it we lost the knowledge pertaining to the other real half of human history that corresponds to some five thousand or more years, much more than twice the time elapsed in our era. In the SECOND CENTURY, according to Aulus Gelius, jurist and writer, the largest library in the world — founded by Alexander the Great in 331 B.C. — already contained 700,000 documents: what remained to be read of classical Greek literature and details of Atlantis; from Egypt, the complete work of Manetho (*The Truth of Thoth*) with the *secrets* of the link between the gods from the stars and the Pharaonic legacy of 11,000 years;[130] the Sumerian clay tablet accounts and the mystery of their relationship with the *Anunnaki*,[131] not to mention the trigonometry, algebra and geometry texts that enabled the Arabian architectural splendor and the illustrated books on medicine, alchemy, astronomy and navigation, not to mention their Greek-inspired philosophy, poetry and literature; all of which apparently went there. Of the Babylonian priest Berossus it is said that he compiled *The History of the World* from its creation to the universal deluge. As far as India and the Himalayas are concerned, we might even have elucidated the mysteries surrounding the eighteen

---

[130] https://es.wikipedia.org/wiki/Canon_Real_de_Tur%C3%ADn.
[131] https://es.wikipedia.org/wiki/Anunnaki.

unknown years of Jesus' life. With the onslaught of war, most of these testimonies disappeared and the damage caused by the earthquake that struck Alexandria on July 21, 365 is not ruled out; let us not forget that the mega-events that for thousands and millions of years have changed the Earth — the movement of the tectonic plates was discovered only in 1967, along with the changes of magnetic polarity and glaciations or the impact of meteorites — have been erasing the physical evidence of the real myths of history.

How deep did we fall? Museums jealously guard fragments, documents, and relics as they appear. For example, the National Archaeological Museum of Athens preserves the Antikythera mechanism rescued from the Aegean Sea at the beginning of the 20TH CENTURY. It is an analog computer that scholars place in Greece in the SECOND century B.C., built to predict astronomical positions and is supposed to have other uses but, more than being an instrument with small gears, it is one of many precision pieces manufactured by the Greeks in metal, and it turns out that this exquisite metallurgy — of small pinions with infinite uses like that of the Antikythera mechanism — simply disappeared and was only seen again with the domestic pendulum clock in the 17TH century. With the passing of the centuries, mankind lost track of things and doubted what it already knew. For example, the criteria for refuting the Inquisition, which arose in France in 1184 and was only dissolved in Spain in 1834, vanished. Not even the fresh ideas of Renaissance humanism in the 15TH CENTURY could prevent the **serious aftermath** of obscurantism from following us to the present day. Therefore, that anyone who dared to challenge its borders would only face a hellish abyss[132]

---

[132] https://www.forbes.com/sites/jimdobson/2019/03/16/flat-earth-supporters-now-plan-an-antarctica-expedition-to-the-edge-of-the-world/?sh=d40136659165

is a myth that persists today in the 21ST century. In the SECOND century B.C., the Greek Eratosthenes had already calculated — with a margin of error of 10% — the circumference of the Earth, and the sphericality of the planets was a standard topic in Mediterranean schools. Now, can you explain why eighteen centuries later, in 1633, Galileo Galilei, in the hands of the Inquisition, had to recant and deny the Earth's orbit around the Sun, in order to save himself from the stake? It went unnoticed that, 350 years after his death, on October 31, 1992, Pope John Paul II asked for his forgiveness at his tomb. This fact shows that, although it is human to impose with cruelty divine ideas created by men, it is also human to know how to ask for forgiveness and to forgive.

The Library of Alexandria housed books that ambitious leaders had to obtain or destroy. Julius Caesar is blamed for the first destruction of the Library of Alexandria in the FIRST century BC. But history agrees that in the year 47 B.C., due to the conflict between Cleopatra and her brother Ptolemy for the throne, a fire broke out and spread to the place where the "royal books" were kept, some 40,000 that the Roman general would have liked to move to Rome: he who has the knowledge has the power. Later, in 297 A.D., Diocletian ordered the burning of the texts of the Hermetic Sciences (such as alchemy) in order to avoid monetary instability in the Empire. But from the 4TH century onwards, with religious fundamentalism, other reasons motivated the aggression. In 391, Coptic Christians razed the Serapeum library in Alexandria to eradicate from history the classical paganism inspired by Plato; and in 415 or 416, a mob of monks incited by Cyril burned the collection of the Neoplatonic scientist and master philosopher Hypatia of Alexandria, who was murdered. Then came the damage caused by the Persians in the 7TH CENTURY in their attempt to conquer Egypt; and, finally, in 642 the Arab-Muslims who professed the Islamic faith destroyed it completely. The note that the caliph Omar sent back to his commander — a learned man who hesitated and preferred to ask questions — read as follows: "If these books agree with the Koran, we have no need of them, and if they oppose the Koran, they must be destroyed". In short: "There is no need for any books but The Book". In the 21ST century, this phrase, without its needing to be uttered, ironically represents those who ground themselves on the sacred books of other religions — the Bible and the Torah — and many like them, immersed in "the book", would be unlikely to read a different text that could provide them with knowledge.

History sometimes hurts. I apologize if you think your faith is being threaten by my words of explanation, which, perhaps, you did not know. But history also makes us wake up because it points out the paths to avoid; those we have traveled and those that lead to the same apocalyptic destinies which our ancestors described and experienced several times. With history I intend to show that humanity is in its adolescence, the precise age at which we begin to know; to know and to learn. In pursuit of maturity and mental development, we have to overcome it to free ourselves from our possible or imminent extinction as a rational species. Because history shows that, when it comes to barbarism, fear takes hold of everyone; knowledge, research laboratories and science are the most vulnerable to any egocentric individual with a craving for total power, for whom it is enough to surround himself with walls, to close borders and pander to militias while eliminating freedoms; his figure grows as a demigod, as did the emperors of old.

Learning about history and recognizing that, perhaps, had it not been for that mental lapse of over a thousand years, our brain capacity would have increased considerably; this situates us and grounds us so that we can get out of the backwardness in which humanity remains. Regarding human development, our pride is based on contemplating the technological advances achieved since the invention of the printing press in 1440. But we do not realize that, alluding to a period of spiritual evolution — which was not so much due to a lack humility or out of simple comfort — we call the period of darkness "Medieval" to justify not yet having been able to overcome the after-effects that prevent us from visualizing what we could be and what we barely are.

According to press reports, for example, from the *Washington Post* of March 21, 2018, which reads, "Some educational institutions plan to withdraw, among other subjects, the chair of history." Will this aggression perhaps be another very bad, non-violent sign of the effects of barbarism? You be the judge.

Those who cannot remember the past are condemned to repeat it.

JORGE AGUSTÍN NICOLÁS RUIZ DE SANTAYANA Y BORRÁS (1863-1952)

But to return to the main topic: when are your next check-up appointment and lab tests scheduled for? Soon, I guess!

GMO, transgenic, and genetically modified organisms

Mother Earth has provided us with all the natural resources we require to subsist; therefore, it may be assumed that agricultural activity did not require money until its appearance in coin, paper or in kind, as the dynamic, practical, and convenient way to trade. Doing without money — as some people propose — is not the real solution to our problem, which, as Aristotle rightly said, lies in the insatiable greed of human beings.

Spontaneous mutation corresponds to the natural selection of species and is the result of thousands or millions of years of evolution. Since Neolithic times, man has been crossing animals of the same species and has adapted plants by grafting to domesticate them, according to his needs or simply for the sake of taste. For more than five thousand years, we have been using forced hybridization methods, but only recently have we been able to **affect** genes to modify organisms. From that moment on, we created genetically modified organisms; this artificial method of selecting species has unleashed great controversy. For example, the first thing we did — out of egocentrism or stupidity — was to play with genes and inoculate people with vaccines that gave them unnatural advantages over the diseases we were trying to eradicate.

We are all in the same experiment. In our own era, more than fifteen hundred Guatemalans were inoculated between 1946 and 1948 with syphilis and gonorrhea "vaccines" to study the ability of penicillin to prevent sexually transmitted infections. In Kenya, women were defiled with UN vaccines which sterilized them, a practice that the Catholic Church denounced in 2014. In March 2019, Dr. Marc Lipsitch — professor of epidemiology at Harvard University — gave an interview to *BBC Mundo*, in which, on behalf of a group of scientists, he warned that were the objective of infecting ferrets with avian flu to be achieved, they could transmit it to another animal, and any human carelessness could unleash another pandemic; this may be what happened with COVID-19 in China. The precedents are set for humanity to be attentive, so that when this happens and it becomes known, if there are any Mengeles[133] of this era, they may be denounced with actual facts and not escape but be severely punished. In the thoughtlessness of those who rule and govern us in these experiments, it is not unreasonable to be dubious about the vaccines they offer for free at each change of season. Without proof, conspiracy theories are nothing more than speculation. But it is suspected that — by means of transgenic foods or by inoculation with vaccines — with these modifications they are very slowly manipulating our DNA in order to control the world's population in the future. Vaccines have been an effective weapon against serious diseases, such as measles, polio and rubella and we should not fear mass inoculation to eradicate lethal viruses with high mortality. However, since the appearance of GMOs in vaccines that contain toxic preservatives, such as mercury, aluminum, propylene glycol, monosodium glutamate (MSG) and formaldehyde — another mutagenic transgressor — complaints and criticisms have increased.

Many people die every year because of the flu; the most vulnerable are old people and sickly, malnourished children, but the rest of the population does not fall into these categories and does not need them. Influenza occurs when it wins the game over a weak immune system and it is nothing more than the consequence of not knowing how to nourish the body, clean its filters and not being clear about what intoxicates and weakens it. Before vaccines, the combination of drinking water, good hygiene, and the habit of washing our hands frequently worked well. A diet that guarantees proteins, essential nutrients, probiotics, and antioxidants shields the immune system in the battle against diseases; except when a pandemic has already been declared and

---

[133] Josef Mengele was a Nazi who conducted genetic experiments on Jewish prisoners in concentration camps and managed to evade human justice: https://es.wikipedia.org/wiki/Josef_Mengele.

the strategy to encircle the virus and control it consists only in the scientific recommendations that we must follow. Thus, without rushing, while we observe the progress of vaccines that do not give extra advantages to viruses, fortifying the body would contribute to reducing mortality from contagious diseases.

Something similar to what happened with vaccines seems to have happened when scientists sought to achieve pre-established objectives in genetically modified seeds. For example, in modified corn seeds, in order for the crop to resist a particular pesticide, the same seed that kills a specific pest always has to be resorted to. While reproducing the plant naturally, they cross genes from other corn varieties with genes from bacteria and animals. This scientific success is, in fact, an artificial advance in evolution that can have unpredictable consequences.

As far as is known, if the organism of the transferred gene and the host share similar metabolisms — the same metabolic pathway — the resulting protein in the GMO we ingest could not affect our organism. But when genes from host organisms are introduced into different species, and especially if a mutagenic effect is intended, the unexpected could be chaotic. With an experiment started in 2007, a Frenchman, Professor Gilles-Eric Séralini, exposed this in the journal *Food & Chemical Toxicology* in September 2012. The published notes of Dr. Séralini and his team, along with photos of rats that developed tumors after being fed with transgenic corn, went round the world as it contradicted the findings of a company that produces and sells seeds and agrochemicals. This study was based on scientific information that Monsanto made available to the European Food Safety Authority (EFSA) to approve three of its GM corn seeds.

Séralini concluded: "The available data reveal hepatorenal toxicity, possibly due to the new pesticides designed for each transgenic corn, and directly or indirectly provoked metabolic consequences are observed, for which genetic modification cannot be excluded". He exposes the possibility that, by consuming foods with rare modifications such as GMOs in the molecules of some vegetables, the Bio-Logic body does not recognize them; consequently, the metabolism assumes them to be foreign elements or free radicals that acidify the interstitial environment of the cells that, to defend themselves, before dying, can mutate and produce cancer. Before the publication of the article in 2012, which the journal later retracted — it became known in 2017, that the retraction was orchestrated by Monsanto — Séralini and his team were already the target of written and verbal attacks. The professor was accused of fraud. Séralini filed two lawsuits: one for libel and the other for defamation against those who accused him of fraud. With the community on edge and his credibility in tatters, the world did not hear about the judgments in the criminal court in Paris. Both in the first case, on January 18, 2011, and in the second, on November 6, 2015, the court found in favor of Séralini. In the first trial it emerged that among the people accusing him — who claimed to be neutral scientists — at least one owned GMO patents in an Israeli company that sold them to large corporations, such as Aventis. Séralini's lawyer also demonstrated links between agribusiness companies and members of the AFBV (French Plant Biotechnology Association) that undermined impartiality. After the trial, Pete Riley of the British organization GM Freeze commented: "The freedom of independent scientists is a vital element of any society. And in the other, the magazine that accused him of fraud was fined twice for repeated libel and the first accuser was shown to be a professional slanderer."

No less worrying is the human crisis triggered by the greed and lack of ethics of GMOs: peasants and farmers, owners of small plots of land around the world, unable to recover their own seed from the harvest and on the verge of bankruptcy, have had to sell their land to pay their debts; some have committed suicide. States convinced of the benefits of GMOs that favor large estates have sided with the industry that sells seeds that work with the same brand of agrochemicals. The company stipulates and dominates prices, this is called a monopoly. Since the comparable costs of producing natural seeds make them unviable, the peasants who persevere and do not yet swell the forced exodus to the cities are forced to buy GMO seeds on the market.

Fortunately, in the struggle for the natural, there are those who obtain their own seedlings or, failing that, share the cutting technique to safeguard native varieties. Catalan farmer and activist Josep Pàmies, promoter of the Slow Food culture, explains in his blog how to do this and recounts the vicissitudes, the siege, and the prohibition he has experienced since he started growing stevia. The genetic contamination caused by GMOs concerns us all, because artificial varieties exterminate natural varieties and unbalance — in favor of monocultures — the ecosystem; and they decimate or eliminate the specific food supply for the animal kingdom, causing the disappearance of species of fauna. They are an attack on biodiversity: bees, vital to the ecosystem, are disappearing. The Netflix series *Our Planet* explains the chilling magnitude of this problem. Farmers affected by genetic contamination who have gone ahead with their crops are then sued for making use of the patent and have had to pay millions.

By 2019, twenty-nine countries allow the cultivation of fourteen GM crops.[134] The list is getting bigger and bigger, in 2016 there were twenty-six. Genetic manipulation has gotten out of hand; there are already allegations of illegal genetic manipulation. The number of products using GMO-derived

---

[134] https://www.isaaa.org/blog/entry/default.asp?BlogDate=1/27/2021.

ingredients in the food industry is staggering. Hence, we have a right to know what the food is hiding. The "NON-GMO" seal does not yet offer full guarantees. The bidding is uneven. Proof of this is the historic Proposition 37, which failed in the November 2012 presidential election, in California, which meant that this state would require specific labeling for food products with genetically modified organisms (GMOs). On October 24, 2012, www.democracynow.org published:

We discuss California's Proposition 37 to label genetically modified foods.

On Presidential Election Day, California voters will also decide whether to accept the so-called Proposition 37, through which their state would be the first in the country to require specific labeling for food products containing genetically modified organisms (GMOs). Under the proposition, the California Department of Public Health would be responsible for labeling everything from baby formula and instant coffee to granola, packaged soups, and soy milk. Many large companies, such as Monsanto, Dow Chemical, Pepsi, and Coca-Cola are spending millions of dollars to prevent passage of this measure, which could have an impact on food labeling rules in the country.

Of course, there are economic interests! They say they are indispensable for the economy to progress. Without objecting to the stock market and free enterprise, it is inevitable to question those behind the "proposed objectives". Incidentally, since 2018, Monsanto belongs to the giant Bayer, which sells aspirin and pharmaceuticals. Even if the brand identity is lost, the problem is not in turning a scientific solution into a lucrative business; it is in that, when the collective interests are gigantic, responsibility is diluted, it becomes intangible and there is no one to complain to or who will answer for what happens. Monopolies are the dynamic part of the mechanism used by mega-companies to own everything. With the pricing of their products, they dominate everything, and the consequences go beyond the environment and ecosystems. With bribes, they achieve their goal of evading regulations or covering up negligence in order to exploit natural and human resources, regardless of whether they are blood diamonds or whether they paint the North Pole black. It is unhealthy for the economy when rivers of money feed a single stream and, when the springs dry up, unbeatable greed, directly or indirectly, transforms free enterprise into a dark and vampiric capitalism that encourages monopolies to generate or sponsor modern slavery.

In a recent interview, the Spanish journalist and writer Juan Luis Cebrián, the soul of the newspaper *El País*, said: "We have to defend capitalism from itself because otherwise it will finish us all off". And regarding what is happening, especially in Latin America — the social violence —, without hesitation, he also said that "not all change is good, sometimes it is for the worse". In business, investments can be of high, medium, and low risk. In the stock market, the universe is immense. Qualitative and technical analysis, based on quarter-to-quarter growth and trading volumes, respectively, depending on whether the market momentum is *bullish* or *bearish*, defines whether bonds or shares of a listed company are a good investment to buy and make a good return, or to buy and sell to make a profit. Although it is about winning, the losses are usually huge, and worse, in seconds. The stock market performance of mega-companies with very low risk is boring because they have already grown enough; their price is too stable and high to satisfy the thirst of the minority investor who wants to see the value of his shares grow vertiginously in a short period of time.

Investing in the stock market is the complete opposite of what, in essence, banks do. In the stock market, you are the one who lends money — yours — to companies or governments. In return, you receive a tiny part in shares of the proportion resulting from dividing their estimated value or in bonds issued by state entities; these papers are quoted, bought, and sold on the stock market. There are three rules that every investor must know: 1. That the money he uses is not needed for daily living. 2. Do not sell at a loss: if you have made a correct analysis, with patience and discipline, you should be alert to the signals that confirm the trend; it is likely that the value will rise again, even exceeding the purchase price. 3. Do not fall in love with any *stock*: "buy on the rumor and sell on the news".

Many are not interested in the subject of GMOs, but every day there are more and more of us who — as with the radiation emitted by cellular devices and microwaves — try to take precautions in this uncertain experiment in which we are involved. Food without genetic manipulation — rightfully so — is an exclusive gift from Mother Earth. Now, if you want to feel responsible for what happens and you are cautious, evaluate better to whom you lend your money. I am firmly convinced of the need to support companies with ecological sense in the emerging market; with your grain of sand and mine, by buying NON-GMO native varieties, we will be avoiding this attack against the ecosystem, human health, biodiversity, and food security.

Regarding this tinkering with plant and animal genes, in a 2019 issue of MIT's *Technology Review*, James Sikela, a geneticist at the University of Colorado, commenting on experiments in China which modify monkeys with human DNA to make them intelligent, warns, "The use of transgenic monkeys to study human genes related to brain evolution is a very risky path. I am concerned that the experiment will show disregard for animals and will soon lead to more extreme modifications."

Chapter VIII

Weight Loss

If you open the book on this page, I suggest that you read it from the beginning, including the introduction, so that you assimilate information and the whole educational process. Having put into practice what you read allows us to find the truth about losing weight and abdominal fat together.

A person has just woken up hungry, passing through the kitchen, he puts a slice of buttered white bread, a waffle with syrup — one of those boxed ones that come ready to pop in the toaster — a doughnut or a cruller in his stomach until breakfast is ready, and without even asking the body, he chooses the wrong solid to start the day off right. This is waking up in the first lane: you've always done it. But in the second, when you have a bite of something in front of you, you wonder, "What am I putting in my mouth?". And later under the shower, "What will I be absorbing into my skin?"; at that very moment, the enlightenment begins that raises more and more questions, and one by one, the answers trigger a series of events that mean *awakening!*

Breakfast is the culmination of the metabolic process of the previous day. Your best option is to quench your thirst first with warm lemon water, without sugar, with tea or an aromatic herbal tea; a coffee, with or without milk, is not the best option at that moment. And fruit so that its pulp can finish cleansing the intestines and alkalinize the body; instead, your unconscious choice acidifies you. After twenty minutes, you proceed to eat your breakfast. Well, it's your choice. You were not born to die.

The acid routine seems more like a suicide that we will achieve between the ages of forty and seventy or, at the most, at eighty. During this period, acid saturation occurs as an orderly process of logical deterioration until some vital organ fails and we die. Regardless of their age, many people "naturally" become overweight, and hypertension develops. They survive but with the diseases produced by excess sugar, such as sclerosis, diabetes, and cancer; or with the internal inflammation that causes cholesterol to clog arteries and produce a heart attack or stroke; in any case, they anticipate budgeting a sum of money greater than that which they have had to spend on the medicines that have long sustained their lives... At any rate, in the end, memory loss, Parkinson's, Alzheimer's, all of these or sudden death await them.

Taking the option to live does not mean that you will not get sick of something and die, but it does mean that you can do it without depending on medicines — just with health check-ups — to be able to reach the age of eighty, or more, with full faculties. According to gerontologists, it is at that age that old age begins, but not necessarily decrepitude. If you want to live, this decision is an excellent introduction to this healthy way of life, which I hope you have assimilated and enjoy reading. Although we may not understand the complicated processes of the mind, among them, believing contains an immeasurable placebo component: faith that moves mountains. And far superior to the alternative that natural and conventional medicine can offer — prevention and healing — ; only the body possesses the ability to heal itself.

Even though you have made progress in your reading, it is likely that you are still avoiding healthy foods and that the wrong foods still persist in your daily intake. There are two explanations for the persistence of the wrong foods; the first appears in the book *Beat Sugar Addiction Now!* written by the renowned American physician Jacob E. Teitelbaum, a graduate of the class of 1977 of Ohio University, and health and alternative medicine journalist Chrystle Fiedler in 2010. Teitelbaum comments, "Eating too much sugar is an addiction: eating sugar early on gives you a *high*, a peak high, from which you will soon fall off, crash within a few hours, and this will leave you craving and craving sugar even more. If you crave sugar so much, telling you to give it up is like telling an addict to stop using or injecting drugs." I mentioned it in Chapter V: sugar is a fast-absorbing carbohydrate closely linked to other refined carbohydrates, such as flours and starches. Because of this addiction, we all — even diabetics and prediabetics, who should not eat sugar — continue to look for that hidden sugar in refined flours. Dr. Mark Hyman, of Cornell University, New York, a proponent of Functional Medicine, hints at the other major problem:

Chips, cookies, ice cream, soda and soft drinks can be as addictive as any other drug. Sugar stimulates the brain's pleasure or reward centers in the same way as addictive drugs. Foods rich in refined carbohydrates also activate the body's internal opioids, which are biochemicals similar to morphine. Just like with alcohol or heroin, you're going to build up a tolerance to processed foods loaded with refined carbohydrates, which means you'll need more and more to be satisfied. Eventually, you have to eat a lot of carbs not just to feel better, but to feel normal.

In any case, regardless of the physical form of living beings and what that body ingests, regardless of the consequences, the metabolism adapts and subsists until it achieves its reproductive capacity. Therefore, the truth about losing weight and abdominal fat rests on the sources available to produce vital energy. What is relevant is that this decision is not made by the body; it comes from the "being", who establishes the paths to follow: the alkaline which has antioxidants and is anti-inflammatory, i.e., the healthy route; or the acidic, oxidizing, and inflammatory route that creates diseases. Unfortunately, the majority adopted the latter in the 20TH CENTURY and became a quasi-relieved, sick humanity.

I will try to guide you to a new life in two weeks. Based on my experience, I will describe sensations and frustrations, because just like you I faced the mirror with my doubts and weaknesses. I will reveal some tricks and especially a recipe that I devised and used to fulfill my purpose. Sporadically, some articles from professionals in the field will reinforce the concepts. The BMR and BMI (basal metabolic rate and body mass index) calculators, which define personal parameters by age, physical activity, height, gender, and current weight, which you can search on the internet, are just a reference point to start this process; do not take them with absolutism, because everything is energy in motion and there is nothing exact or precise, as quantum physics assures us. Reading and rereading the fundamentals and keeping them close will make you believe in yourself; you have an enormous potential in your favor: your accumulated fat and your volume are the source of energy that you are going to use to turn you into a new being.

The **fuel to burn** comes from the foods we choose, and it is certainly a conscious choice that we must make wisely. Mike Geary addressed this topic in the article *How do you know if you're a carb-burner or a fat-burner*, which I have adapted below:

How to tell if you are a carbohydrate burner or a fat burner

For carbohydrate burners their broken-down metabolism robs them of energy and forces them to eat constantly, dulls their mind and generally makes them crave refined carbohydrates like sugar and flours that make them sick and old.

The big problem is that the dictocracy in the last century promoted a diet rich in carbohydrates, up to 60%. From a statement by the Dietary Guidelines Advisory Committee in the United States, which suggested increasing carbohydrate intake by 30 % and decreasing fat intake by 25 % of total calorie intake, a "misunderstanding" arose: the masses listened to wrong advice and destroyed their metabolism. Then everyone who eats a modern diet may be a carbohydrate burner. If they skip breakfast, they crash; if they don't treat themselves to a snack, they get *hangry* (hungry and angry) and even growl; if they don't eat carbs every two hours, their thinking gets sluggish and, come evening, with no strength left, the energy they have left is barely enough to drag themselves home from work.

A carbohydrate burner can only count on a very limited source of energy: 1600 calories in the muscles — glycogen — ; four hundred calories in the liver — glycogen — and a hundred more in the blood — glucose —. Unless you are exercising intensely — something unfeasible and unlikely in the overweight — that energy is deposited as fat in — or around — the muscles, is off-limits and leaves only five hundred calories — four hundred in liver and one hundred in blood — available for the normal activity of the day. Soon enough, you are forced to refuel and eat, guess what, more carbohydrates, more sugar, and more refined flours. No wonder you get so hungry and cranky — so quickly — after devouring a muffin, a piece of buttered white bread, a chocolate roll, some cookies, or your favorite muffin, like that "healthy" wheat bran bagel in North America.

Fortunately, there is a simple solution. The strategy I suggested in the chapter on flours and the ingenious "cheat day" technique, which I detail in this chapter, make it true: "The body is a machine created to burn fat, not store it." This fat-burning adaptation will cause you to use your own fat as an energy source and allow you to develop a supermetabolism that harnesses the energy stored in body fat. From now on, you will be able to go through the day with unlimited stable energy, a well-focused mind, and a sense of humor. This metabolic adaptation allows you to turn first to warm liquids and fruits very early in the morning and — if it is unavoidable — to skip breakfast without craving for white bread, omelets or those pancakes filled with fictitious honey. In return, for snack or lunch, it will allow you to eat those "forbidden" snacks, but loaded with healthy fats, that you already knew when we studied the omega.

So, instead of sitting there inertly sitting on all that untapped energy, you can tap into that reservoir of energy conveniently parked in your belly, hips, thighs, arms, and glutes. Not only that, if you force your body to burn it, that stored fat will provide you with the stable energy conducive to good hormonal balance; in the carbohydrate burner, very unstable energy causes your hormones to go haywire. How is that possible? Potentially speaking, the average person has about 135,000 calories — energy — stored as body fat; that is, 270 times more fat-energy than is available in the five hundred calories of carbo-stored energy.

Fat burners know exactly how they feel when they have adapted to fat and will NEVER give up this change. After a deep, restorative sleep, they wake up refreshed; if they don't want to, they don't need breakfast; at lunch, they gorge themselves on delicious foods rich in healthy fats and, come afternoon, their mind is sharp and stable energy prevents the crashes and crashes sponsored by a carbohydrate-based metabolism. At night, they have no energy crashes, and their mood remains phenomenal. Frequent doctor visits, medications and surgeries are a thing of the past. The best part is that stubborn fat, which they thought would never go away, is gone. In fact, their problem now is resizing their rings and watches and buying new clothes! Another interesting thing is that your monthly grocery bill is reduced by 30—40% or more. So, to enjoy your new fat-burning metabolism, get fat-adapted and stop being a carb-burner.

But it is not about prohibiting. On the contrary, it is about valuing carbohydrates and enjoying them, but not for addiction; take advantage of them at the right time, you can be aware that, without starving, you can lose weight without exercising. It may not be your case, but in fact for many people going to the gym implies a great sacrifice and many even hate it. The reason has been another sophism: "exercise burns fat". But that momentary weight loss is due to sweating. Liquid has weight and, after training, depending on what you eat, the body burns fat. For example, pair proteins — meat, chicken or fish, a boiled egg or tofu — with fibrous vegetables such as broccoli and NOT pasta, potatoes, or rice — flour, starch, or cereal. A study with children and broccoli presented by the BBC in London showed that the taste for the food can change in eleven days: although at the beginning many refused to eat it, on day twelve, the children took the broccoli naturally and ate it with pleasure, without complaining or claiming the reward.

Now for the obvious: it's a fact that you've already eaten huge amounts of everything that hurts you: refined carbohydrates that have been making you sick and aging you. I hope you are no longer one of the people who believe that diet sodas are good for weight loss or claim to eat very healthy and only drink diet soda. It is proven that diet soda is more fattening than regular soda: "Artificial sweeteners containing empty calories create a negative hormonal response that increases the production of fat-storing hormones and creates cravings for more sweets and refined carbohydrates, such as white bread, for example. People believe that by drinking diet sodas — very harmful, by the way — they have more freedom of action, and, at the end of the day, they end up consuming many more calories compared to the regular soda that those who do not care about their health love. Better resort to water with lemon or unsweetened iced tea."[135]

Let's go back to what was left out of the third chapter, the fundamental principle, step three of the elixir that restores health and postpones aging: "It consists of accelerating the metabolism so that the body works at the right speed, burns fat for energy and evacuates waste naturally at least once, twice, or even three times a day. In today's jargon, it means "resetting it": from the outset, these changes will help you to reduce the internal inflammation that causes disease, especially cardiovascular disease, which increases the risk of sudden death.

Let's start by distancing and mixing — as appropriate — the food groups using medium-sized plates and glasses and distributing the food in five or six daily intakes that include fruit and doing what we like: eating all day long. In direct communication with the body and without starving, this change serves to identify early on why some foods don't let us lose weight; at first, I noticed that sodas bloated me and over time I eliminated them completely, and that others — like yogurt with nuts the previous afternoon — were a drag when I weighed myself the

---

[135] https://truthaboutabs.blogspot.com/2014/02/are-you-carb-burner-or-fat-burner-how.html.

next day. But that same yogurt in the middle of the morning helped me eliminate ounces.

Why five or six meals? By eating more frequently, the hormone ghrelin, which makes us feel hungry in the stomach and hungry in the brain, is kept in check. However, in response to general stress, the body produces the hormone cortisol which, among other effects, is linked to flabby muscles and skin: the more cortisol produced, the more fat can lodge in flabby places, such as the belly. A study published by *The New England Journal of Medicine* showed that people who ate five smaller meals than usual, spaced every three hours during the day — 7:00, 10:00, 13:00, 16:00 and 19:00 hours — reduced their cortisol level by 17% compared to those who ate the same distributed in three meals. The study was able to verify that this habit resolved the cortisol dulling in fourteen days. This change allows you to regain control of cortisol. In addition to burning fat, the skin and muscles recover their tempering and support capacity because, in the cells, the proteins collagen and elastin, the antioxidants beta-carotene and vitamin A, and zinc — in pork, beef and crustaceans, brown rice and dark chocolate — work on it. The collagen in vitamin C-rich citrus fruits, such as orange, lemon and grapefruit, and the elastin in the fats of nuts, salmon, avocado and olive oil are ideal for restoring and regaining muscle tone and skin health; most of these foods are fats to include in daily consumption.

Food groups

Protein

Legumes, peas, chickpeas, fava beans, beans, lentils, soybeans, and derivatives
Processed dairy products, such as cheese, yogurt, and butter
Eggs
Tofu
Any kind of fish, crustaceans, mollusks, shellfish
Any type of meat
Meat products, broths, and sausages

Neutral

All vegetables except leguminous plants, and nuts
Walnuts, almonds, hazelnuts, sesame seeds
Olive oil
Seed oil
Flaxseed and chia
Quinoa
Salt
Herbs and spices
Flourless sprouted grain bread
Whole grains
Stevia

Amylaceous

All refined and unrefined rapidly absorbed carbohydrates
Starches and starch derivatives
Cereals and grains:
Wheat
Oats
Papa
Corn
Rice
Rye
Barley
Cassava and sweet potato
Flour
Pasta
White bread
Sugar

Foods in this group

They combine well with foods of the neutral group.
They do not combine well with each other
They should not be combined with those of the starch group.

Foods in this group

Combine well with those of the protein group
Combine with each other
They can be combined with starchy foods.

Source: own elaboration

Foods in this group

May be combined with foods of the neutral group
Can be combined with each other
They should not be combined with those of the protein group.

I have left milk and fruit out of this table because, for trophology, whole cow's milk is a protein food that does not combine with anything, and fruit should be consumed on an empty stomach. As we have already said, trophology should not be taken as a law because we would suffer as with senseless diets. The recommendations of the trophological approach obey scientific considerations and highlight the neutral group as the most important, because by consuming the neutral group and fruit we obtain the ideal arsenal of vitamins, minerals, antioxidants, healthy fats, fiber, and water that accelerates the metabolism to the point of resetting it.

I don't know why but talking about greens — especially with men — is not easy. In my younger years, I didn't eat salads — how awful! An occasional piece of fruit maybe, but greens tasted awful to me. From those trays adorned with lettuce leaves and tomato slices — which for me were only decoration — I liked the combination of hams, sausages, mortadella, salami, pepperoni — stuffed — with cheeses, breads, and crackers. The ham that brushed the lettuce I didn't even turn to look at it because it was contaminated with lettuce. But for health reasons I had to do it. What did I have to do to make me like vegetables and salads? I went back to the books and, among them, one that a friend gave us when we invited her home with her husband and children. With no experience with pots, knives, and pans, like any man who thinks he is a cook, I made them spaghetti to dazzle them. After this first experience, now in private and feeling confident, I started preparing dressings that would make my salads passable. I had a sweet tooth and found that, by mixing a tablespoon of water with pineapple and finely chopped strawberries — no citrus —, a pinch of stevia, salt and cinnamon heated over medium heat in a pan for a few minutes, without drying out, an easy-to-make salad dressing that I had to learn to eat was formed. Something important happened that I understood later: I put in the time.

Soon after, I concluded that to fight addiction, whatever it is, the best thing to do is not to have temptation at hand: I took a trash bag and in it I threw chips, French fries, cookies, pastries, candies, canned fruits, dry flavored broths, dehydrated soups, cereals, white bread, jams; in general, everything processed that comes in boxes, bags, cans, or jars: carbohydrates loaded with toxic preservatives, sugar, salt or questionable oils. Only plums, raisins — without added sugar — ; cocoa, 70% or more dark chocolate and no milk; homemade preserves and a few state-of-the-art canned goods, without toppings containing toxic bisphenols such as BPA, remained. From the fridge, I removed frozen pizzas, packaged juices, sodas, ice cream, mayonnaise, premade dressings. That left butter from cows that walk and graze, mustard, and a low-salt, low-sugar tomato sauce. Don't fool yourself: take them out of your home; it's no use keeping them under lock and key. But didn't this all cost me money? It is worth remembering that when you make these changes of habit you save money and can afford to buy quality: the relevant organic produce, a good wine and, if you eat meat, better quality; and all this on a smaller budget than you needed before.

Then I remembered the two cruets that some restaurants put next to the plate of rabbit food, which got in my way, and I immediately removed from the table: extra virgin olive oil and balsamic vinegar. In my cupboard, I installed the disguises that make you like vegetables and salads. The appropriate ones, according to nutritionists, are edible olive, pistachio, macadamia oils; sesame, chia, or flax seeds; quinoa, Himalayan, or unrefined sea salt; dates, cranberries, walnuts, prunes, and raisins; natural mixed herbs — without monosodium glutamate — and balsamic vinegar — without preservatives or additives —. When we ask ourselves "What are we eating today?", we almost always answer: "I've already defrosted the meat" or "Don't worry, I'll pick up a roast chicken on the way home" — not fried —. Rarely do we say, "What do you want me to add to the salad? Don't forget to bring the avocados! Today's dressing has olive oil, walnuts and a few drops of balsamic."

Who hasn't been offered celery and carrot sticks with hummus, blue cheese, or ranch dressing on a tray at a gathering? They don't taste so bad; however, in the end, all that's left on the tray is green. Another tricky issue I also had to overcome. Steamed vegetables don't taste good because their essential nutrients, minerals and flavor-giving salts are diluted and lost when overcooked. Ideally, they should be washed and eaten crisp. For hygiene, blanch cauliflower and broccoli in a bowl of boiling water, which instantly kills any germs.

To break the curse that hangs over the net carnivore who only accompanies meat with pale colors: rice, yucca, corn, and potato, I remember a trick I used. It is not very orthodox with fat consumption, but it works wonders as long as you manage to change your sense of taste: sauté vegetables in the fat — the flavor — left in the pan after roasting meat; peppers, carrots, scallions, zucchini, miniature tomatoes, asparagus, celery, olives and mushrooms — on medium-low heat —, sprinkled with garlic powder, wheat flour and soy sauce. Include the diced cooked potato left over from the roast in the sauté. After a couple of minutes, pour a splash of white wine, stir, and remove from the heat so that the vegetables do not continue cooking. The alcohol evaporates and results in a slightly thick juice with the wine, which leaves a special seasoning. To make it look well-presented and provocative, sprinkle it with toasted sesame seeds. They are the other ideal companion for the protein and to give you a break from salads. Since then, I've been learning to cook and what I like the most: I prepare my own food.

It seemed that everything was going well, but I needed to solve something more complex: I had to do something that would guarantee me at least four times a day to eat bright colored foods, including fruit, vegetables, and greens, to give the alkaline balance that the body requires. A situation led me to something that I then took advantage of to create a versatile dish, easy to prepare, with different versions, so as not to become boring and with the colors of the complete *vegetable* rainbow: *cherry* tomatoes, carrots, red, yellow, or green peppers, celery, radishes, olives, and eggplant, for example. It is a sandwich as a main meal. In my personal environment and to my friends I have taught them to prepare my favorite recipe. This creation I called:

The Hippocratic sandwich

Sometimes, in fast food restaurants, diners put aside the top of the hamburger or sandwich bun and ask to replace it with an extra slice of tomato, onion, and lettuce. For health reasons, this is a favorable choice, known as an *open sandwich*.

Years ago, I had breakfast with my family at the Hyatt hotel in Key West. From the menu — and for pursuing omega-3 fat and fluoride in V-tailed fish — a "rare" pesto salmon sandwich caught my eye. My surprise was an open-faced sandwich of carpaccio — thin cuts — of fresh salmon, marinated with onions on a green coating that I deduced was basil pesto and, moreover, cold. I'm still scratching my head wondering how the chefs manage to intersperse squares of tomato and melon on top of that salmon that I craved when I saw it at the next table. Wow, what did I order! Embarked and half bored, I thought I would have preferred scrambled eggs, hamburger or a regular toasted ham and cheese sandwich, between two pieces of bread, and tons of fries. I might as well keep exploring. When the waiter suggested adding oil and balsamic vinegar, I agreed and, upon tasting it, those "horrible flavors" I had imagined did not appear. On the contrary, it was one of the best breakfasts I have ever had. I tried to recreate it when I got home. I didn't succeed, but the enthusiasm was enough for me to create my own version of an open sandwich perfect for breakfast, lunch, or dinner; versatile, variable and, best of all, with the specific Hippocratic characteristics for you to enjoy at any time, any day: FOOD and MEDICINE.

Start with a really healthy bread that provides, in addition to nutrients, two, three or more grams of fiber per serving. In the United States, the popular Ezequiel brand — a refrigerated whole grain — protein — and sprouted grains bread with a sweet touch of raisins, and NO flours —, is great fresh for this sandwich. Some artisan bakeries have already cloned it. Alone and cold it is not tasty, but if you toast it lightly, it is delicious with any of these sauces that keep well for many days in the fridge.

Salmon or trout sauce (dip)

Pour into the food processor a medium steak cut into chunks; a handful of well-washed uncooked spinach; four tablespoons of cream cheese, kefir or yogurt — with the live bacilli, *live cultures* — ; a drizzle of honey or some stevia if you are diabetic; a clove or two of garlic; a pinch of salt — I prefer Himalayan and you know why —, finally, a tablespoon of olive or sesame oil — whichever you like — ; process, pour into a wide-mouthed glass container and put in the fridge. Garnish with capers.

Basil pesto

Pour into the processor a handful of basil, two or three cloves of garlic, ¼ cup of unroasted pine nuts or macadamia nuts for their natural oil flavor, ½ cup of Parmesan cheese, a pinch of unrefined salt and ¼ cup of olive oil. Process and refrigerate in a glass container. This sauce for spreading on French toast with ham and fresh vegetables can be thinned with more olive oil to dress salads, rice dishes or to make pesto pasta.

Chickpea hummus

Pour into the processor 15 ounces of cooked chickpeas — 1½ cups — ; two tablespoons of *tahini* — sesame or sesame paste —. Add the juice of a lemon, a large clove of garlic, three or four tablespoons of cold-pressed extra virgin olive oil and a pinch of salt. The recipe also contains sweet paprika, parsley and cumin. Process and that's it.

You can also vary it with aioli — garlic —, egg, olive oil and salt, or with cilantro dip; both recipes include a raw egg. In essence, you will be preparing a nutritious mayonnaise with different flavors. Preparing it in advance saves time.

Let's go back to the sandwich. You can put some spinach or lettuce leaves. To ensure iodine, put dried leaves of nori seaweed (sushi seaweed), which easily adheres to the cream on the bread already spread with the dip. In its original packaging, this sea vegetable keeps well in the refrigerator tray.

From the refrigerator, choose vegetables of different colors and separately, on the large cutting board, chop some peppers — green, red, and yellow —, celery, a broccoli head, carrots, two olives — remove excess sodium by squeezing them a little under the running tap —, cilantro or parsley, artichoke if you have one, and a clove of garlic. Add a touch of another dip to give it more flavor and consistency. You can vary the mixture every season to take advantage of mushrooms, white asparagus, Brussels sprouts, peas.

After nightfall, your breakfast should include protein and fat because both satiate and fat ignites the body in the morning. Which one? The one you did NOT consume yesterday and the one you need at that moment to maintain the balance in your weekly fat intake: unsaturated, from salmon or tuna with omega 3; if you need saturated, two strips of bacon or pancetta — previously defatted in the pan —, ham or prosciutto — without nitrites or nitrates —. If your idea of breakfast is still an egg, it looks good on the plate cooked and sliced and it tastes delicious with *gomasio*. Then add onion, one of the natural remedies for infections. (The red ones are spicier.) Next, add thin slices of tomato and basil in small or leafy pieces. So that you don't make a mountain of stuff, when setting the picadillo on this bed, chop and stir with the wide-bladed knife and press the vegetable rainbow well. Garnish with fresh farmer's cheese, curds or whatever you have on hand. Mature goat cheese or aromatics, blue cheese, or Roquefort, go well with a few drops of honey or maple syrup. Then, decorate with chia seeds, flaxseed, quinoa, or another superfood; if you want a delicacy, add the caviar that came in that gift basket you got and, to firm up the cheese, give it a few minutes in the oven.

When plating, do not forget the drizzle of olive oil; to give order and aesthetics to the plate of food. There are hundreds of ideas with design and creativity. A good concept is that different foods should not touch, as it helps to moderate portions and to make food the main topic at the table and not the problems that usually emerge when eating in company. Discussions that turn a gathering into a nightmare lead to indigestion. Chewing your food well is healthy and invites you to take it easy.

If you opt for the sandwich for lunch, you can complement the dish with asparagus, which you previously sautéed in butter and garlic, and cross them over the boiled egg, broken in half. Add acorn ham to the bread, for example, and accompany it with wild brown rice with multicolored grains — organic — and red fruit tea.

In short, the recipe consists of toasting the bread, on which you spread the dip while the egg is cooking, and put nori seaweed, some spinach leaves, kale, or lettuce. On top of the protein, then tomato and onion, basil and gomasio salt, sprinkle the seven colors and cheese with sesame, flaxseed or chia seeds and bake in the oven for a few minutes. When serving, a drizzle of olive oil and, if you like, a few drops of balsamic vinegar: and that's it. Or if you prefer, eat it cold.

This *gourmet* Sunday breakfast or lunch, which became ideal any time, any day, changed my life. I know it involves dedication and time, but it offers endless variety. Given its health benefits, you will optimize the preparation time and include in your almost daily intake the colors you need to alkalize the body and heal.

If you have time, prepare, so it's ready in the fridge, the dip of your choice and use leftovers from the weekend barbecue. Thinly slice leftover chicken, pork, lamb, turkey, or beef to be the protein for the open Hippocratic breakfast sandwich. Start tomorrow.

Fluid intake

The idea that every person needs at least eight glasses of water a day was based on scientific studies which, at the end of the 20TH CENTURY, gave a very particular boost to water bottled in plastic.

And it turns out that it is not so crucial to drink so much water; the finely tuned body warns us in advance of the need to drink liquids, and the fact that we do not feel thirsty and do not drink water does not mean that we are dehydrated. This myth arose in 1945 from a recommendation by the U.S. Food and Nutrition Service (FNS): "People need to drink about 5 pints of water," something like eight ten-ounce glasses a day. In the area of health, nutrition and food, short phrases taken out of context have been used to misinform and create myths. People ignored the sentence that followed: ignored it completely: "Most of this amount is contained in the food we prepare and consume".

The article *Medical Myths*, by Rachel C. Vreeman and Aaron E. Carroll, published by the *British Medical Journal* in 2007, dismantled this myth. These professionals argue that there is no evidence that drinking a lot more water keeps the skin hydrated; nor does it "cure" wrinkles; nor does it make the skin look healthier in healthy people. In conclusion, the volume of water contained in fruits, vegetables, fresh vegetables — 95% — and in other foods, such as meats, soups, juices, teas, aromatic herbs, coffee, chocolate, plus what we normally ingest, corresponds to the 5 pints of water that the human body requires daily to stay hydrated. Then another popular myth: drinking coffee dehydrates is not true either. Short phrases with dissuasive powers. And another one: saying that sea water makes us crazy was enough to make us not even think about trying to drink salt water. In human plasma, nine out of every thousand grams are salt; in seawater, thirty-five out of every thousand grams are salt. So, if you dilute one part seawater in three parts fresh water with lemon, you get a complete alkalizing juice with trace minerals that is healthy and tasty. I have noticed that roofers — who work under a scorching sun — recreate this formula: they pour a tablespoon of Himalayan salt into 2 pints of water to prevent dehydration.

The Scottish physician Gordon Latto (1911-1998), former president of the International Vegetarian Union and promoter of the campaign for real bread in Great Britain in 1976, has always maintained that ingesting liquids during meals dilutes digestive enzymes and hinders digestion. This is understandable: to treat severe intoxications that require washing out the intestines, six pints of water distributed in up to ten doses orally are used in this gastric cleansing and, to wash out the colon, *a maximum of two pints rectally. In* other words, ingesting four pints of water alone in a day is excessive since it washes out the digestive process and prevents the absorption of nutrients.

However, it is proven that people with kidney problems need to drink twelve ounces of water — one or two glasses — extra to prevent the appearance of stones. Fluid intake should be increased if the body requires it. When you exercise, the ideal is to drink water; but if you feel dehydrated due to daily activity or even illness, you should drink broth, tea or, if you prefer, non-alcoholic beer, which provide more water and nutrients. The belief is that only cold drinks quench thirst, but it is the liquid — not its temperature — that hydrates and quenches thirst. According to a study by the University of Montana,[136] the exception is when you exercise — the most efficient and fastest way to lower body temperature in hot conditions is to drink cold liquids — because at room temperature or lukewarm you would require twice as much liquid. The only reasonable purpose of any cold drink is to lower body temperature faster, and yet hot or cold, under normal conditions, both hydrate the body and quench thirst. Otherwise, it is a matter of taste whether to add ice or alcohol. But drinking

---

[136] Walter S. Hailes, John S. Cuddy, Kyle Cochrane & Brent C. Ruby (2016). *"Thermoregulation during extended exercise in the heat: comparisons of fluid volume and temperature"*. *Wilderness & Environmental Medicine*, *27*(3), 386-392. doi: 10.1016/j.wem.2016.06.004.

ice-cold liquids involves a risk because, in order to counteract this instantaneous drop in temperature and bring warm blood flow to the brain, the body suddenly expands the anterior artery located in the forehead. Among other discomforts it causes, this reaction — in addition to being painful — could be dangerous.

The tendency to drink warm or hot beverages is on the rise. In restaurants, many people already ask for water with lemon peel without ice, a glass of red wine at room temperature, tea, or aromatic herbal tea for lunch. This healthy digestive habit sustains the average longevity in the East, which is lower in the West. The aging process is accelerated if one has the bad habit of passing food with cold drinks: just as it is easier to wash the fat off the dishes with hot water, the same happens in the stomach, which finds it more difficult to digest the food bolus solidified by cold drinks and has to work twice as hard. Something similar happens with milk: the opaque layer that remains on the walls of the glass is more difficult to wash off with cold water; for this reason, milky liquids — which contain fat — should be drunk alone; when combined with other foods, the absorption of nutrients becomes more difficult, and the metabolism slows down.

Another bad eating habit, perhaps the worst, is that after lunch we eat dessert. This mistake is tripled if we have a fruit juice with lunch and, even more so if it is cold. The ideal is an aromatic water. When you mix carbohydrates with sweet, the enzymes involved in their digestion counteract each other because they are opposite and the metabolic process is inhibited; immediately, fermentation appears, which produces gases. If the bad combination of foods persists, the toxicity produced by the constant decomposition causes allergies, gastritis, headaches, reflux, stomach discomfort, nausea. To give the body time to digest the other foods properly, that refreshing fruit juice, milk or dessert should be drunk or eaten alone.

Up to now, we have considered that lunch consists of a starter, main course, and dessert, accompanied by cold or iced drinks, and we top it off with hot coffee or tea, even in hot climates. The point is to adapt the habit by omitting the cold drink and changing the order: drink hot tea or aromatic herbs with lunch — or after — and drink the juice only in the middle of the afternoon or to lower the body temperature when you exercise. You will notice the difference in your stomach and in your well-being. Breaking routines is healthy for the mind and it's the same with food. If we are talking about ordering — when I mentioned the tricks to like greens —, I had already realized that habits and the scale of values change when you define what is important: yourself and what you love, your family and your children, if you have them. At home, for example, before grilling the steaks, which are ready in minutes, we spend time preparing the tea and the salad or the vegetables, because hungry or not — if we do not respect this order — the smell of the meat won't even let us think, and it ends up being easier to take the rice and a soda out of the fridge, to heat the rice with the meat and abandon the idea of making a salad. Many may think, "That's the way I like it, with rice and soda, just like always!". But if you jump on my bandwagon, you will experience a rewarding weight loss, healthy fitness and, best of all, you're going to boost a super metabolism that ensures a stable weight.

Today is Monday. When you woke up, I suppose you had hot water or tea with lemon and then fruit. Now, if you don't have time for breakfast, plan the mid-morning snack and the afternoon hors d'oeuvre and, with the leftovers from yesterday's barbecue, for lunch, prepare the Hippocratic Sandwich I suggested. For now, avoid eating in restaurants, because after these two weeks — educated and without bragging —, you will be ready and trained to choose the accompaniments of any menu you are presented with. You know that's where we've made the simple, but harmful mistakes that have led us to accumulate body fat. Although soon I will expose the conceptual part of this proposal that stimulates the good use of carbohydrates later, just for these days, with the sole purpose of refining communication with the body, get on the scale at the same time each day, and be prepared to observe what happens with the "cheat days".

Nervous about your final exam? Use common sense, be moderate, don't go hungry and invest your calorie budget wisely. With the knowledge gained, I know you will pass the test, because broadening your perspective has allowed you to see that changing everything that revolves around the health of the body and the planet also depends on your attitude and your being.

The hen's egg

In the 1960s, the warning that "eggs play a major role in heart disease" fueled the myth that whole eggs trigger cholesterol, which demonized them, especially the yolks. It was not known what actually happens: the fats in the foods we eat impact the quality of total cholesterol: specifically, their higher or lower proportion of omega 3 and 6 may or may NOT contribute to inflammation in the body and arteries. When we eat foods with good "dietary" cholesterol (HDL lipoprotein), which sweeps bad cholesterol (LDL) out of the bloodstream, to balance, the liver lowers the production of triglycerides, which are the result of the molecular bonding of the three fatty acids omega 3, 6 and 9 into glycerin, the most efficient way the body has to store energy. Eating whole eggs — yolk and white — is NOT bad and does not increase the risk of cardiovascular disease.

It is worth remembering that organic eggs contain a more even ratio — from 1:1 to a maximum of 1:4 — between omegas 3 and 6, which determines the inflammatory capacity and which is higher in other eggs — from 1:19 up to 1:25. The inflammation of the arteries causes the cholesterol to get stuck and the blood does not flow well and produces circulatory problems; the real problem is that processed foods have a huge disproportion of omega-6 fatty acids that end up inflaming the entire system. So, consuming eggs does not increase the risk of clogged arteries, but the internal inflammation of the body also definitely depends, on the egg you consume. You are what you eat and so are the hens. Let's clarify something else: although the genetics of the animal determines the color of the shell, the color of the yolks depends exclusively on the hen's diet. The yolks of eggs from "industrial" hens, barn hens fed grain-based animal feed or vegetarian hens usually range from yellow to orange with faint shades. Eggs from free-range (cage free) hens that graze and eat earthworms, tiny farm-raised fingerlings, natural foods, airborne insects, and worms under trees, due to the concentration of the carotenoids lutein and zeaxanthin, combined with the red pigment from dried leaves falling from trees, are brightly colored and the shades range up to reddish.

To become a fat burner and not have problems with total cholesterol — triglycerides — and your bad cholesterol, simply try to avoid processed foods and increase your intake of natural foods high in omega 3 and 9 — anti-inflammatory —. This way you can enjoy the perfect food.

A whole egg contains antioxidants, vitamins A, D, E and K and those of the B complex, including thiamine, which converts food into energy, biotin, and pantothenic acid, crucial in the production of growth hormones; all of them are water-soluble and essential as omegas, but since the body does not store them, we must consume them daily, and the best and cheapest source is a hen's egg. The yolk contains the nutrients choline and folic acid — its major source with 125 mg per unit —, essential for maintaining the structural integrity of the cell membrane and the proper development and performance of the nervous system. Fundamental in the brain development of the fetus and infants, choline favors increased attention and memory and protects them from mental illness, stress, and hypertension. A single egg contains 166 micrograms of lutein and zeaxanthin, antimutagenic and anticarcinogenic super-antioxidants that prevent the formation of free radicals and prevent cataracts and blindness in general. The balanced amino acid, nutrient and mineral profile of calcium, iron, phosphorus, zinc contained in a single egg — capable of giving rise to a living creature — makes it the highest yielding bioavailable food, the cheapest and most valuable protein available. The egg white — 88% water — among other nutrients, provides us with albumin, which protects kidney function, and above all collagen, a protein without which the body would not be a body, because its vital function is to hold together all the structures of the organism.

That's not all. We already said that illegitimate fats from and breaded foods and foods fried in refined oils and partially hydrogenated fats tend to become saturated with free radicals and produce dangerous trans fats. But among the legitimate fats, saturated fats, such as those from hens' eggs, free-range acorn-fed pigs, butter from free-range cows or coconut oil are the raw material, "the host in the production of androgens — testosterone, androsterone; estrogen and progesterone; the male and female sex hormones," as Mary G. Enig states in her article on saturated fats. In addition, the consumption of — healthy — saturated fats ensures that the liver can produce the right number of ketones — from triglycerides — which brain cells use as an ideal alternative to insulin to produce glucose in the brain. The problem with insulin is that it prevents brain cells from absorbing glucose, and, without glucose, they die. For this reason — due to their deficiency of glucose in the brain — diabetic patients are prone to develop Alzheimer's and other mental illnesses: "Dementia in the elderly is like having diabetes in the head. Before one has the symptoms of diabetes or Alzheimer's, the body has already had problems for ten or twenty years", that is the conclusion of writer and physician Mary Newport — with more than twenty years of practice — from the University of Cincinnati, who studied her husband — an Alzheimer's patient — and achieved progressive intellectual, emotional, and physical successes by giving him coconut oil regularly.

These reasons are significant for you to limit the consumption of processed foods; the corrective is to choose well the origin of fats and consume saturated fat in the right proportion: fifty-fifty with the unsaturated and omega 3 you need: olive oil, avocados, nuts, flaxseeds, chia. One or two boiled organic eggs provide the protein you need to start the day and are a great investment because they are low in calories. And if you don't have time, they go well at lunch or in the afternoon with the Hippocratic Sandwich. To complement your intake and balance the fats from the snacks — yogurt, nuts, and seeds — that you have used to get through the day without going hungry, remember to eat salads or fresh, crunchy vegetables, which accompany the proteins in the main course. Favor fish that have a lot of omega 3. The important thing on this second and third day — Tuesday and Wednesday — is that you have the strength and discipline to reduce dairy products, replace sugar with stevia or monk fruit and reduce flours and carbohydrates — the starchy group — to a minimum. To better understand what happened with them, let's talk about oils.

Oils for human consumption

The study of nutrition in the 21ST CENTURY encompasses the absorption of nutrients by skin and hair; natural oils, of animal and vegetable origin, which are suitable for human consumption also fulfill this function. Oils of mineral origin, which are the product of petroleum distillation, are toxic and therefore unhealthy to use on the skin. Vaseline and oils containing *petrolatum* or *kerosene* that are sold as protective lubricants do NOT nourish and act as an insulator that prevents perspiration. On the contrary, coconut, grape, macadamia, almond, olive, or arnica oils — compatible with body fat —, which deflate, soothe, and provide the right form of vitamin E -alpha tocopherol, not gamma tocopherol, which in excess affects the respiratory tract —, are ideal for the health of skin, hair, and nails. I am reminded of the testimony of many people who, to overcome their incurable disease, opted to include the controversial cannabis oil in their naturopathic treatment; as they were already legally dead, they preferred to remain "illegally alive". In the 21ST CENTURY, the use of this prodigious oil is already permitted in many places. Much of science welcomes the use of the medicinal properties — as shamans have done — of natural substances in plasters or massages with oils extracted cold-pressed from plants that only release psychoactive elements by the action of heat and intense fire, i.e., smoked, or cooked. Its direct competitor is science, which has entered the multi-million dollar business of producing different varieties of cannabis sold in legal dispensaries and is developing substances and other ways of ingesting marijuana: in drops under the tongue — which the body absorbs in seconds through the sublingual artery — or smoked in cigarettes — which, according to them, with specific doses — produces the necessary hallucinogenic effects that contribute to the physical and mental health of the patient. Or, without the medicinal argument, to enjoy it recreationally.

As for the oils for human consumption invented in the 20TH CENTURY, we have all been faced with the dilemma of which fat to use in cooking. How do 20TH century industrial oils relate to the processed carbohydrates sold to us as a source of vital energy to the detriment of natural fats?

At the turn of the 19TH CENTURY, whale oil was the preferred fuel for lighting all kinds of lanterns. But with the advent of electricity, the production of lamps of all kinds and the nascent automobile industry, the need arose to satisfy this demand with more economical oils, and heat-refined oils were produced from olive bagasse and rapeseed. Later, with more complex processes such as deodorization, these same oils were modified and made suitable for human consumption. Today, they also come from other vegetable blends and seeds of genetically modified organisms, whose refining process considerably affects any qualities they may have. The problem is that, in the middle of the last century, the mainstream insisted so much on carbohydrate consumption that we ended up ingesting refined oils by the bucketload in fried foods, breaded foods, fast foods, baked goods and preparations of the modern Western diet. The boost given to biofuels, the sponsorship of the agricultural sector that generated their development and the consequent economic success, which meant an additional push to monocultures of corn, soybean, cotton, sugar cane, rapeseed, palm, sunflower, barley, wheat — which only in a minimum percentage are used to produce food —, unintentionally unleashed the ecologically disastrous perfect storm that is sweeping the planet.

The other industrial paradigm, according to which world food supply can only be guaranteed by expanding agricultural and livestock land, is also false. The United Nations Conference on Trade and Development, UNCTAD, in its search for ways to eradicate hunger in the world, insists that: "Developed and developing countries need a paradigm shift: **from the green revolution to a genuine intensification of organic agriculture**". In the modern model of rural development, the protagonist must be the local ecological agro-industry and by no means the expansive industrial agriculture. Researchers at Washington State University[137] demonstrate that its financial viability benefits producers and workers in the rural sector and the environment, and conclude: "Efficiently used organic agriculture can feed the entire world population". FAO states that "31% of average daily protein consumption comes from just five animal species". It adds: "Diversifying production stabilizes household incomes and increases resilience to climate change and natural disasters. It also reduces vulnerability to possible drastic events, such as a sudden increase in food prices, which can be fatal for poor people, given their limited access to credit and savings".[138]

The concepts of self-sufficient whole farm and urban agriculture are evolving around the world. For example, many restaurants already produce organic food — even fish and shellfish — in their basements and on their roofs. Agriculture is changing and so are the numbers. With the economy set to change patterns, the state could support smallholder farmers and micro — enterprises that generate more direct, and indirect employment, and better distribute wealth. **Food security is**

---

[137] John P. Reganold & Jonathan M. Wachter (2016). "*Organic Agriculture in the Twenty-First Century.*" *Nature Plants, 2* (2), 15221. https://www.nature.com/articles/nplants2015221

[138] Food and Agriculture Organization of the United Nations, FAO (2018): *Transforming food and agriculture to achieve the Sustainable Development Goals*, SDGs. 20 interconnected actions to guide decision makers. Rome. http://www.fao.org/3/i9900es/I9900ES.PDF

NOT only about health; it also depends on changing our tastes and beliefs.

Let's move on to cooking. The first thing to consider is the temperature of the grill and on the standard stove to know what they are used for: low, medium, and high. For cooking and grilling, low: between 140 °F and 210 °F (60 °C and 98.8 °C); for cooking and sautéing, medium: between 210 °F and 300 °F (98.8 °C and 148.8 °C); for frying and searing meats, high: between 300 °F and 500 °F (148.8 °C and 260 °C). The smoke point of oils is the temperature they can withstand before smoking and burning. The smoke points of some refined oils are shown in the table below.

Smoke points of some oils	
Corn	450 °F
Sunflower	450 °F
Cotton	420 °F
Peanut	450 °F
Extra light olive	468 °F
Soybeans	450 °F
Safflower	511 °F

Fried foods are delicious. But consuming fried and breaded foods is the fastest way to inflame and acidify the body because they invade it with oxidants and trans fats in a single meal! To consume refined oils **wisely**, it is best to use them as little as possible in cooking. Canola oil, for example, at the end of the refining process contains 62% of monounsaturated fatty acids and looks very similar to cold-pressed virgin or extra virgin olive oil — our best healthy reference; although they offer it unrefined, cold-pressed, and "organic", this is a fallacy that sounds wonderful because they get it from genetically modified seeds.

Joel Marion, an expert nutritionist certified by the National Academy of Sports Medicine in 2001, comments on canola oil and the refining process:

> Canola oil, which is actually rapeseed oil, a successful marketing triumph that was renamed for obvious reasons (CANadian Oil Low Acids)... to turn it into something edible they remove the erucic acid and bleach and deodorize it with chemical solvents, including hexane — a hydrocarbon used to dilute paints or the sticky adhesive of labels, among other industrial purposes. Approximately 30% of canola oil is composed of polyunsaturated fats, very fragile fatty acids that can be easily damaged by the high heat treatment to which they are subjected, which is the method of processing and refining virtually all forms of commercial oils.

Because of the bad taste of most refined oils and because of what we know about the refining process that can make them unhealthy, the choice is to throw them out after two heating because they spoil more than they are and produce or contain trans fats. "Most of the trans fats in our diet come from partially hydrogenated vegetable oils produced in industry."[139]

Refined or unrefined, vegetable fats contain no cholesterol and coconut and avocado oils — raw and unrefined can be consumed directly — are the most versatile, ideal for recipes that require a lot of oven or stove time. Avocado oil, whose proportion — between 10 and 19% — of saturated fatty acids depends on the

---

[139] Tiffany N. Stodtko & Wendy J. Dahl (2018): *Facts about fats and oils.* Florida University. Institute of Food and Agricultural Sciences (IFAS). Publication #FSHN16-3S. https://edis.ifas.ufl.edu/fs292, https://edis.ifas.ufl.edu/fs281.

variety and maturity of the fruit, contains a good load of omega 9 monounsaturated fat that can reach up to 80% and an acceptable level — from 11 to 15% — of omega 3 and 6 polyunsaturated fats; cold pressed, its smoke point is 380 °F (195°C) and, among the refined ones, avocado oil can withstand up to 518 °F (270°C) without burning. The densest oil is the one that is least absorbed by food, and for frying — on high — coconut oil is the one that best meets this condition. It is very stable and resistant due to the 92 % saturated fat content in its tightly packed molecules. And make no mistake: at room temperature, coconut oil is solid. It belongs to the *medium chain triglycerides* (MCT) group, which the body metabolizes to lower cholesterol and stay healthy. Cold-pressed *virgin coconut oil* (VCO) — obtained from milk or shredding — has a smoke point of 351 °F (177 °C) and that of RBD coconut — refined, bleached, and deodorized coconut used industrially — 450 °F (232 °C) —.

Undoubtedly, fat consumption is a sensitive issue. Although saturated fats are some of the healthiest fats available, from the standpoint of alkalinity propensity, the best way to frequently ingest the various oils that provide essential fats for the body is also the most delicious: eating them directly in raw nuts, dried fruits, and seeds. Almost all of them have a pH between 5 and 6 — almonds have pH 8 — and, in addition to fiber, they provide enzymes, vitamins and minerals. To get the best out of them and extract their flavors, store them mixed in a jar with a few drops of olive oil and a pinch of Himalayan salt. At night, they go well with herbal tea — chamomile and valerian — before bedtime. Sometimes, we give in to the taste of fried foods. For example, peanut oil gives fried turkey an unmistakable flavor on Thanksgiving Day — the last Thursday of November — in the United States; peanuts are a legume — like lentils — and have proteins, but because of their high acidity with pH 2, I consume them with caution. Highly refined peanut oil — not cold-pressed, expelled, or extruded — does not contain the protein that causes the allergic reaction.

Apart from coconut or avocado oil, cold extracted unrefined vegetable oils are not very stable, their molecules are not as tightly packed, and they are NOT for frying. Because of their "virgin" state, minimal processing allows their potent healthful qualities to be obtained from them; as a true nutritional option, they are excellent for sautéing and cooking at medium to medium-low heat. We also have other flavors, such as *walnut*, pistachio, almond, grape seeds; in them, there is a different universe that will give an exquisite, healthy, and nutritious taste to your salads and vegetables. It depends on your taste. And another saturated fat: real cow's butter, *grass-fed cows,* with its delicious characteristic flavor — smoke point of 349 °F (176 °C), is perfect for sautéing vegetables.

On the net, I found tables that illustrate the composition of fats in the most representative oils. However, they do not include exotic oils such as Brazil nut — which provides selenium — ; macadamia — which provides potassium, phosphorus and calcium — ; avocado, which regulates cholesterol, is a friend of the skin and hair, prevents wrinkles, stretch marks, and fights gray hair. In addition, avocado stone, peel, or leaves are used to make teas — with anti-inflammatory and antibiotic properties — that prevent irritation and eliminate parasites from the gastrointestinal tract. In the tables, pay attention to flaxseed, which has the best ratio of fats: with little omega 6, it provides the highest amount of omega 3. Organic flaxseed, which can be used in a poultice to treat skin allergies, restores vital energy; many bioenergetic practitioners have obtained excellent results in terminally ill patients by treating them with highly alkalizing diets that focus on this seed and its derivatives.

Another fact to observe in these tables is lard, which with little inflammatory omega 6 — something like 9 or 10% — has in equal proportions 45% of omega 9 monounsaturated fats and 45% saturated fats that do contain cholesterol, but which are only bad if you consume them in excess or burned. Before the commercialization of oils, frying after frying, we accumulated these fats in a cauldron and later, for economic reasons — in industrial food production or in our kitchens — we continue to do the same: we accumulate the residue of these fats in the cauldron. This burnt cholesterol has been and continues to be the biggest killer in history. However, animal fat has a great advantage: with the stove on high, its smoke point is 350 to 370 °F (177 °C to 182 °C); this allows sealing and cooking meats in their own fat, without burning them. The trick is to put the fillets or loin, on the fatty side, in a very hot frying pan with tongs; wait until the fat melts, sealing each side of the meat, and when it browns, you don't use it anymore. **The residues should not be reused:** discard them in a covered glass jar until they can go in the garbage. Keep in mind that, for frying, you do not need a "pool of oil", because it is wasteful. Unless at medium or medium-low temperature — which should not exceed 195 °F nor be less than 140 °F —, taking care not to burn the oil — duck fat, lard, clarified butter — what you are doing is confit: an ancient cooking technique that prevents food from absorbing too much oil, because — with the pan covered — it cooks without browning and acquires a special flavor.

The 21ST CENTURY nutritional perspective avoids frying as much as possible, uses the minimum amount of cooking oil and, on the contrary, increases the direct daily consumption of healthy fats and oils. The favorable impact on the pocketbook is such that the consumer can afford to choose the finest oils, which, because of their qualities, are the correct source of energy required by the body for its vital functions.

Virgin, extra virgin or unfiltered oils are for direct consumption and the fact that they are first cold *pressed* guarantees that they have not been processed at high temperatures. However, there is a special condition for those that contain healthy residues from fruits: unfiltered oils must be young, recently harvested and should be consumed soon because they are "alive" and are still maturing. They are select. The best way to preserve any oil is in dark-colored glass containers that block the passage of light in the darkest, coolest place in the kitchen.

For many people, talking about oils makes their livers churn, and I think it is a convenient moment to think of the refreshing foods that burn fat. The apple burns more calories than it provides. Fruit: pumpkin, peppers, tomatoes, pickles, kiwi, lemons, blueberries, avocados, prunes and raisins, coconut, banana, watermelon, grapefruit, and red wine. Vegetables and legumes: Brussels sprouts, mushrooms, spinach, beets, kale, fennel, asparagus, black beans and peanuts or peanut butter. Spices and beverages: cinnamon, turmeric, black pepper, cayenne, tea — white, green, gray, such as *oolong* — ; fermented, such as *kombucha*; and red *pu-erh* —. Proteins: salmon, tuna, herring, *mahi-mahi*, tofu, and eggs. Grains and cereals: rice and whole — grain breads, sprouted grain bread and quinoa. Dairy products: kefir, cheese, and Greek yogurt. Dried fruits: nuts, seeds. Natural oils: pistachio, flax, almond, sunflower, olive, dark chocolate. Baked or roasted potatoes, when eaten alone, also help burn fat.

When I talked about trophology and the anger that comes with change, I asked you to save some of that anger for this chapter. This is a good time to remember how important it is to adopt a green day at least twice a month; the body listens, the metabolism notices and uses this vegetarian day more effectively to detoxify the body. It can be Friday and the weekend is perfect, because Sunday can coincide with the second cheat day, when you can eat whatever you want; it is convenient to be free of the concept so you can relax and continue the process next week.

What about potatoes and white foods?

In the chapter on flours, I mentioned that rice, pasta, and potatoes are white foods with which we have problems because practically every day we put them on the plate to accompany protein. According to trophology, the enzymes that process and metabolize them oppose each other and eating them at the same time makes digestion disastrous. Later, we gave milk, flours, sugar and salt a fair trial and concluded that, for example, refined sugar and its laboratory-invented substitutes, white bread — full of preservatives and without fiber —, white rice without nutrients — not organic, with traces of arsenic — [140] or French fries cooked in suspect oils are some of the worst things we can eat: the real white killers. However, they are all carbohydrates, and it is not true that we should avoid white foods. We also talked about the vegetable rainbow but failed to mention that the glycemic index of gluten-free and white foods, such as potatoes and cassava, should not matter to us either, because what determines whether the body loses weight is the right combination of foods. Potatoes, cassava, and bananas belong to the starchy group; since they are starchy, they should not be mixed with proteins and among fruits, for example — which should be eaten alone —, you would have to eat a lot of watermelon — which has a high glycemic index — for you to notice that you have gained ounces.

---

[140] https://www.ewg.org/foodscores/content/arsenic-contamination
-in-rice/.

Let us clarify, the white foods of the starchy group are in no case accompaniments; they alone can be the protagonist of the dish and be accompanied with fresh vegetables, whole grains, and nuts of the neutral group. For example, a delicious way to enjoy two large potatoes is to peel them and cut them into sticks, then fry them and once drained, put them in a medium saucepan over low heat with almond milk that barely covers them, butter, salt and a pinch of cinnamon and icing sugar, stir them for a while and that's it. You will love it. Or accompany it cooked, cut in cubes peel and all, with thickly sliced sautéed vegetables; if you like, you can cover the potatoes with guacamole, which is macerated avocado; with white and green onion, chopped tomatoes, cilantro, lemon, and salt, which can also accompany fried plantain chips — another white food — from time to time. Potatoes eaten correctly are a healthy carbohydrate that contains vitamins, minerals, and a long list of nutrients. The skin provides fiber. A medium-sized potato has only about one hundred to one hundred and twenty calories and does not sabotage your weight loss efforts, especially when accompanied by fibrous vegetables and perhaps some healthy fats — a little tuna, for example — and NOT, on the contrary, when it accompany meats.

Foods from the neutral group should always be the companions. And among them, certain white foods require special attention. Onions and garlic can be found almost everywhere. Full of protective and anticarcinogenic antioxidants, they are unique in that they possess anti-inflammatory and antibacterial nutrients allicin, quercetin, chromium, selenium, and other antiviral agents. Garlic and onions, perhaps magical, are also antibiotics.

Another important example is cauliflower: loaded with vitamin C, fiber, and minerals, like broccoli, it contains special compounds such as glucosinolates that protect us from infections and cancer,[141] and thiocyanates, which are attributed with a potent antibacterial function in the body. Among pale foods, mushrooms and white asparagus have high levels of unique nutrients and antioxidants; mushrooms are high in polyphenols and ergothioneine, two different types of antioxidants; asparagus, rich in fiber, iron, potassium, phosphorus, and iodine, provides vitamins C and E, folates, and beta-carotene. The list of white foods is longer; it is made up of bamboo shoots, alfalfa, hearts of palm, artichoke, and others that, although colorful — such as eggplant, radish and cucumber — are white on the inside.

It's Wednesday of this first week and since last Sunday's barbecue the craving for *pizza* or beans with everything or hamburger with the bun top — not the open sandwich — is rising like foam to your head! But, in these three days that you have eaten differently from usual, perhaps because of discipline, healthy intention or curiosity to eat differently and fulfill the promise you made to yourself, you can't say that you have not been hungry either. Well, the time has come to dream about tomorrow's breakfast. How about French toast, waffles with butter, honey and strawberries or a full omelet; then, for lunch, the all-you-can-eat burger, and fries; and in the evening you can calm your craving for pistachio ice cream with blackberry sauce. Tomorrow is your first cheat day! I synthesized two papers by Joel Marion, a professional trainer and nutritionist certified by the International Society of Sports Nutrition, that make clear how leptin, cheat days and convenient carbohydrate use work.

---

[141] Maria Traka & Richard Mithen (2009): "*Glucosinolates, isothiocyanates and human health*". *Phytochemistry Reviews*, *8* (1), 269-282.

The most important hormone you probably haven't heard of

Its name is leptin, derived from the Greek word *leptos*, meaning 'thin', 'fine'. Leptin was first isolated in 1994 and is the most important hormone for weight loss — a discovery of the 21ST CENTURY. Its function is to communicate nutritional status to the body and brain. Leptin levels depend on two things that are equally true for all people: the level of body fat and calorie intake. Fat cells secrete leptin; people with more body fat have higher leptin levels and vice versa. Under normal conditions, the correlation between leptin levels and the amount of body fat makes sense. Unfortunately, when you restrict calories to try to lose fat, conditions are anything but normal and the body responds by reducing leptin levels. This is because the other mediator of leptin levels in the blood is calorie intake. If you decrease your calorie intake, the leptin level drops, and this is independent of body fat. So, if you are overweight and still want to suffer from the effects of low leptin levels, just go on a diet!

What happens when leptin levels drop, why should we care?

Normally, when leptin is at a good level, the brain receives a clear signal that nutrient intake is adequate; metabolism is high, and the body's internal environment is conducive to fat burning. Even when you start dieting!

If you diet, leptin levels drop precipitously — 50% or more after a week — ; the body receives the starvation signal and creates the hormonal environment conducive to fat storage: the metabolism slows down with the sudden drop in thyroid hormones — fundamental for metabolism —, becomes disrupted and, at the same time, responds by triggering cortisol

— the hormone of stress and abdominal fat storage — in a perceptible way: hello, abdominal fat!

And if that wasn't enough, the appetite-stimulating hormone ghrelin, neuropeptide Y and anandamide also jump on board to make your life even more miserable. Don't struggle to remember all the names, just remember that, when leptin drops, you get "hungry" for real. Even though you have the healthy intention of losing weight, it's ironic that, although the body is always primed for fat loss, the exception is when you start burning fat by dieting. Ideally, we should keep leptin levels high while trying to lose those extra pounds.

And how do we do it?

Leptin is a protein-based hormone; thus, leptin pills as an oral dietary supplement would not be viable because they would simply be digested by the body. This leaves the method of leptin injections, which work well because, even if you continue to restrict calories, they succeed in reversing the metabolic maladaptation that arises in response to dieting and starvation. Experiments by Rexford S. Ahima in 1996 in mice, Steven Heymsfield in 1999 in humans, Michael Rosenbaum in 2002, A. J. Fogteloo in 2003, K. Welt in 2004 and, again, Rosenbaum in 2005 and their respective teams of specialists and researchers demonstrated that daily leptin injections are successful in weight loss. The problem is that leptin injections are expensive and, moreover — at least for pleasure — many of us would not be willing to inject ourselves every day.

After a week of dieting, leptin levels can drop by as much as 50%; but fortunately, with a sudden and substantial increase in calories, it would only take twelve to twenty-four hours for leptin to return to its level. Therefore, the real solution — which does not involve needles or hundreds of dollars' worth of squirts — is to consume high-calorie foods to naturally manipulate leptin production and trick the brain in a way we love by eating carbohydrates.

What is special about carbohydrates?

Research by Guenther H. Boden and his team at Temple University School of Medicine revealed that leptin levels would not drop, even when fasting, if insulin and blood sugar are maintained by intravenous drips. It sounds crazy, but it highlights the strong relationship between insulin and sugar — carbohydrates — with leptin — which is produced by fats. And it has been determined that, to reverse the negative variations caused by diet, overfeeding with protein and fat has little effect on leptin, so based on Boden's research — since calories alone don't get the job done and insulin takes time to respond — it makes sense to think that foods that combine carbohydrates and fats work best because of the strong link between them and leptin. To get a strong leptin response from overeating, the mix needs to involve a lot of carbohydrates.

In the middle of the diet, you can give leptin and metabolism a big boost with high calorie foods by "cheating" with *pizza*, ice cream, cookies, chicken wings, soups and rice with everything or with burgers and fries and return the body to the conditions necessary for subsequent fat loss; this does not mean that the fat will magically melt away if we do not adopt the strategy that, after leptin is extremely high and the body is on fat burning priority, we will then go with a low carbohydrate approach. Realistically, this is the best sustainable way to lose weight. The unfortunate thing is that, with this immediate low-carb goal, the dominance of the fat-loss friendly environment — which we set out to achieve at the beginning of the week — soon declines with the drop in leptin due to the absence of carbs. When you diet, leptin and ghrelin — the hormone that makes you feel hungry in the stomach and hungry in the brain —

drop; but, if we gradually add carbs, blood glucose and insulin push them back up and communicate to the brain that all is well. This means that to make the most of the environment created in our body and burn fat we must adopt a "strategic carbohydrate cycle" during the week, which is that once the body begins to adapt and burn more fat, we will increase carbs from zero or very low — again — the first day; moderate the next day — or the next two — and high on the first cheat day in the middle of the week and repeat the same until the second cheat day at the end of the week. Renewing the cycle ensures that you will never go a single day without the body feeling the priority of burning fat. For the most part, diets are boring because the foods are repeated every day and the best thing about the cycle is that you can use a wide variety of carbohydrates.

Have you experienced guilt, failure, anxiety, discouragement, and low motivation with dieting before? Never again! Now that you know this, every time you do it, you'll get away from the "guilt"; you'll notice that you're accelerating your progress and you'll feel better knowing that you've used your favorite dessert to accelerate fat loss. When you have cravings, remember that, in a few days, when your next cheat session arrives, you'll be able to enjoy that food you crave. Simply put, strategic cheats solve the dieting dilemma by providing powerful metabolic benefits and, best of all, a powerful psychological benefit.

JOEL MARION, CISSN, NSCA-CPT
https://thealivexperienceonline.com/
the-most-important-hormone-youve-never-heard-of/
http://www.cheatyourwaythin.com/launch_members/
carb-cycling.html

I know some of you may be thinking what I said earlier: that these are the wrong foods. From Geary and others, we already knew about the traps, but I would not hesitate to say that the strategy proposed by Joel Marion to make the body always ready to burn fat and lose weight is the best way to take advantage of and enjoy the delicious recipes based on cereals, grains and milk that we made essential — but which only appeared less than ten thousand years ago in the Paleolithic Age — that include in large proportions the acidifying ingredients that we invented in the last century: fast-absorbing carbohydrates, refined sugars and white flours; refined or hydrogenated margarines and oils; synthetic flavorings, colorings and sugars; refined salt and industrial preservatives, along with antibiotics, growth hormones and genetically modified organisms involved in food production, with a tendency to be loaded with inflammatory omega-6. Those who have accompanied me, and have already included the vegetarian day, have learned to eat, know the foods, and know well how they work mixed in the body. They understand that the most important thing is to eat natural foods regularly, and they have experienced that, over time, carbohydrates — which are part of the past associated with memories and, which you now use in the diet and on cheat days — become cravings. Consuming them from time to time is the reward of having become a fat burner, not a carb burner. In other words, all this is not a diet, because the educational process has allowed you to adapt to a new healthy life by changing your habits and beliefs.

Right after the cheat day, with the carbohydrate strategy, you will gain at least one pound, but the cycle is so dynamic and works so well that, when you return to the low-calorie eating regimen, the next day you will notice that you have already lost three, or almost three, pounds. This means you've lost more net fat and one less pound of weight to get the body you want and deserve.

Tomorrow, you start the second week and I leave you free to fine-tune your communication with the body. Learn to read its messages: if you are just getting used to drinking tea and your body responds with constipation, do not give up tea; what you need is the "fiber" provided by legumes, vegetables, whole grains and, above all, fruits such as pitahaya, kiwi, prunes, figs, or figs, which have moderate laxative effects. To lose weight, fibrous fruits, such as oranges, pears, grapefruit, pineapple; and red fruits, such as strawberries and raspberries, which, in addition to providing water and minerals, load you with antioxidants. By the end of the next week, you'll be on this train and the weight loss will increase as the conversation with your body becomes more fluid. Over time, you'll notice that your body will invite you to exercise to achieve fullness.

For this week, I propose — as cravings — octopus tapas a la botija, which consists of cooking the mollusk, slicing its tentacles, and bathing them with a mayonnaise based on botija olives; they are purple and their characteristic flavor is because, in Peru, they are harvested at a specific point of maturation. The base of this mayonnaise is a whole egg, fifteen pitted olives, olive oil, salt, and pepper to taste mixed in the processor; and it is served over the octopus and accompanied with soda crackers or French bread. Or how about...?

Soups and rice dishes with everything

There is no region on Earth where we have not mixed the leftovers and cuts of meat left in the pots with the seasonings and herbs of the place to prepare with water and rice — or without it — traditional recipes that over time became part of each culture. These recipes mix in the same dish the three food groups contrary to trophology — the science of combining foods — and we love them.

In the past, when we did not have air-conditioned environments, in the inns of the oldest cities, cold most of the year, it was customary to welcome travelers with light and hearty broths to warm them up and comfort them. In Europe, for example, the French consommé — which in Spanish means 'consumed' or 'reduced meat', usually chicken (in England, chicken broth); the Italian minestrone with pasta and vegetables or the delicious Dutch soup *groentesoep,* which contains meatballs, became familiar. Diners — for a fee — could also enjoy other heavier creamy soups, such as cream of broccoli with cheddar cheese, which are part of the heritage of the English and French; or clam chowder — a great favorite in the United States —, which mixes clams in their juice with potatoes, onion, celery, bacon, butter, and cream.

In summer, for example, in Spain, the custom is to have cold soups such as the elegant pine nut gazpacho; or the popular gazpacho with green bell pepper, onion, garlic, tomato, vinegar and olive oil, or salmorejo with more garlic and without paprika, neither containing bread; or ajoblanco with almonds, which does have stale bread. Some soups and rice dishes have also become famous around the world: *ramen* — with noodles and pork — or *miso* with tofu; tripe soup a la madrileña; the discreet and humble Greek lentil soup or *fakí soúpa*; Chinese rice, Valencian paella or *maqluba* or Arab rice and eggplant paella. In Mexico, chili con carne is very well known; in Colombia, *sancochos* (stews), rice soup with meatballs or mondongo — beef belly with potato similar to Mexican pozole, which has white corn — flavored with coriander. Many of them escape me, but they are recipes that remind us of our parents' house and even more so those of us who are far away, because ever since we were children, they have brought us the longing for that special ingredient: the love of mother or father. Fortunately, during the pandemic we have been getting rid of the taint that cooking is only for women, becoming usual for both genders to cook.

Although, in many cases, the complement may seem null and void and one of the two may not be there afterwards, these apparently opposite relationships are complementary and vital for the formation of the individual; every child has the right to receive the formative contribution of the polarity between the genders. My principle focuses exclusively on the welfare of the child; orphaned and abandoned children are being denied these reference values in the modern experiment of cohabitation, in which couples of the same gender adopt or conceive them to form a family. Couples of women who want children or the transgender man, who also has the biological capacity to give birth, should think that their attitude of being only moms or dads-moms is selfish and raises precisely the thesis of what it means to be an orphan. Being mothers corresponds to the gender capable of giving birth, but for the sake of the infant, if there are not two people who match — at least physically — the roles of father and mother — and even less, if there is no couple —, it is impossible to configure a **family,** since it requires both, so that between the father and the mother the child be the nucleus that represents the foundation of society: the family, which has always saved us from many circumstances.

The article "Sex beyond the Genitalia"[142], consistent with previous studies, argues that regardless of human anatomy, the

---

[142] Daphna Joel, Zohar Berman, Ido Tavor, Nadav Wexler, Olga Gaber, Yaniv Stein, Nisan Shefi, Jared Pool, Sebastian Urchs, Daniel S. Margulies, Franziskus Liem, Jürgen Hänggi, Lutz Jäncke & Yaniv Assaf (2015): *"Sex Beyond the Genitalia: The Human Brain Mosaic"*. *Proceedings of the National Academy of Sciences, PNAS, 112* (50), 15468-15473. https://www.pnas.org/content/112/50/15468.

brain — starting at conception, obviously — has male and female "parts" and there is no true dimorphism. The study suggests that there is no purely male or female brain and that not only female and male hormones — estrogens and testosterone — are responsible for shaping the brain: during its development, a set of genetic, environmental and epigenetic factors — traits not pre-formed in the fertilized egg and that emerge over time in the living being — define the patterns of behavior and conduct that will determine the identity of the "being" with its gender, understood from a sociocultural point of view, not a biological sex. I said it before: "Taking into account that there may be male or female gender identity in a non-corresponding body...", the feeling of the individual is what really invites to ratify the gender to which he or she belongs.

When during the consolidation or transition the feminine or masculine self-concept — which sometimes worries us parents — does not match the packaging, the tendency is to think that they are aberrations. They are not, and they give us the reasons to think that there is a God other than the one who humiliates, punishes and is to be feared. At the top of evolution, although in countries like Saudi Arabia, Brunei, Iraq, Iran, Mauritania, Nigeria, Syria, Somalia, Sudan, Yemen, and many others, they are judged and imprisoned or killed, these persecuted beings have come to fulfill the mission of teaching us the meaning of coexistence. That we have not yet accepted it is another thing, but the word "aberration" clarifies things: in biology, aberration means an extreme morphological or physiological anomaly; on this basis some assume that they do not identify with their genitalia; others simply cannot stand it and to escape reprobation decide to change sex through surgery. In social terms, aberration designates a depraved or perverse act or conduct which deviates from what is accepted as licit and, although there is still a long way to go, the defenders of the rights of these communities have been doing a great job. But what is clearer is its main meaning in Spanish: "Aberration is a serious error of understanding" (RAE).

We believe that sexual organs must necessarily correspond to a specific gender or being; if this is not the case, there are already countless diseases or mental disorders that categorize them as aberrations. Body and being are not the same, they are two different entities; and in something as personal as genitalia, regardless of size or shape, eunuch, or hermaphrodite, "normality does not exist": they are a particularity, an endowment, and a natural, epigenetic, physical attribute. It is incorrect that they are aberrations, and it turns out that there are more mentally ill people among those who believe that they are not. And if they were, for transgender people to feel comfortable and for there to be inclusion — because otherwise there would not be —, by function and design, without complicating our lives, we must accept that they use the public rest-room they want — according to their appearance —, with an extra toilet, allowing them to live in their body with dignity, in correspondence with the gender with which they identify.

"Gay" is the favorite label that society uses to discriminate against men and women who prefer same-sex partners. And the tendency to label them as aberrant because we believe that they have "sexual tastes" different from ours, is unfair because they do not affect the physical integrity of other people, and more so because, when it comes to tastes, everyone has his or her own. From the legal point of view, in some countries, they can get married; gay marriage is a fair achievement because it guarantees inheritance and economic rights to the couple when one of them dies and to decide rights over their assets and retirement funds if they have them.

However, adopted children now surprise us, because they let us know that, if every family intends to protect innocence and naivety in infants and that sex is something private between adults, the physical appearance of the parents DOES matter, because it is NOT about sex; it is about gender identity, which can be explained without major trauma during the upbringing of the children. From their point of view, that "other side of the rainbow", some children raised by same-gender couples claim to have grown up with a dissident idea of what a family structure means; the necessary reference to the opposite gender in the couple is that irreplaceable bond of love that they claim not to have had: a father or a mother, "something strange happens with either of them and I don't know what it is", and they disagree because, growing up, they felt a natural restlessness that has no explanation. Some say that, by knowing the identity of their absent fathers or mothers, they somehow achieved behavioral and emotional stability. Others feel deceived because they were led to believe that at some point a seed took the place of a father or mother. And they mention that some are single and live alone. But ask their children when they grow up and they will tell you that they had a grandparent, uncle, grandmother, or aunt as a reference of the opposite gender, and in many cases, the nanny or the butler. No matter how much love there is, that space is not filled, the objective is NOT met, and they continue to feel orphaned.

On the other hand, whenever children are present, expressions of affection are welcome. But some people have turned sexual tastes into ideology and others — not necessarily of the same gender — over-express sexual desire in inappropriate places; this constitutes an abuse; the serious thing is that now they pretend to make them part of the children's curriculum. As art, *drag* and *queer* expressions in theaters are fine, because that subject is for adults, but not in schools and libraries to make pedagogy and in stories specifically written for children: tolerance is taught, and the sexual too, but sexuality is NOT. To induce it to children is an attack on their innocence and is a great aberration: a serious error of understanding. Naturally, sexuality is felt with puberty; in most of us, sexuality, personal and specific sexual tastes are defined from adolescence onwards. They do not fall under anyone's judgment if they remain exclusively in intimacy where they surface and where — speaking of pleasure — love and sex are not the same thing: attraction is inherent to love; however, love, its entire spectrum, only goes so far to ignite the passion that unleashes the human animal within us. Hence the subtlety of a good love, which depends on the couple's sex growing, maturing and being their great complement. Exotic means strange, shocking, or extravagant and, in a world as convulsed as ours, some exotic expressions violate reason and, for there to be inclusion and understanding, prudence and respect must come from both parties. For example, people with excessive tattoos, full of piercings or unkempt long beards can be intimidating, but only when there has been no communication with them.

Let's go back to soups. The concept of lunch can be reevaluated with changes in habits that favor us; for example, hot soups should go at the end, not at the beginning. When we eat soup, we think of saving space for the main course; but, if instead, we think of saving space for the broth, we would be more cautious with the main course. If they are soups with everything, the appropriate thing to do is to make them the only dish and set aside the peripherals to be your next intakes. The point is that by habit those peripherals have become part of the lunch and many of us like to include in the same dish chicken or meat, avocado, even rice or pasta, chips, soda crackers, which we take from the peripheral dishes to give weight to the soup when the meal is served; the same happens when we mix rice with everything.

The habit of holding out to eat everything at lunch made us forget about snacking. You are right, it is better to divide the meal into five or six intakes: mid-afternoon or after a nap, something light from the neutral group with flours, a yogurt, a dessert with stevia or oatmeal with chia seeds and raisins. When you come back from work, you can eat the meat or chicken that you left in the peripheral dishes at lunch — the extra protein —, accompanied by a good salad with nuts or a Hippocratic Sandwich and a warm aromatic to help you digest the food. You can be sure that you will not eat it all, because you have already eaten less than two hours ago, and your body will tell you that it is satisfied. In the evening, you can enjoy a slice of cheese with honey and a hot green tea.

We are already understanding part of the secret to change everything: eliminate or correct old customs and beliefs. When that irresistible stew with chickpeas, ajiaco[143] or rice with everything appear on the menu, wisely, include only what fits in that one dish. Here comes the point: do not eat even a single additional peripheral, such as croutons or banana chips, potatoes, another piece of ham or more rice, chicken... With this practice of distancing the meals and including snacks, we will put the new eating habits to work in our favor to burn those extra fats that affect us. Without going hungry, you will encourage your mind to readapt and value the foods that you did not include in your diet before. For example, take advantage of soups and rice with everything, loaded with carbohydrates and fats, to increase leptin levels or, better, one at a time on cheat days. Keep in mind that part of personal hygiene includes brushing our teeth frequently;

---

[143] Soup with shredded chicken, three types of potatoes, corn on the cob and an herb called guasca served with cream and capers.

flossing helps control anxiety. Without so much study, it stands to reason that this habit can give you what some studies say: on average four more years of life. Let's move on to exercise.

Physical exercise

The cycle of life is common to every embryo that manages to gestate and survives the change of environment. With its birth, the spirit is established in the creature: the being exists and the body subsists on what mother earth can offer... However, for us to enjoy the intellect and the spirit — the divine gift —, humans pay the price of years of vulnerability until the brain develops and the body — from the animal instinct — acquires agility and motor capacity to communicate, move and flee.

Exercise is vital, and when we exercise outdoors, the sun recharges us with vitamin D, which is essential for strengthening bones, for muscle movement, for nerves to transmit messages between the brain and other parts of the body, and for the immune system to fight off the bacteria and viruses that attack it. As children, the natural tendency is to play. However, in schools, interest in physical exercise and sports has declined. Interest in physical exercise and sports tends to decline for three basic reasons; the first is the little time parents have to be with their families and take care of their children, who end up being innocent victims of the TV or tablets. Thus, the addiction to violent virtual games arises. The second is the bad approach to the competition factor, as teenagers feel they have no chance of winning and, for fear of losing, they massively exclude themselves from participating in amateur sports. I commented earlier that the concept of educating groups and not individuals is obsolete. It is true that "everyone is a genius. But if you judge a fish by its ability to climb trees, it will live its whole life thinking that it is useless". And if we add to this the "competition" factor, our educational system as it stands is a disaster. This is the third reason why physical exercise — the self-taught alternative — does not appeal to young people in the face of the interest that smartphones arouse in them, because they determine their priority from a very early age: to be considered and to be someone recognized in the cyberspace of social networks.

In any case, exercise is disappearing from our lives. At university, the social aspect is displacing the practice of sports, which is limited to a small elite group of very exclusive, high competition athletes, and to the few who understand that "sport is health". Then, with the same creativity that smartphones have awakened, we must be able to develop applications that equitably involve distraction factors so that today's children from an early age do not feel like losers and that physical exercise is a passion that means "health" rather than competition.

Because of bad eating habits, many people gain weight, but not from lack of exercise. For that reason, I left it to the end of the chapter: physical exercise, the gym and a "good diet" that restricts calories do NOT have an inexorable relationship with losing weight; due to that bad approach, thousands of people who walk or jog habitually, with effort and will, continue with the same muffin top and do not lose a single ounce. We have believed that it is the exercise that burns fat, but after training, when the body is ready to recover the energy consumed during exercise, it is the body that burns it according to what you eat in the following forty-five minutes. Fat loss is definitive if you eat protein accompanied with crunchy vegetables, avoid flour and, with the metabolic function actively normal, the enzymes act in time so that the muscles and skin are toned. Therefore, the relationship between weight loss and physical exercise is usually an illusion for dieters and is, however, a reality for those who change their habits and beliefs. I would like to explain what happens and tell you not to waste your time with diets that restrict calories; it is true that you lose some pounds due to the intense expenditure of energy at a given time, but you gain them back easily, and more due to the action and reaction effect; even if you do not want to, the body will claim more calories than you lost. When you go for a walk, wearing girdles serves to loosen a little accumulated fat and, although this makes you lose weight momentarily, over time, this ill-planned struggle will wear you down physically and mentally; without deserving it, you will blame it on your lack of willpower, you will disown the girdles, you will stop exercising and, instead of enjoying it, you will end up hating it.

However, it is not at all advisable to exercise sporadically when you are overweight; moreover, if you have stopped doing it for a long time, it is dangerous. Professionals in sports such as baseball, sumo, shot put, discus or football exceed their weight, because it suits their performance, and they make a living out of it. But they are prone to diabetes and do not take into account the impact of 9 pounds for every extra pound they acquire, which is transferred to the lower joints — knees, ankles, and feet. Then there are the people who believe that full, pot-bellied babies are healthy children; no, their parents start doing things wrong from the beginning. Can you imagine a bent ankle with a bad step? Many people with a lot of belly fat are decalcified and don't know it. But if they exercise, what can happen to all that pressure on their hips or their heart as their heart rate increases? These people should have medical monitoring.

People without regular training, overweight and at constant risk of suffering from something should not attempt to make great physical efforts from one moment to the next; this is an absurdity and an attack on their health. Although they wish to walk, joint pain does not allow them to do so. It is irresponsible to expect them to exercise because it damages their joints, their bones, and their heart. It is not about encouraging them or lying to them. If they lose five pounds instead, they will get rid of at least twenty pounds of percussion in their knees every time they walk. To lose weight, you don't need to exercise, but to achieve a higher end of fulfillment, exercise IS strictly necessary.

Walking under the sun with a good rhythm, contemplating the landscape and breathing fresh air is a great pleasure; and finishing your exercise routine at the gym after the walk is to meet your body again: your vigor reappears, and you feel you can do whatever you want. With your new holistic attitude that turns body, mind and soul into one, you have already realized that mental age does not correspond to the paradigm that limits "having to carry the weight of years"; without the sophism that exercise is the condition to lose weight, to make the last adjustments and reach fullness, enjoy exercise and the gym, you only need to lose those few pounds that are left over to make your weight and proportion optimal.

Have you ever wondered why, since you learned to eat, at the end of the weight loss process you have experienced, the body is the one that is practically forcing you to exercise. Due to pollution, stress, medications, infections, radiation or poor diet, the genetic factor, psychological trauma and, above all, having stopped exercising, the body's production of hormones and enzymes is decreasing; for example, melatonin connects the environment — day and night — with the neural in the brain and facilitates sleep, because when it is dark it invites us to sleep. Melanin, responsible for skin and hair coloration, resists pH variations and acts as a filter to protect us from the sun, especially from ultraviolet rays and the damage they could cause to the deep layers of the skin. Over time, these substances are depleted and, as a direct consequence, the hours of sleep tend to decrease, the skin and hair become discolored and spots and gray hair appear. As a result of insufficient sleep, among other things, the levels of the hormones estrogen and testosterone decrease, and sexual desire diminishes. We call this chain reaction — in which oxidizing free radicals participate — aging, and it is precisely the antioxidants that are responsible for reducing and mitigating the aging action in the body. Exercise is health! Scientific observation in the 21ST CENTURY has revealed that, at any age, with an adequate diet containing sulfur and with the practice of exercise, glutathione, the most important antioxidant molecule in relation to longevity, recovers quickly.

Early research agreed that if acidification increases in the body and the toxic load is too great, the liver becomes overloaded and clogged. When this detoxification becomes more difficult as we lose this glutathione molecule, we become susceptible to oxidative stress, free radicals, infections, and uncontrolled cell growth: cancer. The study *"Glutathione: in sickness and in health"*,[144] published in 1998 in the prestigious British medical journal *The Lancet*, found a lower glutathione count in hospitalized elderly; minimal levels in the elderly and somewhat better in healthy elderly compared to a high level in young, healthy people. Today it has been discovered that — unlike the other antioxidants ingested with food — in the process of building proteins, the body produces glutathione (GSH) by the simple combination of three groups of amino acids: cysteine, glycine, and glutamine. Dr. Mark Hyman tells how in his article "Essential glutathione

---

[144] S. L. Nuttall, U. Martin, A. J. Sinclair & M. J. Kendall (1998): *"Glutathione: in sickness and in health"*. *The Lancet*, *351* (9103) 645-646. https://www.thelancet.com/journals/lancet/article/PIIS0140-6736 (05)78428-2/fulltext.

is the mother of all antioxidants."[145] The sulfur in garlic, onions, cruciferous vegetables such as broccoli, kale, cabbage, cauliflower, watercress, mustard greens, gives glutathione "the ability to regenerate and recover the other antioxidants; the most critical part of the detoxification system." Sulfur molecules act as a blotting paper to which free radicals, toxins, heavy metals such as mercury, and other harmful products adhere and are then carried into the bile and feces to be excreted from the body. For example, the antioxidants in vitamins C and E and alpha lipoic acid, which in the first instance protect us against chronic diseases, neutralize free radicals, are released from an electron, and oxidized. The magic of glutathione lies in the fact that, before regenerating itself, it recycles the molecules of the other antioxidants to then produce or not — the key is in the exercise — one more molecule of glutathione and recover its own levels. Thus, glutathione is the highest-ranking detoxifying agent in the body that protects our cells and promotes immune function in them that fights infection and inflammation. Logically, it prevents cancer. Studies show that glutathione is a great recycler of antioxidants and influences the metabolism to function energetically independent; therefore, it has been vital in the search for and development of treatments against AIDS.

Age is just a number in the mind and the body does NOT have a clock that counts the minutes in reverse. Many people over fifty-five, sixty-five and seventy-five — who used to look ninety — have proven to the world that exercise builds muscle and, with enough tone, reverses a haggard appearance. It's a fact: with a healthy diet loaded with antioxidants, glutathione to complete the cycle pushes you to exercise to fully regenerate and quickly resume its rightful place, because it increases the strength

---

[145] https://drhyman.com/blog/2010/05/19/glutathione-the-mother-of-all-antioxidants/.

and physical endurance of muscles and directly influences the metabolism to produce the fats involved in muscle development and thus work specifically to reduce the body's recovery time.

Only in this 21ST CENTURY have we discovered the reason why the human body, to survive — from its animal instinct — makes us exercise. This fact corroborates that, without the need to force us, the will to exercise is born in us as something natural. If you have been attentive to the body's messages, the reciprocity with the being is cordial; once you have gotten rid of the excess weight that sabotaged your will, without haste and making use of your caloric investment without starving, the body will reward you. Now that you know that emotional stability does not only depend on exercise, whose objective is different, you understand that the path is different, and that longevity can be achieved; it is only a matter of time before the body invites you to walk. For you, who want to rejuvenate, and for pre-diabetics and type 2 diabetics, who must change their lifestyle to reverse the disease, these are the steps:

Learn to eat.

Stop being a burner of simple absorption carbohydrates — white bread, pasta, rice, flours, and starches — and become a burner of healthy fats. Keep in mind that fried and breaded foods are bad for you.

Focus on obtaining from fruit, vegetables, and greens — the complex carbohydrates of the neutral group — the minerals, enzymes, vitamins, and antioxidants that ensure the body is always prone to alkalinity.

Eat vegetarian one day a week and take good care of your protein intake.

Get used to aromatic infusions such as cow's foot, dandelion, plantain and licorice, green tea, or fenugreek, which restore pancreatic function by increasing the activity of insulin-secreting cells, and no more cold drinks to get through meals.

Sleep well, but if you have not yet achieved it — for example, because you suffer from apnea —, it is urgent that you let them help you with a device that provides you with oxygen; otherwise, your brain function will soon be very compromised, or help yourself with one milligram melatonin, which invites you to sleep and is not addictive. Do not sleep more than eight hours a day.

In your alcove, balcony, or terrace, before breakfast, but after the warm water with lemon and fruit, do gentle exercises, preferably in the sun. Sweating is a clear sign of detoxification, and the sun synthesizes the vitamin D that your bones require. Focus on breathing. You can find many examples of light floor exercises on the internet.

In short, with weight loss and the habit of eating five or six times a day — as long as the pancreas is not too impaired — ; with cortisol controlled and sleep regulated; with glutathione at the ready and antioxidants recovered, the metabolism is "reset" and accelerated so that the conditions that favor the way to break insulin resistance are reinstalled in the body.

Personal trainers for years have tested a modern method of exercise and recommend that you structure your own exercise plan that combines aerobic oxygenation-running, swimming, cycling, walking... — with anaerobic intensity-weights, speed workouts and exercises that require great effort in a short time — without the long hours in the gym of the previous century. The concept has changed: focus on three or four routines per week to provide muscle tone and, when exercising, invest 75% of the time in cardiovascular — aerobic — exercise; walking at a demanding pace requires seven minutes to reach the heart rate and to run between two and a half to three miles, thirty-five to forty minutes more. Then, in the gym, without resting, add the fifteen to twenty minutes to complete the hour with anaerobic exercise: do ten to fifteen repetitions per machine — four to five different ones — ; alternate with ten to fifteen sit-ups until you complete one hundred or one hundred and twenty-five, which is enough to complete the hour of exercise. According to your particular needs, don't forget to include some discipline, such as yoga, that requires relaxation or some sport; even golf requires inner focus, and its challenge is to beat yourself.

Chapter IX

The Intelligent Consumer

On October 26, 2015, the World Health Organization, and the United Nations International Agency for Research on Cancer (IARC) declared that processed meats — hamburgers, sausages or sausages with preservatives and other unnatural substances — are carcinogenic, and that red meat is probably carcinogenic.[146] Expressions of support or rejection on social networks were not long in coming. This bewilderment highlights the fact that most people are uprooted from the truth. The reason for popular disenchantment is unknowledgeable and denotes that disinformation or silence has been used as a tool to manipulate our thinking and actions; however, when the intelligent consumer — which we all are — learns the facts, he/she decides to take control of his/her life: the first thing he/she does is to investigate and maintain a cautious attitude.

The TWENTIETH CENTURY brought together all the development of our history, which came upon us, and we began the mad race we are in today. The elites: intellectuals, governments, and the clergy, benefiting from fear and ignorance, have always manipulated and doctored multiple truths to suit their own interests. For example, learned Christians such as Basil the Great, Ambrose Aurelianus and Augustine of Hippo knew the hidden truth about the myth of the flat earth. Or, as happened with the

---

[146] https://www.iarc.fr/wp-content/uploads/2018/07/pr240_E.pdf.

Dark Ages and the Inquisition, dogmas have had sedative effects; after centuries and with the increase of ignorance — which is not calmed just by learning to read and write —, since the Middle Ages, the clergy preferred to remain silent or were silenced so that myths and legends, such as the flat earth, Adam and Eve — the first parents — or that heaven, hell and purgatory were a physical place, could spread. The delicate thing is that, even in the present, with additional fears generated by uncertainty, because it is recorded in the sacred books, each side interprets their sacred books with the solemnity of when they were written and still invoke, in their own way and with different names — for example El, Yahweh, Elohim, Abba, Adonai, Jehovah, Allah and hundreds of other names that identify their qualities —, a god, produced out of our arrogance, that dictates rules and laws, humiliates and segregates and punishes the infidels. And in the political arena, those who invoke fear through populist ideas use the concept of God to inflame or appease passions so as to manipulate the people in their favor.

Fear and ignorance have always played their part. For example, the republican model of Rome, with a division of public powers — the separation of powers in the Roman Republic disappeared when the Roman Empire was established — succeeded in defending the democracy that was later lost under Augustus Caesar. But the unusual thing is that, hand in hand with the fanaticism that spread over the centuries, fear, ignorance and fanaticism widened a gap that has served in the modern era for today's ultra-right politicians — who support those who instill more fear among their followers with the holy scriptures — to gain followers; and on the other side, to the left, give way to those who, disguised as a communism that banished God by decree but beyond that, manage their kidnapped peoples with violence and at will. To achieve this, both extremes trample democracy and claim to love the poor, but just make the people poorer while enriching themselves. In the antagonism of political and economic ideas, the tremendous novelty of the TWENTIETH CENTURY was that of mutually exclusive extreme thinking. They have brought us to the limit of our own extinction: in the 21ST CENTURY, with absolute maturity, we must decide where to go.

This extreme thinking has tested us for more than a century! It was unheard of that Greta Thunberg,[147] then sixteen years old, on September 23, 2019, had to raise her voice in protest at the United Nations on behalf of the very young: "Here and now is where we draw the line. The world is waking up and change is coming, like it or not! We are at the beginning of a mass extinction and all you can talk about is money and fairy tales of eternal economic growth. How dare you!".

The extreme left still tries to make social classes clash and does not notice that these confrontations are increasingly rare, but that street protests against inconsistent governments or corrupt narco-governments incapable of serving everyone, rich and poor alike, are on the rise around the world. To destabilize, it easily manipulates the most ignorant, because, according to it — it does not avoid it —, the only way to protest is to create chaos with violence and destroy public and private property; looting is its reward. But the worst damage done by the left, especially for the Western world, is that it prostituted the truth about a form of government that, besides overcoming trials and errors and being economically successful, allows free enterprise and private property and, socially, guarantees the people universal education and health. This form of government is not perfect, because it obviously requires honest management of the treasury, but it motivates the most advanced societies in the world. The right-wingers, and the spheres of power with control over information,

---

[147] https://news.un.org/es/story/2019/09/1462622.

dare to ridicule the press and label as fake news any palpable truth, even if it is undeniable. Disinformation is becoming a habit: in cyber warfare, they are making use of our data to disrupt social networks and to influence, and alter the people's decisions in their favor, at the time of election. The short film *The Great Hack* (Netflix, 2019) documents this fully.

Either we continue in inertia, destroy the world, and disappear. Or we stop to examine the manipulations of extreme thinking and learn to navigate in two lanes: the one that leads us at high speed in everyday life and the one that allows us to broaden our criteria and contribute to change. In the 21ST CENTURY, the dilemma is that, before protesting and demanding everything, we must carefully verify the information that reaches us on our cell phones and that which is just a click away. The network is full of harmful and malicious information that encourages us to act incorrectly. Among other things, we have discovered that nothing is free and that we comprise 70% or more of the engine of the economy.

The reality we live in every day is still a very persistent illusion, as Albert Einstein pointed out: extreme thoughts benefit from justifying the perfect framing of the mainstream in which we live, where ignorance persists, and the slower walking second reality is distorted. Consequently, that "real" world we perceive of paradigm-adjusted, dismayed, and guideless money does not even know where to go today. We look everywhere and the firmament intrigues us, the stars attract us, and we are always trying to search in the darkness for the light they emit. The irony is that darkness is precisely what we know most about the human universe. At this point, I am reminded of the saying of a Californian, Marianne Deborah Williamson: "Only when we have found the monsters within us, will we stop trying to kill them in the outside world. And we will realize that we can't, because all the darkness in the world comes from the darkness in the heart, and that is where we must work."

Of course, we cannot discard the spiritual reality; when the three realities — the high-speed one in which we live daily, its antipode, which allows us to stop and think, and the spiritual one — confront each other and openly coincide with the maturity of the individual, positive changes for humanity emerge: thus, was democracy born. The other outstanding fact in relation to spiritual reality and extreme thoughts — which denote ignorance and lead to chaos — is that they possess nothing of Jesus, because in complicit silence they brand him and use him as the most subversive being of all times. Facundo Cabral (1937-2011), Argentine poet and singer-songwriter, said: "In an eternity for that reason, because TIME is a human invention, you can always start again!". It is not by chance that the theories of Einstein and others assure us that past, present, and future events all coexist in the same space-time. If this were not so, we could not be pondering the human quantum universe. We know that, in the cosmos, the gravitational effect of an object — a galaxy, for example — can deform the surrounding space-time, and it turns out that, depending on the speed with which that object rotates — acting as a lens — it can even magnify and project its own or reflected light backwards. Since we are matter or — better — light that transcends space-time — Einstein said that they are inseparable and exist as a fourth dimension —, the light that illuminates the world, that from year zero illuminates us all, is real: the light of that beacon of time — which turns backwards to illuminate the followers of Buddha and forwards, for the same almost six hundred years, to the followers of Mohammed, for it is said that Siddhartha Gautama was born in 563 BC and the prophet Mohammed in 570 AD — does not come alone; to bring us its greatest brightness, its intensity is generated by the energy that created itself and that identifies us and has always been there in the human universe. Human darkness is so overwhelming that, as a consequence of the devastating damage done by wars and atomic bombs, in 1947 the *Bulletin of Atomic Scientists*[148] (BAS) created the symbolic apocalypse clock to measure year by year the time we have left. Between 2018 and 2019, the clock remained at two minutes to midnight (23:58), but in January 2020, due to the ineptitude to address climate change, cyber warfare misinformation and nuclear proliferation, scientists moved the countdown forward and we are only one minute and forty seconds away from the end of our existence. And what about the light?

The laws of classical physics — the established measurement patterns, calendars, clocks, and aspects such as time and temperature, which correspond to the macro — are valid for measuring the extent and spectra of the universe. However, these principles are not valid when applied to the submicroscopic systems of quantum physics and, in particular, to photons or particles of light. The German theoretical physicist Werner Karl Heisenberg (1901-1976) — winner of the Nobel Prize in Physics in 1932 for formulating the uncertainty principle: it is impossible to measure simultaneously and precisely the position and linear momentum of a particle — stated: "The first sip from the cup of science makes you an atheist, but at the bottom of the cup God awaits you". Now, I know and can tell you that never before have religion and science been so close. Quantum physics is not as complicated a subject as you might think.

Before that, history had already given us Einstein (1879-1955), winner of the Nobel Prize in Physics in 1921, who before his death reviewed and shared the earlier theories of Max Planck — his friend and mentor, Dean at the University of Berlin, when

---

[148] https://thebulletin.org/.

Einstein was just a professor —, who discovered the quantum and proposed the quantum theory. Already, today, in laboratories, advanced experiments confirm the statement Planck made when he received his Nobel Prize in Physics in 1918: "There is no such thing as matter as such. All matter originates and exists only by virtue of a force, which brings the particle of an atom into vibration and keeps the shortest distance of the solar system from the atom together. We must assume that behind this force there is a conscious and intelligent mind. This mind is the matrix of all matter". Let us remember that we are energy and that in itself that photon — that tiny invisible particle — indifferently possesses a great power; the foundation of quantum physics clarifies the other truth that is confirmed by that particle of light that we do not see, but that we feel, is enough to ignite the spirit in every creature — that is what childbirth is all about.

However, in humans, this spiritual baptism — the divine blessing — lacking in frequency — unlike other creatures —, is not enough to enlighten the individual, who needs to constantly ingest sips of wisdom consecrated with knowledge — not with dogma — to invigorate the brain, which summarizes the source of illumination that forges criteria. With a broad mind, the point of equilibrium expands. In order not to extinguish the original fire and to avoid the slow and painful extinction of its intelligence, it is with faith and spirituality — the food of the soul — that, without fear, together with others — in physics, an illuminated body is a body that receives the light that illuminates it from a different source, which can pass through it or not —, we will find the path that leads to the truth and to the change through which it leads us. And it is said that, having fulfilled this precept, the force that identifies us all will shine in us, is God: Love, which flows inevitably through the eternal lighthouse: "It is light, due to its constant frequency that is thus related, that manages to transport electromagnetic energy in the waves of magnetism and heat which light also possesses"; this is the basic principle, the law of quantum physics that science books explain step by step.

Conversely, in the macroscopic, mankind has for centuries searched the dark with telescopes. We know that the light from stars was emitted in the past and, the farther away an object is, the further back in time we see. For example — even if the linear distance is enormous — when we see a star a thousand light years away through a telescope, this star is as it was a thousand years ago. Well, it turns out, that faith, that light of hope, that force that makes us persist until we find that star, and makes us stare through the telescope for hours until, when it appears, we see its shine; that light of constant frequency, was already within you from birth and, although in itself it contains its own opposite of repulsion and negative polarity, it is part of our cosmogony: the Love that constantly surrounds, grows, evolves and that emerged from our feelings long ago.

The 20TH CENTURY has been the most dynamic and significant in the history of human development. At the beginning of the chapter, I mentioned meat consumption. To put it in perspective for the intelligent consumer, we cannot overlook a detail that characterized us and led us to greater excesses of accumulation, squandering everything, and, perhaps without realizing it, wasting food and, without hesitation, consuming all types of meat, especially red and processed meats.

It was by eating so much meat that the kings of the past died of gout. History and, in general, literature and the arts were in charge of narrating and portraying how the kings enjoyed their bacchanals and banquets, and all the luxury and daily excesses of their courts. Little mention is made of the pages and lackeys, whom they describe as "hungry and opportunistic" who knew how to cleverly hide a piece of ham; but logically, they were healthier than those they served. And it so happens that this frustration of lacking the excesses of the aristocracy and the desire to live like kings was reinforced by advertising and the movie boom at the beginning of the 20TH CENTURY. Thus, for centuries humanity has carried the subliminal message of the "commoner complex" that leads some to eat and drink at dizzying speeds: we should be like them and, moreover, full, and "healthy". After World War I (1914-1918) and the 1918 flu pandemic — misnamed Spanish flu, an outbreak of the influenza A virus (subtype H1N1) — which around the world killed between twenty and forty million of the proletariat that had grown up with the industrial revolution and had been oblivious to monarchies and empires in conflict. In his novel *The Great Gatsby*, the American, Scott Fitzgerald, reminds us how in the 1920s it was usual for the ruling class and the new middle class — formerly proletarian — with greater purchasing power to recreate those feasts and match their excesses. And for all that, sometimes, being full, that subconscious something still compels and demands to ravage everything; the "commoner" who believes that this could be his last abundant meal.

Would the proposed changes — to stop consuming cereals loaded with harmful sugars, industrial food with preservatives, excessive red meat, colas and energy drinks, unhealthy fats, avoiding unnecessary drugs and pharmaceuticals and, on the contrary, consuming more vegetables to maintain the alkaline pH — give a blow to the economy that could mean massive job losses, including yours? No.

The loss of jobs caused by addressing climate change is already a central theme in the speeches of denialist politicians, who propose deregulating the production of fossil fuels to generate employment and keep the economy stable. In short, they sell you the idea of keeping things as they are, because it is supposedly in your interest. They are not afraid of novelty, constant development, or progress; their fear is something else. Meanwhile, many politicians protect the interests of the mega-corporations and corporations with which they are involved so that they will sponsor them again and thus remain in Congress. In effect, the companies pass quietly — their voice is money — to continue their monopolizing pace; with strategic mergers, they collect assets and job cuts are on the rise. The thirst for money is so serious that — while issuing banknotes — the economic gurus make us believe that companies that achieve "normal" yields and profits and that guarantee fair salaries and benefits to their employees cannot be considered successful unless they comply with the stock market norm of pursuing extravagant growth.

Industry, in constant production, plans but, even so, does not always have someone to sell things to; it assesses the risks. But whether it prevails or disappears, the labor variable in that equation — the human factor — is the least important. Due to the impoverishment of the middle class, the base of the social pyramid has widened further; the big difference is that we are adaptable to the daily onslaught of the economy; by force majeure, we learned to reinvent ourselves; the owners of power do not reinvent themselves, because they do not need to! Communism and capitalism see the "people" as their slaves or as numbers, productive objects. Companies are born, grow or stagnate, cease, and die at the pace of development, technology, advances in science, communications. An example is Kodak, which opened its doors in 1892 to produce photographic material, equipment, and film; in 2012 it went bankrupt and is not even a shadow of the multinational emporium it once was. In the digital era, coal is gone; soon oil and gas, which are fossil fuels that leave a carbon footprint, will be gone as energy sources, as well as the internal combustion engine. Hiroshima, Nagasaki, Three Mile Island, Chernobyl, Mururoa, Fangataufa, Fukushima... have shown how devastating atomic energy can be. There are more than 400 nuclear power plants in the world; but what are we to do with all that radioactive waste? Germany and other developed countries have started to close all their plants. Photovoltaic cells are now an affordable option and large solar power farms have been appearing. All these developments correspond to the natural development of societies. The New York futurist writer Alvin Toffler (1928-2016) skillfully compared civilization to waves that have been coming: first the agricultural revolution and then the industrial revolution; in his book *The Third Wave* he described — with some predictions — the post-industrial society that was already pounding the 20TH CENTURY. What better metaphor to explain what is happening!

When the wave hits, there is the momentary trauma of change, but it passes quickly; then — like the money vital to the economy — the fluid slowly and gently washes up on the beach. After prosperity comes the hangover and there we are: under a burning sun that does not let us think. As happened with the rise of the monopolies, countries and their communities have begun to contemplate isolationism again in order to be big and successful; in emulating the empires, they have not realized that this is precisely what the receding waves are all about. The fourth wave took us by surprise and brought with it the technology that will allow us to no longer depend on oil and that is already beginning to change things. The third wave had made it possible for the political hegemony to control dirty energy sources; this is what those who did not see the fourth wave coming are afraid of: inexhaustible clean energies — cheaper than oil, coming from the sun, wind, tides, volcanoes, and from the air — just as it sounds —, they are almost free and difficult to quantify and control. The elite do not know how to own them, they cannot, and they fear losing the pooled power that the empires have fought over.

In the United States and around the world, despite the creation of businesses and jobs, everyday stores, supermarkets, factories, shopping malls and other stores are closing; people are losing their jobs massively. There is greater invisible poverty than ever in the homeless population: the homeless, single mothers, the disabled, students and veterans who cannot get jobs, or immigrants who have not yet learnt the language.[149]

It is not only for the sake of the planet that the intelligent consumer should question the extreme ideologies that opt for isolationism, sponsored by patriots who think that the enemy is their neighbor. They do not share the idea of a world without borders, without limits, without flags. Due to competition — which requires them to win I don't know what — they do not believe in or, rather, are not interested in, a consolidated global economy that would facilitate the redistribution of wealth and social mobility and prefer to continue dreaming of the bonanza that the exploitation and control of dirty energy sources has brought them. The signals we are receiving are more significant than any wall of the past, because they actually isolate and warn us now to be prepared for the armed conflicts that will gain strength in the new spiral of empires that the world will not be able to withstand: Brexit, which on January 31, 2020 took the United Kingdom out of the European Union; the suspension of the ban on anti-personnel mines by the U.S. military and its deployment of a low-yield nuclear weapon on a submarine to deter friendly and rival powers from using similar weapons without having to respond to each other with mega-bombs; — I thought we were about to grow out of adolescence — the emergence of the coronavirus in mysterious and totalitarian China, which spread

---

[149] https://www.youtube.com/watch?v=JHDkALRz5Rk
https://blogs.msn.com/es-us/pobrezaquenovemos/
acerca-de-la-pobreza-que-no-vemos/.

panic, locked us all up and weakened the world economy. No wonder that in 2019 global military spending had its biggest rise in ten years[150] and that, despite the pandemic, in 2020 it rose another 2.6%.

We talk about religion, science, and energy. Prophecies — good or bad, positive, or negative — are fulfilled because we implement them. Yet, those who divide to rule also fear the other reality that makes money: wars, which we almost always enter to resolve conflicts. Extreme and exclusionary thinking is harmful to the awakening of humanity. Abraham Lincoln, President of the United States, in his Union Address to the Congress "of the people" in 1862, said:

The dogmas of the quiet past are inadequate to the stormy present. The occasion is piled high with difficulty, and we must rise with the occasion. As our case is new, so we must think anew and act anew. We must disenthrall ourselves, and then we shall save our country.

Fellow citizens, we cannot escape history...The fiery trial through which we pass will light us down in honor or dishonor, to the latest generation. We say we are for the Union. The world will not forget that we say this. We know how to save the Union. In giving freedom to the slave, we assure freedom to the free — honorable alike in what we give and what we preserve. We will nobly save or meanly lose the last, best hope of earth...

---

[150] https://www.sipri.org/media/press-release/2021/world-military-spending-rises-almost-2-trillion-2020#:~:text=(Stockholm%2C%20 26%20April%202021),Peace%20Research%20Institute%20(SIPRI).

Synthetic coatings continue to be endocrine disruptors

This is a good time for the intelligent consumer to be on his guard against the continuous and constant experiment we have been in since the 20TH CENTURY with regard to the products and devices we buy to enjoy a more comfortable and, perhaps, more convenient life... Faced with the facts, the intelligent consumer maintains a cautious attitude towards the strange names that appear on food ingredients and on the labels of new mass consumer products. Read and verify the information when making your purchases; supply, demand and put pressure on industry to stop producing what is not good for the planet and its inhabitants.

Since the end of the 20TH CENTURY, a group of scientists, led by Tegan S. Horan, have warned about the potential risk of bisphenol A (BPA), which is used to prevent corroded metal from touching food in cans, and discovered that the malformations of fertilized eggs in female mice were due to a sudden increase in chromosomes produced by this polymer which was being released by the plastic cages in which these animals lived in the laboratory. This led to a new generation of bisphenols: bisphenols F and S (BPF and BPS), which now coat the inside of the aluminum in 58% of soda cans. And again, in 2018, this same group of scientists warned about the replacement F and S bisphenols.[151] BPA is still used in canned goods, in car parts, and in thermal paper for printing receipts at cash registers.

---

[151] Tegan S. Horan, Hannah Pulcastro, Crystal Lawson, Roy Gerona, Spencer Martin, Mary C. Gieske, Caroline V. Sartain & Patricia A. Hunt (2018): *"Replacement bisphenols adversely affect mouse gametogenesis with consequences for subsequent generations"*. Current Biology, 28, 2948-2954. https://www.cell.com/current-biology/pdf/S0960-9822(18)30861-3.pdf.

Canned goods are a useful invention attributed to Nicolas Appert, who developed them between 1795 and 1810 so that soldiers would have clean and safe food rations at any time. They save lives but were designed for casual consumption in case of emergency or necessity. EWG, based on research by Hiroshi Masuno[152] and others in 2002, says, "They show that low doses of BPA in combination with insulin stimulate both the formation and growth of fat cells." This is bad news, especially for diabetics and people who are used to eating and drinking canned food.

A 2014 investigation found BPA, BPF or BPS in urine samples from 95% of participants in the United States.[153] The Environmental Working Group (EWG) noted:

It's a problem that's not just limited to Americans, it's worldwide; analysis of our tests reveals that in one in five cans tested and in one-third of all vegetables and pasta — ravioli and noodles with tomato sauce — a single serving, one can, would expose a pregnant woman to BPA at levels entering a factor of five times the dose linked to birth defects and permanent damage to developing male reproductive organs.

Bisphenol A (BPA), bisphenols S (BPS) and F (BPF) used in canned foods, perfluorinated non-stick agents (PFOA and PFOS) in Teflon — polytetrafluoroethylene (PTFE) —,

---

[152] Hiroshi Masuno, Teruki Kidani, Keizo Sekiya, Kenshi Sakayama, Takahiko Shiosaka, Haruyasu Yamamoto & Katsuhisa Honda (2002): *"Bisphenol A in combination with insulin can accelerate the conversion of 3T3-L1 fibroblasts to adipocytes"*. Journal of Lipid Research, 43 (5), 676-684. https://www.ncbi.nlm.nih.gov/pubmed/11971937.

[153] Hans-Joachim Lehmler, Buyun Liu, Manuel Gadogbe & Wei Bao (2018). *"Exposure to Bisphenol A, Bisphenol F, and Bisphenol S in U. S. adults and children: The National Health and Nutrition Examination Survey 2013-2014"*. ACS Omega, 3 (6), 6523-6532. doi: 10.1021/acsomega.8b00824. https://www.ncbi.nlm.nih.gov/pmc/articles/PMC6028148/.

parabens, and phthalates — among other chemical compounds — are xenohormones that accumulate in the liver and kidneys, cause obesity and ruin the immune system. They are known as xenoestrogens, and their main characteristic is that they are active endocrine disruptors. "Xeno-" means 'foreign', 'foreign', 'from the outside'; and "endo-" means 'within', 'inside'; endogenous originates or is born inside, like the cell that forms inside another cell. Estrogens are naturally produced by the ovaries; they are endogenous. Xenoestrogens behave like endogenous estrogens, in essence usurping the function of carrying the physical and chemical message to the reproductive system and the brain at the receptor of these synthetic hormones. The problem is that they interfere in many ways in the functions of the endocrine system, as they vary the way they behave, and one of them is that they increase the synthesis of estrogens, purely feminine hormones. Much research remains to be done.

Animal studies with surprisingly small doses of xenoestrogens have linked these chemicals to the development of heart disease, diabetes, infertility, birth defects, miscarriages, and cancers. They have also found that the BPS that replaces bisphenol A leaches into the placenta of mice, transfers to the blood and affects the brain development of those babies.[154] It causes early puberty in girls; as for breast cancer, it affects oncogenesis and has generationally transmissible mutagenic effects. For all these reasons, experts recommend handling shopping receipts as little as possible,

---

[154] Jiude Mao, Ashish Jain, Nancy D. Denslow, Mohammad-Zaman Nouri, Sixue Cheng, Tingting Wang, Ning Zhuh, Jin Kohh, Saurav J. Sarma, Barbara W. Sumner, Zhentian Lei, Lloyd W. Sumner, Nathan J. Bivensk, R. Michael Roberts, Geetu Tuteja & Cheryl S. Rosenfeld (2020): "*Bisphenol A and bisphenol S disruptions of the mouse placenta and potential effects on the placenta-brain axis*". *Proceedings of the National Academy of Sciences, PNAS, 117* (9), 4642-4652. https://www.pnas.org/content/pnas/117/9/4642.full.pdf.

because bisphenol stays on your hands, and you absorb it. Do not crumple or accumulate receipts; if you pay by credit card, the purchase is automatically registered in the electronic reports provided by banks, and they are usually sufficient for tax support or for any claim.

After years of scientific research — as happened with the endocrine disruptors triclosan and triclocarban, protected by the FDA for forty years — the industry began to avoid bisphenol A in canned goods and PFOA and PFOS in its products. Have you heard "let your car breathe"? Yes, BPA is also in the dashboard and interior trim of most cars which, when closed, heat up, expelling it and it's in the air; open it up, don't turn on the air conditioning and let it breathe before you get in the car.

The report *A Toxic Issue*,[155] collated over ten years by the French journalist Stéphane Horel, denounces how the chemical industry lobbied the European Commission that deals with these issues and managed to block the adoption of measures against endocrine disruptors that "surround us" and are an attack on the health of people, who by habit or lack of time, utilize canned food, sachet soups, precooked or frozen food in their diet. They are even in personal hygiene products. Around the world, when the establishment tries to hide the truth at all costs, it murders ecologists; in the United States, in recent years, at least ninety people, including researchers, doctors and specialists, who promoted holistic or alternative medicine practices which went against the establishment, have died, or disappeared in very strange circumstances.[156]

---

[155] Stéphane Horel & Corporate Europe Observatory (2015): *A toxic affair: how the chemical industry lobby blocked action against endocrine disruptors.* https://www.ecologistasenaccion.org/wp-content/uploads/adjuntos-spip/pdf/info_un-asunto-toxico.pdf.

[156] https://nexusnewsfeed.com/article/human-rights/mysterious-deaths-of-holistic-doctors-around-the-country/.

Labels that say "free of BPA, PFOA, PFOS or parabens" do not guarantee that the product is safe, as the replacement ingredients could still be potentially harmful. Concerning obesity, for example, Melanie Jacobson, M.D., at New York University School of Medicine, has advanced a study linking BPS and BPF to increased childhood obesity.[157] The indications that microwave ovens have negative health effects are very serious. If, for some reason, you decide to cook food in a microwave oven, do not use plastic containers because they increase the release of chemicals including BPA.

In a study published in *The Lancet, Diabetes & Endocrinology*,[158] researchers developed a more accurate method for measuring toxicity levels from bisphenols and other endocrine disruptors — BPA, PFOA, PFOS, triclosan, benzophenone, parabens, phthalates — present in mass consumer products such as food packaging, personal hygiene products, toys and even food. They have found that measurements previously used by regulatory agencies such as the FDA are seriously flawed and may be underestimating our exposure by as much as forty-four times. Another study[159] states:

---

[157] Melanie H. Jacobson, Miriam Woodward, Wei Bao, Buyun Liu & Leonardo Trasande (2019). *"Urinary bisphenols and obesity prevalence among U. S. children and adolescents"*. *Journal of the Endocrine Society*, JES, 3 (9), 1715-1726, https://doi.org/10.1210/js.2019-00201. https://academic.oup.com/jes/article/3/9/1715/5537531.

[158] Roy Gerona, Frederick S. vom Saal & Patricia A. Hunt (2020): *"BPA: have flawed analytical techniques compromised risk assessments?"*. *The Lancet, Diabetes & Endocrinology*, 8 (1), 11-13. doi: 10.1016/S2213-8587(19)30381-X. https://www.thelancet.com/journals/landia/article/PIIS2213-8587(19)30381-X/fulltext.

[159] Linda G. Kahn, Claire Philippat, Shoji F. Nakayama, Rémy Slama & Leonardo Trasande (2020): *"Endocrine-disrupting chemicals: implications for human health"*. *The Lancet, Diabetes & Endocrinology*, 8 (8), 703-718. https://www.thelancet.com/journals/landia/article/PIIS2213-8587(20)30129-7/fulltext.

Mounting evidence supports urgent action to reduce exposure to endocrine disruptors. Unfortunately, some of the chemicals that manufacturers have used in BPA-free products, particularly BPS and BPF, have been shown to have BPA-like effects. Plastic items that have recycling numbers 3 and 7 likely contain one of these chemicals, but the best approach is to avoid plastic altogether, particularly when it comes to food packaging.

PFOA and PFOS — the old Teflons — in frying pans, pots and utensils containing lead, copper or non-anodized aluminum deteriorate and, with the slightest scratch, are no longer safe; due to the effect of heat, the particles of these chemicals are released, and we end up ingesting them along with the food. There are already safer options: earthenware pots, lead-free glazed ceramic, or borosilicate glass — Corning, Pyrex, Duran, Kimax — are a durable option of inert materials to use in the oven. And on the stovetop, the trendiest cookware is stainless steel, ceramic, anodized aluminum, or titanium with nonstick coatings. To avoid peeling these frying pans, pots and pans, wooden utensils should be used and soft sponges to wash them. Although certified silicone baking sheets and molds are nonstick and withstand low and high temperatures at the same time — up to 500 °F in the heat and 140 °F in the cold — they are likely to react with fatty or highly acidic foods and ordinary silicone is likely to deteriorate or melt and mix with the baked goods. Mineral iron pans tend to rust. Cast iron pans, which is sometimes enameled — lead-free — are the heaviest; because of their versatility on the stove top, stove or oven, professional chefs prefer them, even if washing them is not easy.

Let's move on to another topic. From accumulating everything, consuming and feeling "I can do it too!", predation has made garbage and waste on Earth limitless, so learning to recycle is a priority: it consists of adopting practices and behaviors so that recycling and reusing organic and inorganic waste becomes a habit. It seems that we have already begun to make sense of this: we do it, but only half-heartedly.

Recycling culture and other issues

Use and throw away has become a habit. Let's not deny it: there is something inside that makes us indifferent to what no longer represents a possession, a monetary tangible; we despise what we believe has no value and it seems to hurt us to recycle. "Despise" means 'to look down on with disrespect or aversion', 'to regard as negligible, worthless, or distasteful' (Merriam Webster) and we quite like it. We scorn what no longer contributes anything: friendships and old loves; obsolete things that we no longer like or that fulfill their function; the leftovers on the plate, the cupboard, the closet; the playroom in whose production many hands intervened, and huge resources were invested.

"There isn't enough food for so many people!". False. They have us convinced that, to alleviate hunger in the world, we must expand the land for cultivation and animal husbandry to produce more food. The food we throw away, which often ends up in lakes, rivers, the sea... already exceeds 45% worldwide. Due to the 'commoner complex', the eagerness to produce money and the abundance of dishes that are cultural factors, this percentage is higher in the United States. Take-out food involves dosing it in individual packages; sauces in sachets that are not used and food that is not consumed add up to tons of food that does not go to the stomach of those who need it. Opulence and lack are two sides of the same coin: especially in developed and rich countries, where young people play and throw food on the table while in developing countries — such as those in Latin America — or even in Spain, not only among the poor, but it is also considered a great sin to waste food. Malnutrition is serious: the underlying cause of the death of millions of children is hunger. NGOs that find a space in the chain of waste, and organizations that creatively give another destination to waste and garbage, make a positive note, and make a difference, because in addition to working for the health of the planet, they have become an engine that generates lots of jobs; a different model that, without the excessive profit motive, discards predation.

In the United States, *Clean the World* recycles bars of soap that are only used for one or two days in hotels, processes them, and distributes them in countries, where water and soap are a luxury, and death from viruses and gastrointestinal diseases such as dysentery — which kills 1,450 children a day and used to cause more deaths among soldiers than the war itself — is rife. The social commitment objective of the ECOALF foundation in Spain (ecoalf.com), is to collect garbage from the sea with the help of fishermen: it recycles it and, selectively, with new scientific and technological knowledge, gives it back its value by using it as raw material to create garments with great design; 10% of the value of what you buy supports the project of cleaning the oceans. Have you ever thought about why Japan looks so clean and impeccable? Change makes a difference, and it has to do with cultural issues. The Japanese at the FIFA World Cup Russia 2018 caused surprise because, before leaving the stadium, they cleaned the area where they were watching their national team play. And it is culture: from a young age, they have the habit of leaving the place of study or work tidy and clean because they were taught to do so at school before the end of the day. Why is it that in Finland the one who arrives first at work, without questioning the motives of the any other, parks their vehicle in the most secluded place in the building? It is so that the one who arrives later wastes less time. In the 21ST CENTURY, we must unlearn what we learned by mistake in the last century and start anew. It is time for us to overcome the complex that led to excesses and to undo the culture of contempt for what is of no use to us.

It is a fact: due to the natural development of societies, the size of families has reduced, and house design is starting to obviate the formal space of the large dining room to use this area for bathrooms, kitchen and living room, the places where we "live" the most. And if, on a large scale, farmers use organic waste to produce gas for their stoves and compost to fertilize the fields, we could do the same at home on a smaller scale and produce more soil or compost for plants. As for recycling, we already more or less separate what is recyclable and what "isn't" by putting things in different bins for the garbage truck to pick up. Taking advantage of the novelty, builders and planners can include in the exterior of the houses a plate similar to the one we use to install the external unit of the air conditioning with its electrical point which would serve to locate the organic waste digester. The biodigester can be installed on the terraces or on the first floors of buildings, next to the garbage containers, it does not produce odors and can be found in several brands and models. In size and price, they are similar to the dishwashers, which tend to disappear in small families, and the more affordable, smaller indoor biodigesters consume less energy than the microwave; this eco-friendly solution converts organic waste into nutrient-rich compost and, unlike compost, which involves manure, is new soil that is pathogen-free and can be stored for month before being used to revitalize soils and fertilize plants, almost for free. It is a simple solution that would alleviate much of the environmental impact of landfills. By exchanging the dishwasher for the biodigester, we expand the available kitchen space and unleash the collector gene within us. These solutions to obsolete answers would solve something urgent: in your vegetable garden, in your backyard or on any exterior wall of your house, the building's terrace or in your kitchen, you can install a hydroponic drip channel and grow fruits, vegetables, spices and flowers to exchange or share the harvest with family and neighbors. Dustin Fedako, a young entrepreneur in Austin, Texas, created a company with adapted bicycles — Compost Pedallers @compedallers — that produce compost while pedaling.

While not exempt from suffering from misinformation, the news that reports the developments that contribute to the intellect — available at www.AlternativeNewsProject.org or similar channels — informs you about many things that do not appear on television. And on television, half the news, even if it involves constant recycling about ourselves, is generally information that scares, that evil takes advantage of as propaganda to spread the fear that makes us afraid of even a good neighbor. The other thing is that, on television, the transcription of events is biased information where the establishment defends its interests and industries sponsor everything, or almost everything. Those little boxes we put in our homes with colored news about ourselves, help to lull the intelligent consumer with the promise of being rewarded for working hard during the week. They invite him to feed on fast food; to enjoy the football game on Sunday afternoon with beer and chips... but with one condition: having been in church in the morning. That is what the old American dream was all about.

Sleeping more than eight hours is not healthy, because it is known that the body becomes ankylosed and the being becomes accustomed to it. And it turns out that since July 1, 1941 — in the middle of World War II —, with the first television broadcast in New York, the world has lived a deep sleep that worked very well because we made progress, but the time has come to wake up.

Do you remember *The Jetsons*, the cartoon characters whose cars flew? Since the 1970s, we dreamed that, by the year 2000, we would be living in an advanced world without pollution. And the most we did — to usher in the new millennium — was to first mass-produce a couple of hybrid vehicles — electric and gasoline — between 1997 and 2000. Far from fulfilling the promise of NO pollution, the closest we apparently came to taking free energy from the air, based on Nikola Tesla's work, was the reactionless synchronous generator (RLG) — which produces up to 250% more energy than it needs to function —, which the electrical engineer Paramahamsa Tewari (1937-2017) managed to develop for India at a time when the BRIC countries — Brazil, Russia, India and China — in 2001 began to ally themselves in the struggle for energy supremacy. Tewari's invention, which was ready for testing in 2014, did not hit the market. But the technology had eluded the United States long before that.

The third wave — which had already been growing in the 1970s and reached its maximum elongation and wavelength in the 1980s — reached the beach in the digital age of the 1990s and, apparently, the establishment preferred to wait, because between 1989 and 1993, under the presidency of George H. W. Bush (1924-2018), this event took place: just before the physicist and inventor Adam Trombly was to present a Tesla-inspired generator — consisting of a dynamo that harnesses magnetism to transform air energy into direct current — before a Congressional committee the meeting was abruptly cancelled and the FBI seized the scientific material from his laboratory. Earlier, the Canadian inventor John Hutchison, who in 1971 — using Tesla's theories

— succeeded in counteracting gravity and making objects float; but to silence science, he was harassed for decades by the police. John Bedini, who also worked on Tesla's radiant energy theories, in 1974 created several devices and battery chargers that generate more energy than they need to function; but he had to put aside the idea of producing and distributing them cheaply when he was attacked and threatened in his laboratory. And Eugene Mallove, a Harvard engineer and editor of *Infinite Energy* magazine, *was* beaten to death in 2004. Foster Gamble, in his multilingual film *Thrive*,[160], features and interviews Adam Trombly, and makes these allegations.

Because it was clean, free energy taken from the air, little was left of Tesla's legacy. At his death in 1943 it was learned that his room was ransacked, and many things were lost, and that the FBI seized his important documents: his notebook and technical drawings. To Tesla we owe the invention of the alternating current circuit. He was not only obsessed with electricity because he knew that magnetism held the key to anti-gravity and the operation of electric motors. Among many other things, his theories were a precursor to the invention of X-rays and wireless telecommunications; he operated wireless devices that took energy from the air to light bulbs. What happened to his legacy in these areas has always been a mystery. From prototypes, inventors claim that his theories work; in 2007, this was endorsed at MIT, by means of a relatively simple experiment, in which they managed to transmit energy through the air and light a light bulb at seven meters. The goal is to trap, with appliances or devices, the energy that vibrates — although it sounds redundant — with the help of the wind, the tides or the heat of the Earth that heats the groundwater; or the sun,

---

[160] www.thrivemovement.com.

with photovoltaic cells [161][162] that can be connected to the power grid or not. The truly revolutionary thing would be to be able to connect Tesla-inspired perpetual motion machines to houses that defy the utopia of producing energy from air that we thought was empty:

> All perceptible matter comes from a primary substance, or tenuity beyond conception, filling all space, the *akasha* or luminiferous ether acts upon the *Prana*, life-giving or creative force, calling into existence, in endless cycles, all things and phenomena.
>
> NIKOLA TESLA. Excerpt from *Man's Greatest Achievement*

As happened to Greece, Rome, and the Mediterranean city-states in the classical period; with the evolution of the cultural waves, prosperity, and population increase, but when education and health cease to be a singular priority of the State and become a business, it is only a matter of time before decadence sets in. We believe that the generational clash occurs because new proposals result in every generation criticizing its predecessor; history confirms that this tendency corresponds more with decadence than with the flourishing of cultures. It is evident from the humanism of the Renaissance (15TH and 16TH CENTURIES), which opened every possibility of artistic expression over these last five hundred years, that past cycles repeat themselves in waves. Take, for example, the *zarzuela*, the cultured and classical musical genre of the 17TH century stage, which then appeared with great success — with short versions — as the basest but most popular entertainment in the following centuries. Since the 90's, in the cities, social deterioration and the lack of culture

---

[161] https://www.worldenergytrade.com/energias-alternativas/energia-solar/barcelona-instala-el-primer-pavimento-de-energia-solar-de-espana.

[162] https://eldefinido.cl/actualidad/mundo/4989/Holanda-abre-al-publico-primera-ciclovia-solar-del-mundo/.

in music — regardless of the morality of the songs of the urban genres, which recycle and mix rhythms in interesting ways — have made us think that badly written lyrics, which distort every language, prevail; it is another example, a sign that the decadence is becoming more and more acute. Culture is built on education.

It is worth noting that, as a result of trivialization, we are living in one of the lowest moments, in every sense, which corresponds to painting, sculpture, theater, literature, philosophy... With the receding wave and a deliberately misguided education, in response to ignorance, what we call "culture" is already indifferent to that part of society that matters to many of us who have children; the youth, which we misguided, has lost its way. Our young people do not read, or read little, unless they are text messages. The worthless paintings, sculptures and chants that sell and bring millions to "new" art — with a few exceptions — are a coven of vulgar rudeness that once again demonstrates the aimlessness of the human species. Through fashion or inertia, good or bad, the examples of the leaders are copied. The prolific Russian writer and naturalized American, Isaac Asimov (1920-1992), said: "There is a cult of ignorance in America that has always existed: the pressure of anti-intellectualism has been working its way through our political and cultural life, nurtured by the false notion that democracy means that 'my ignorance is as valid as your knowledge'.".

When in February 2016 the LIGO (Laser Interferometer Gravitational-Wave Observatory) team captured the gravitational waves passing through space, Einstein's theory of special relativity was definitively proven; with this fact it is also confirmed that all information is constantly transmitted and retransmitted in the quantum universe. In the introduction, I mentioned that we are about to conclude the stage of evolutionary development that will allow our senses to focus on the perception of total information.

But the world is not resolved by adjusting the antenna and communicating through emotions with the energetic whole of collective consciousness theorized by Max Planck; it depends on that quantum leap towards the light being made with knowledge and education, so as to NOT let us fall deeper into the black hole left by obscurantism. *Déjà vu*: those difficult to understand moments in which, without having ever been there, you feel you have been or think you have already lived in those same places, which the mainstream dismisses on the basis of a 19TH CENTURY psychology essay that erroneously defines them as "imaginary assumptions produced by the false sensation of familiarity with past events". But those *déjà vu* moments are "the light" that connects and shares with you, in a timeless span, past, present, and future visualizations in the fourth dimension. In the case of generally joyful events, it wants to tell you to be alert and to watch for other signs that could be nearby: nothing bad is happening; on the contrary, if you see them, take advantage of them, because they could signify the road ahead that you were — or were not — looking for.

If you "discover" that the radiation produced by 5G devices and technology affects the cyclical appearance of viruses, and thus also affects our immune system; or that the UFO evidence is irrefutable; read well, research, but do not shout it to the four winds lest you are treated as a crazy, a witch, or in cahoots with the devil — as happened to Galileo —, and you are advised to go see a priest or a psychiatrist. This is your awakening; enable others who also walk the path but do NOT flaunt the moments of connection. It has helped me to find the origin of some things, and it is not fortuitous that on the way to the light you learn of certain revelations. It took me almost eleven years to put the pieces together, to demonstrate with science and history that everything is connected, that nothing is coincidence, and that the universe is pure energy in constant movement. The first thing you grasp is that the power of the mind is the most powerful, inexhaustible force, and that the force of love can do anything. What the books, *The Cosmic Serpent. DNA and the Origins of Knowledge,* by the Canadian Jeremy Narby — a scientific text that interrelates hallucinogenic concoctions, shamans, and medicinal plants with the DNA language of nature — and the novel *The Celestine Prophecy,* by James Redfield — which was made into a movie —, have in common is that they are not just theory and prophecy. It is true that the strong thing that connects us in the common prayer: the energy that you emit plus that of another, and another, and others, which, if shared, expands, and moves the whole, and is capable of moving mountains and planets. This energy flow depends on you, because feelings (A) can affect the DNA of living beings (B) and things (C): A → B → C; therefore, A → C: it is definite that feelings could eventually affect the matter of things.

We cannot deny that after the second wave, which brought with it the industrial revolution, the third wave was also phenomenal! Since the digital era of the 1990s, the progress and advancement we have made has been immeasurable, but we know what it all comes down to: even though there has been progress and development, fear and ignorance persist. Regardless of which extreme they belong to, both the current corporatocracy that collects the money scattered on the beach, and the populists that lead the receding wave, are leaving us adrift. And the issue, over which politicians — whom we can already call of yesteryear — have aired fears, is the much-feared loss of jobs, which was effortlessly produced by the global COVID-19 crisis. In spite of this, between natural tensions in adjustment, we already know what to do, because with what happened with the coronavirus: "three little drops of snot made us think that our pyramid of values was inverted; that it is worth more to value science over economy; that not only the indigent bring plagues; that hospitals are more important than a missile or that, at the risk of losing ourselves in isolation, the alternative is to be better together" — words of the Colombian psychiatrist and writer Edna Rueda Abrahams, in *Empatía viral* —.

Fear is that great disease of society that Love heals. So, let us take this opportunity to fight that fatal virus — and COVID19 —, and while we restructure things, let us stop supporting autocratic, xenophobic leaders who believe they are above science and people, and, even less so, the little emperors of totalitarian regimes that end up not trusting any citizen. The intelligent consumer, who is used to the lurches of the economy and is not afraid of progress, would rather think that, since the first edition of Karl Marx's *Capital*, it took a century and a half to understand that the extreme ideas of total antagonism generated by that ideology have been the worst thing for society, because they have left us with a deep social abyss and an enormous "poverty". And while we are talking about poverty, in contrast, the *First Global Atlas of Childhood Obesity*, by the World Obesity Federation,[163] points out that in 2019 there were 158 million obese school-age young people in the world and estimates that by 2030 there will be more than 250 million. I believe that, for the time being, with sufficient maturity, we have know-how to demonstrate to Einstein that he was wrong in the saying attributed to him that "there are two infinite things: the universe and human stupidity"; he doubted the first statement, and was right because

---

[163] World Obesity Federation, WOF. *The First Global Atlas on Childhood Obesity*. https://www.worldobesity.org/membersarea/global-atlas-on-childhood-obesity#:~:text=The%20first%20global%20atlas%20on,target%20for%20tackling%20childhood%20obesity.

the expansion of the universe is accelerating, but in the future it will do the opposite.

The answer is to end our dependence on carbon-based fuels. If we succeed, we will create a boom of new industries, wealth, clean and safe energy that can perhaps avert the greatest disaster we know of so far in human history, saving millions of lives while improving billions more. If we continue as we are while things slowly get worse all around us, we basically fail.

AL GORE, 2006

And secondly, human stupidity.

The power of one

It consists of rescuing and asserting true democracy.

The assimilation of modern concepts on health and nutrition in the 21ST CENTURY is giving "power" back to the intelligent consumer, who learns, educates himself, pauses and reflects, because with his decision to change his habits, the alternative that each one has to change things is glimpsed, and perhaps also the course of humanity. That's right. It is up to us, to each individual, to clarify the concepts. This decision does NOT belong to the religious currents NOR to the political parties, which conspired with the corporations to protect their vested interests without thinking about, or for, the people; parties which have ruled us this way for decades. Since the consolidation of the "single thought" in the economic sphere in the 80s,[164] in which "the welfare economy disappears; the individual thus becomes once again entirely responsible for his own fate. *Homo economicus* re-emerges in full force and the economy takes precedence over the political", the resulting new order, as it stubbornly seeks the god of money and every man for himself, has led to the reign of inhumanity. The intelligent consumer, who defies destiny in a peaceful way and yearns with every awakening to change the world, awaits the next elections to assert and rescue democracy, knowing that with his daily consumption his power is in his pocket when he makes purchases.

Politicians believed that, with the mere exponential growth of large corporations, enough jobs could be generated to guarantee the full sustenance of humanity but have not understood that this end-of-century dream was not fulfilled because those who promoted irresponsible globalization did not anticipate the implications of promoting it. For more than a decade, economic theories have been failing and it has been demonstrated that, despite all attempts, one by one the known strategies have only served to inflate the pockets of the richest. Based on actual figures or not, globalization was supposed to support job creation; but since the great recession of 2008, formal employment has become a utopia and is a mirage that was diluted in the face of global economic recovery. In its 2019 report, the International Labor Organization (ILO) declares that the quality of employment fell, and that informal employment grew: 61% of the world's workforce — two billion people — have informal jobs, typically

---

[164] Mario Rapoport (2002): "Origen y actualidad del "pensamiento único"". In *La globalización económicofinanciera. Su impacto en América Latina*, 357-363. Buenos Aires: Consejo Latinoamericano de Ciencias Sociales, CLACSO. http://biblioteca.clacso.edu.ar/clacso/gt/20101004010747/22.pdf.

vulnerable jobs with low wages and no social protection;[165] the 2020 report,[166] will undoubtedly confirm that things got much worse with the pandemic.

The breeding ground for corruption to make its way into the corporate will and for us to go beyond the point of NO return was when the monopolies reduced the flow of money to the pyramid base, introduced unhealthy competition and mixed politics and lobbying to twist everything to point at money: jobs are not the reason or the object for the State to support the industries, but jobs are the reason and the object to support the new industry that is already generating the fourth wave.

We are squandering money by the bucketload; immediate interests are stronger than long-term global needs and we are not attending to basic needs in exchange for attending to futile and useless things.

PEPE MUJICA

So said the ex-guerrilla, ex-communist, former president of Uruguay who later became an equanimous thinker, who affirms that for the State to comply with a true social approach, it requires a lot of money and zero corruption. It is no longer as before: the intelligent consumer, in order to beat the system, focuses on the health of his family, and for economy only buys what he needs and avoids waste. Let's understand that we are the 99% that surpasses that 1% that believes it rules the economy; and let's face the reality

---

[165] https://www.ambito.com/economia/desempleo/oit-advierte-que-cae-la-calidad-los-empleos-nivel-mundial-n5015806.

[166] ILO Observatory: *COVID19 and the world of work*. Seventh edition. Updated estimates and analysis January 25, 2021. https://www.ilo.org/wcmsp5/groups/public/---dgreports/---dcomm/documents/briefingnote/wcms_767045.pdf.

that it is we who rule the economy and not the economy that rules our wallet, because with what we decide to buy, we are the engine that changes the ways of thinking. This is the moment that is needed if we are not to miss out on every opportunity. We have to embrace and protect democracy by electing people with new ideals who are capable of providing solutions to today's problems; not false leaders without discourse or conversation, who are incapable of facing the real reasons for the current problems, but flaunting their ignorance, insist on defending the mistakes of the past, because, given the circumstances, we would be setting a deadly trap for true democracy.

The "power of one" sustained over time is more fragile than you thought. True democracy has only been experienced in a few places, for relatively short periods in two different eras, which lie in very distant history. It is useful to know the short version of the history of this common good that belongs to all of us.

If we resort to the definition, power can be summarized as "to be able" or "to be capable of". However, in human settlements, the usual use of the term refers to the control, empire, dominion, and jurisdiction that a man has at his disposal to accomplish something or impose a mandate. Power is not just associated with physical force, but can also be political, economic, intellectual, legal, or all of these. In any case, it was usual for experienced elders to make the most important decisions for communities. In the early days of classical Greece, around the 5TH CENTURY BC in Athens, with the dismantling of the timocratic system — in which only landowning citizens ruled — Solon's Constitution in 594, to which Clístenes made reforms in 508, gave birth to the Athenian democracy. Pericles was its greatest promoter. An educated Greek people who conversed while enjoying a free thermal bath and debated with philosophers was normal for two or three centuries; that was the pillar of democracy and the "power of one" which held firm in the city-states that spread throughout the Mediterranean. Although the august Alexander the Great defended democracy in Greece and contained the war until his death in 323 B.C., it only lasted until in 322, when the Macedonian hegemony eliminated the democratic institutions. In Rome, in the republican period — from 509 to 27 B.C. — the power of the people was entrusted to regional representatives descended from noble families who made up the Senate, which made the laws, the administration; to consuls, proconsuls and military commanders who acted as dictators; and to magistrates, the judicial system supposedly being faithful to the truth. And the terrible thing happened: the power of the people and democracy withered to near death with the dictatorship granted to Julius Caesar — yes, the one who was heard to say, "Divide and conquer"; the last ruler of the Roman republic from a patrician family, who increased the Senate to nine hundred members — and died under Augustus, the first emperor, who ruled from 27 B.C. until his death in A.D. 14, and his successors, Tiberius, Caligula, Claudius, Nero and the other seven emperors in the FIRST CENTURY of our era.

With the borders under siege, it was costly for Rome to pay mercenaries to protect them, and this forced them to raise taxes to cover defense expenses. With a growing number of inhabitants and an inflation rate of 1000%, when it comes to cutting the budget — as always, the defense bill is always the first to be paid —, free education for all was only provided from the top down to the children of the centurions — the captains of today —. And so, at a time when Rome and its military were expanding their dominion over the conquered territories, the same cancer that consumes society today reappeared — behind the backs of the emperors, who sprang up as a greedy, independent lineage — : corruption crept in through those with deep enough pockets. And then, between empires and monarchies, republics, and more empires, it took more than seventeen centuries for democracy to have a less brilliant resurgence in a bloody moment with the French Revolution. And yet, with the full yearning of the colonies for freedom, it was reborn pure as the form of government that the liberators were able to offer to the peoples of America. And only since 1945 — between the post-war period and the Korean War in 1950 —, in a second, tiny moment of peace, its seed managed to spread and prosper in different places of the Earth.

In England, in the SEVENTEENTH CENTURY, people spoke of *Whigs* and *Tories* — Liberals and Conservatives —, with the French Revolution in the EIGHTEENTH CENTURY they began to speak of Left, Center and Right, and with the Industrial Revolution in the NINETEENTH CENTURY, the quarrels between social classes increased. The intelligent consumer has noticed that, from the 20TH CENTURY onwards, the trends polarized — like two devilish snakes — poisonous socialism, which injects communism at the slightest slip of the tongue, and exploitative capitalism, which constrains, launched themselves in frenzied coils in pursuit of their extremes. If in the West you were caught reading Marx, it was the same as if you were found looking through the Koran — frowned upon for being different from your faith —, and the logical reaction was that they stopped seeing you as a socialist and considered you a communist of the worst kind, because you were also an atheist. Then, without fear, we can speak in retrospect of what happened with communism.

For many on the left who found the answers in *The Communist Manifesto* and *Capital*, believing became an esoteric feeling that validates their utopia of atheism, for like religions, they enthroned them as sacred books; without mentioning the word "faith" and denying God, they still believe they feel that inexplicable "something". The truth is that, while *Capital* was a simple treatise that follows the trail of money, in *The Communist Manifesto*, Engels and Marx did not predict anything different or additional to what already happened in the TWENTIETH CENTURY. Except for the prediction in 1950 of the Russian writer Alissa Zinovievna — a graduate in history and philosophy from the University of St. Petersburg in 1924 —, who in 1931 wrote under the pseudonym of Ayn Rand (1905-1982):

> When you realize that in order to produce you need to obtain authorization from those who produce nothing; when you realize that money flows to those who do not deal in goods, but in favors; when you perceive that many become rich by bribery and influence rather than by their work; and that the laws do not protect you against them, but, on the contrary, it is they who are protected against you; when you discover that corruption is rewarded and honesty becomes a self-sacrifice, then you can affirm, without fear of being wrong, that your society is doomed.

After Marx's death in 1883, communism was hit by schisms: Stalin's version, which at no time contemplated coexisting peacefully with capitalism, which Lenin had intended, clashed with Leon Trotsky and Eduard Bernstein. And the latter — "redder" than the former — inspired Mao Zedong to impose an authentic and unusual communism in China with revisionism. While — in the civil war from 1927 to 1949 — his peasant movement gradually got rid of the Nationalists and the British — who kept Hong Kong until returning it in 1997 — and tried to repel the Japanese Empire, which invaded Manchuria from 1931 to 1945. After the war, Mao took great leap forward with the novel task of burning books and all vestiges of the millenary habits, customs, and cultures of the Chinese past. From Russia to China and its neighbors, it was easy for communism to use the immense natural fence they share to expand and delimit itself. However, after fifty years of communist coercion, there were border incidents between them in the 1960s, but this is a brief history and, in truth, they were not always communist.

Isolated for millennia, between barriers as high as the Himalayas or the Great Wall of China or the immense steppes next to the North Pole, which served as a boundary to their nations, the only form of government they always knew — the countries of the Silk Road on the Eurasian slope that shared cultures — was the imperial monarchic system. That is why, for example, after achieving an incipient and immature democracy infected by the greed and corruption of the world, Russia, with a totalitarian leader, tends to be the same. This is not the case for China which, with a market socialism that I prefer to call an internally militarized State capitalism, has never known democracy. China has tried to convince the world that its "economic and educational" model works, but, has not taken into account that — as with dogmas — the mind can only be curtailed to the point of indoctrination: those who supply the world by "occupying their people" disregard the freedom of the self in the power of one. History has fully demonstrated that walls have served States to exercise total dominion over their inhabitants rather than to protect and defend their territories against external threat.

Faced with the atomic brake imposed by the West in 1945 at the end of World War II, the bloc of the Union of Soviet Socialist Republics, USSR, put the bolt on the central European plain and, taking advantage of the geographical barriers, with the Caucasus to the north, the Balkans to the south and the rivers descending from the Alps that encircle it, it was enough to build something new and "symbolic" in Germany and complete the communist grip until time to judge who was right. We were left without knowing what happened in Russia and China for decades. But we saw on television how, for trying to escape by crossing the wall of infamy — which split Berlin in two —, right there, in the barbed wire barrier of the death zone, they were easy prey for the Soviet soldiers who, without thinking and without mercy, gave them the coup de grace. The song *Libre*, by José Luis Armenteros and Pablo Herrero, performed by Spanish singer Nino Bravo[167] (1944-1973), tells this story. Walls, which in the past helped isolate regions to forge empires, were later a **tangible** threat to democracy; a misfortune that can happen today to any society. But the absolute worst is the other terrible and **intangible** threat that emerged from the darkness: it is that accursed corruption that we must defeat.

When governments fail to convince, in the midst of political and economic intricacies, they take on powers, either by the use of force or little by little through their support base. In Republican Rome, given the generalized ignorance that made the people manipulable, dictators who exceeded the term of their office arose to snatch from the people "the power of one", and the emperors, thanks to the special powers granted to them by the corrupt Senate, definitively put an end to democracy. And so, they meddled in religious matters, anointing themselves with divine power so that the people would never doubt the *imperium*:

And we have that, not counting on the decisions, the people — every time more ignorant and apathetic — did not count anymore, they do not even remember that once they deposited their vote of confidence in those who always have to bear the total responsibility of democracy: the congressmen who, since Rome, were, the original ones, thirty and have been turning

---

[167] https://www.youtube.com/watch?v=Xa68YjqWTJM.

into simple stone guests, but not all of them, of course. And it only takes six out of ten to blame them for having been directly responsible for the vote being disregarded, losing its total virtue and importance, not understanding that with this ignorant abstentionist attitude their "corrupt buffoonery" continues to be sponsored. The people must always be dominated by the political decisions of only **6** or **6** more. This is the exact successive factor that is required: **6** out of **10**, and **18** out of **30**, required to deliberate in favor of corruption, as in the beginning, since the other sessions they do not even attend, charging equally without honor their fees. Then thus, in this way, we will be destined to survive without living, always ignoring what happens where it originates. And "always serving evil" with our conduct, the control over the people, for obvious reasons, will have to fall on a huge and necessary repressive police or military apparatus, from where also "emerged" as then many emperors.

When the ideas come, I write and write, but after researching and ordering them, it's different. Undoubtedly, there is something from above that tells you what to write, the muses perhaps. But when that, which I saw so tellingly, appeared before me — the sign of the three sixes in the previous paragraph —, I cannot deny it, it so happens that my first name is also Juan and I got goose bumps. I leave the text as it came to my mind; that is how I wrote it about ten years ago, and that is how ideas come when you are connected to the divine matrix, and you write without thinking for yourself. Then, without the blindness produced by the fear of the sacred — which I mentioned before —, what I had to do was to read John, including the Gospel, 'see' in his Apocalypse what happens, and continue with the explanation.

"Seeing him [John], Peter said to Jesus, 'What about him, Lord?' Jesus answered, 'If I want him to stay behind until, I come, what does it matter to you? You are to follow me.' The rumour then went out among the brothers that this disciple would not die. Yet Jesus had not said to Peter, 'He will not die,' but 'If I want him to stay behind until I come.' This disciple is the one who vouches for these things and has written them down, and we know that his testimony is true. (Jn 21:22-24)[168].

With a recent history in which democracy had gone to the dogs, in 30 AD the expanding Roman Empire had already conquered the Mediterranean world, parts of Europe and Egypt. Due to ruthless persecution by some emperors, which helped Jews and Christians drift apart, abstracted, sharpening his senses, and having much to say from exile, a man standing on the sand of the island of Patmos in Greece, in the Aegean Sea, describes the gravest thing he saw in the civilized world in which he knew, and "lived". John constantly brings up the decadence of Babylon — six hundred years earlier — and makes one think that he was a learned man who knew his history, the history of Greece and, of course, the history of Rome very well. He feared for his life. But without losing faith in humanity, he elaborated his Apocalypse with wisdom — it is said, between the years 80 and 120 — in a prophetic language full of metaphors. And of his world, which he saw collapsing, he warns us in Revelation 13 of a beast that "was like a leopard, with paws like a bear and a mouth like a lion" to focus us. Centuries later, we need to understand his words in order not to be the cause of our extinction and to be able to evolve. "There is need for shrewdness here: anyone clever may interpret the number of the beast: it is the number of a human being, the number 666." John, for obvious reasons, hides the

---

[168] https://www.bibliacatolica.com.br/new-jerusalem-bible/john/21/.

clue that was missing, the pattern — 6 of 10 and 18 of 30 — that unveils the mystery to describe masterfully in the beasts what happened before and during the empire; the tangible and intangible correlation of the beasts with the institutions of the State[169] and its consequences: what it is, what happens and how the great beast was affecting human coexistence. Very early in the direct lineage of Romulus and Remus — the founders of Rome in 753 BC —, the patricians were organized by curiae — the *gens* that relate several families — and each of the three ancient tribes "had ten curiae and these, in turn, one hundred men", but only one patrician for each of the first **thirty** curiae could vote in the *comitia curiata*: the Roman assembly. 666 by now "might" mean nothing, but eighteen as we saw. The six and the ten — with which John insists —, together, are the factor that defines the representative proportional majority: 6 out of 10, **18** out of **30**; 60 out of 100, again — the original Senate — ; 180 out of 300 in the republic — until the first century BC —, and so on up to 540 out of 900, the maximum number of senators that Rome had under the dictator Julius Caesar. What John was talking about was democracy.

We already have two clues. And the third are the ten diadems on the ten horns that identify with a man's number — 10 x 10 = 100 and 10 x 30 = 300 — the *noble patritii* senators of Rome, and among them those who head the profane majority that make part of the beast, the first **6** individuals of each **10** — the number of their name —, with a blasphemous name of ten letters on their heads, which are seven. Now, by double proof, without any error, let us use the number 10 of the diadems and 18 and 30 — the simple clues and the multiplying factor — : 10 x 18 and 30; 180 out of 300 equals the exact exponential proportion of the democratic principle (50 % +1) — more than enough in

---

[169] https://en.wikipedia.org/wiki/State_(polity)

the Senate of the republic of the FIRST CENTURY — to help to upset everything in favor of the dictatorship. If that's not shady, I don't know what is! Anyway, from the beginning the beast was already roaming intangibly in the human. In 509 B.C., the Senate — to protect itself, externally or internally in case of danger, or to maintain its hegemony over other magistrates — created the figure of the dictator to alone fulfill, or as the case may be, his irrevocable mandate, to act — in theory — for a maximum period of **six** months. The usual thing was to choose prominent figures, such as consuls, proconsuls, or the best military commander; with the almost total power granted to them, it was normal for them to abuse their *imperium* — the term of the six months — and, in this way, paved the way for the monarchical figure of the emperor to emerge again. By definition, because of its unique and independent character — a brilliant misdirection in the riddle —, the dictatorship or empire is the seventh head of the beast that does not count in the numerical factor of democracy.

But what happened with Julius Caesar, the greatest dictator in history, who was also "allowed to mouth its boasts and blasphemies and to be active for forty-two months; and it mouthed its blasphemies against God, against his name, his heavenly Tent and all those who are sheltered there" (Rev 13: 5-6)? In 49 B.C., after returning from his campaigns in Gaul — today's France — he exercised dictatorship for the first time, then resigned eleven days later to be elected consul; then, in 48, when he was appointed for one year, the six-month limit was definitely broken, and he was given authority to act for forty-two months. From then on, he manipulated the Senate, which appointed him dictator for ten years. After he had held the legal office of dictator for the third time (666) — for three and a half years which was only to be for six months —, before his death on March 15, 44 B.C., he proclaimed himself in perpetuity; but the people hated him and, in the midst of a plot by the senators, he was assassinated, twelve hundred and sixty days — or forty-two months — after he had been elected to the formal office of dictator, on December 15, 48 B.C., for the second time that he broke the six-month limit.

The common Roman calendar was of 304 days divided into ten months — six of 30 days and four of 31. However, in the year 46 B.C., which was called "the last year of confusion; the year of fifteen months", something crucial happened. To correct the major solar lag, Julius Caesar ordered that, in that year alone, 445 days were to be counted, with two *Merkedinus* months of 33 and 34 days between November and December — which were used from time to time to compensate for the lags produced in the seasons —. This is a retrograde increase of slightly more than two months — almost three —, plus one day in February of the year 44 — which was a leap year —, in the countdown, which was then adjusted to the seasons and years. The Julian calendar of 365.25 days with twelve months — like the present one, which included leap years in February every four years and kept *Januarius* as the first month of the year — came into effect in 45, or between 45 and 44, towards year 0.

History relates that Julius Caesar definitively repealed the six-month limit when he was appointed dictator for the second time at the end of the year, in December 48 B.C. By military logistics, since 153 B.C., the first of January had been taken as the beginning of the year. But the time lag was real; for example, spring came to be dated in the astronomical winter, which lends itself to confusion and further misdirection. From the earliest calendar of the classical world, despite all the reforms and trials they made, they always used the lunar calendar, which is inaccurate. The first month of the year was *Martius* with thirty-one days, NOT January, because the beginning of the year had to coincide with the "rebirth of spring". The year 46 B.C., which began in January, had fifteen months of 29.66 days on average or 445 days. According to the distribution of months and days in the previous classical world,[170] from the 1st of *Martius* (which marked the beginning of the year) to the end of *December* (which had thirty days, in 47), in the winter — the cold season of vital importance for the preparation of the invasions — there were 304 days distributed over ten months. It would be necessary to count the two months of the year 48: *Februarius* with twenty-eight and *Januarius* with twenty-nine — that Numa Pompilius[171] (centuries vii-vi B.C.) included in the original calendar —, and half a month more, until the 15 of *Decembris of* twenty-nine days, when the dictator Julius Caesar definitively broke the six-month limit. If we strictly follow the Roman calendar — reformed from 153 B.C., which comprised 355 days over twelve months —, it would be the 9th day, but still in December. The only known clue that history offers us. Let us bear in mind that his death took place exactly two and a half months after the beginning of the year 44 — on March 15 —, forty-two months after the start of his second dictatorship, when he began to use his total power to bring the end of democracy.

John saw and lived through the persecution and martyrdom of Jews and Christians by the Caesars: from Gaius Julius Caesar to Domitian. Regarding the beast and the *imperium* in Revelation 13: "It was allowed to make war against the saints and conquer them, and given power over every race, people, language and nation"; he refers to the murder at the hands of Nero of the apostles crucified with the inverted cross of Peter and Paul — or Paul beheaded, it is not known —, according to him, to overcome them; "and all people of the world will worship it, that

---

[170] https://es.wikipedia.org/wiki/Calendario_juliano.
[171] https://es.wikipedia.org/wiki/Calendario_romano.

is, everybody whose name has not been written down since the foundation of the world in the sacrificial Lamb's book of life." John is referring to Genesis and Adam and Eve: a mockery of the people who worshipped gods and the ignorance of the world for not having recognized the Judeo-Christian God from the beginning.

The blood is the light of Jesus, the lamb sacrificed for men. And let us remember that John obfuscates to protect his life. In Revelation 12: "The woman was delivered of a boy, the son who was to rule all the nations with an iron sceptre, and the child was taken straight up to God and to his throne" — to be judged? — is not the is not the same as the woman in Revelation 17, "the famous Harlot": Rome, city of the seven kings, almost eight. The wondrous woman, who, in her crown, holds the rights, duties and civil liberties that act day and night, "...escaped into the desert, where God had prepared a place for her to be looked after for twelve hundred and sixty days" (that is, forty-two months), during which time, in the midst of her solitude, she was unable to act; she is the beautiful lady DEMOCRACY that gave birth to the dictatorship represented by Julius Caesar — a male child — who autocratically abused his term. And that winged hodgepodge of fear and ignorance in the fiery red banner — which identified the Empire with the acronym SPQR: *Senātus Populusque Rōmānus* (the Senate and the People of Rome) —, sometimes, eagle; sometimes, serpent or both, which for the Romans symbolized power and wisdom; it is that fastidious dragon that makes part of the beast on which have ridden many who were born to raze and who knew something more than the others.

John was a Jew and, at the time, when referring to the four horsemen, he did NOT emphasis the horses, which was another necessary oversight. Remember that Julius Caesar's horse, Genitor, was not white, but black, — there are no green horses, as correctly rendered in English Bibles[172] —, and among the twelve Caesars, starting with Julius Caesar, "and its rider was holding a bow; he was given a victor's crown and he went away, to go from victory to victory....", in chronological order from the FIRST century, he pointed out the next three emperors of the Julio-Claudian dynasty and the Flavian — the successor — dynasty, who had been assiduous Judeo-Christian persecutors: Caligula (37-41) who, "to take away peace from the earth and set people killing each other..." — in the coliseum — "...was given a huge sword.", and by edict he raged against the Jews; Nero (64-68) who had in his hand "a pair of scales", for it is well known that in matters of the Empire he was a great administrator. And that tyrant, the cruel and paranoid Domitian (81-96), who apparently banished John to the island of Patmos, was the little mentioned fourth horseman, whose "rider was called Death", the most heinous and last Caesar. The next persecutors were the emperors Trajan (109-111) and Marcus Aurelius (161-180), but John — of whom Jesus said to Peter: "If I want him to stay behind till, I come" — was already in exile or had passed away. And if there is any doubt, all of them "...were given authority over a quarter of the earth, to kill by the sword, by famine, by plague and through wild beasts." (Rev. 6:8b).[173]

I clarify that evil itself is not the beast, which has always required the dragon to reign in the unlettered, unwary, and fearful man. Evil is the ideal incognito complement of intangible

---

[172] The Greek word St John used to describe the 4th horse is χλωρός (chlorós), which means green (as in the first part of chlorophyl). Therefore, the English translations which use 'green' are actually more accurate than those which use 'pale' instead of green -doing reference to the color of the horse, who's the rider is Death- the color of a decaying corpse-, or, the Bibles in Spanish which use "yellow" instead green, which in Biblical Greek would have been ξουθόν (xouthón).

[173] https://www.bibliacatolica.com.br/new-jerusalem-bible/revelation/6/

CORRUPTION — the united act of men — which, in the form of a beast, efficiently does the worst of all harm. To sustain the great beast, in the Empire — as an extension of the State — another would be lacking, which would emerge as a tangible, represented by the soldier, who also fears the power that his weapon gives him. For the State, its power is based on the militias, which use their strength to expand the corroded in the people with the cruelty of their horns. "It had two horns like a lamb but made a noise like a dragon."; the apparently small horns are here the indicator of meekness, the absent-mindedness. In the analogy, the first thing is to describe the geography of the empire with the head and horns of the lamb, which is clearly drawn from the Mediterranean world, the *Mare Internum*: on one side, northwest to the Rhine River, the provinces of Germania and Belgium, the first horn, which, with the other, on the other side, to the east, the province of Armenia and up to the Tigris and Euphrates, make up the entire territory of the Empire: the "lamb's face". John is concerned to see in the young ram how its horns flow and twist, which close to delimit the Empire, which deploys its power to exercise authority. And just as the mountains rise, what "rose from the earth" are the walls built by men — Julius Caesar built his own to encircle the Gallic leader Vercingetorix at the siege of Alesia —. The second is to typify human ego and arrogance, which, yesterday out of necessity and today out of ignorance, are monumental; without the horns of the tame lamb, the empire would cease to function as such. The analogy is the brute power that receives orders: **the militias**, the military apparatus that by order served the empire and project its image to the conquered cultures, which is anyone who carries weapons authorized by the beast. "And it worked great miracles, even to calling down fire from heaven onto the earth while people watched." Without further explanation, let us remember, as the story goes, that they assaulted each other with thousands of flaming spears and arrows and, terrified, saw fire fall from heaven before their feet. To count how many live and die in the name of the beast within, and the slaves, every four years, the *census* of individuals identified the "being" by virtue of their purpose with a number or with the name of the beast to then claim from them the payment of their taxes for what they have always traded for better or worse. The title of censor for life was granted to Julius Caesar long before he pretended to be king.

Having unveiled the mystery, let us bear in mind that the number of the beast ten — with the ten diadems, symbolizing its legacy — identifies the senators. And among them the six unnecessary exponential ones plus one — the dictator who gave way to the emperor — are false leaders; the seven destructive heads that put an end to democracy. John knew beforehand and mentioned the wound three times. "I saw that one of its heads seemed to have had a fatal wound but that this deadly injury had healed..."; and "...that had been wounded by the sword and still lived": after a virtuous past in which democracy had prevailed, monarchies revived over time. And of dictatorship, John refers specifically to the blow it received when the office of dictator was suspended for more than a century — from the end of the Second Punic War in 201 B.C. — until Sulla restored it; then, when Julius Caesar made serious modifications to it, the office died with him; democracy faltered, and Octavian Augustus, his putative son, emerged with the title of emperor. As far as we can figure, the beast came to stay in power and inspire those he called for evil to reign in Rome. Since then, in any society claiming to be democratic, he who brazenly or unashamedly hides his name, bears in past participle the blasphemous word *katasapeís* -κατασαπείς- in ancient Greek 'CORRUPTED' over their heads: *corrumpĕre* in in the original language, Latin, or in three different

Romance languages it has ten letters, and the other meanings are 'rotten', 'putrid' or 'putrefied'. For almost two thousand years, the number of the corrupt, six hundred and sixty-six, about evil or the evil one, inspired people to make all kinds of conjectures. And I clarify, once again, that evil itself is not the great beast, whose name is CORRUPTION.

We tend to believe that individual good is absolute, and that evil is something external that tempts or invades us. However, the worst evil is that which "I" do; the time has come to recognize that to remove evil from man — as the Inquisition pretended with torture — is impossible, because good and evil — both — are a constitutive part of our permanent essence in human reason. For it turns out that "and lead us not into temptation but deliver us from evil" praises the reality of God and his manifestations; for Christianity, doxology becomes an absolute objective and is directed to "being". It is worth saying here, "let anyone of you who has no sin throw the first stone...". Who has never thought of tripping someone? Yet in the presence of good, evil disappears; magnetism is tacit, it unites or repels, and good would not exist without evil either. Let us remember that in man the essential energies — without being able to detach themselves, constantly tied together — rotate with an intensity that makes it possible for hatred to become love in the same instant, and vice versa. In the end, fear and ignorance have made, from the beginning, the evil that is lovelessness and the negative energies that we have been accumulating do us much harm. To go one step further in evolution, always in the human universe, in our energetic polarity, evil is a matter of the absence of good, and negative energy is something that we can change! Let's face once and for all the evil that, without realizing it, we also carry within us and that tempts us.

Even if the good is good for some and the bad is good for others, in any case, corrupt actions are not justified, but they have defenders. Democracy is the perfect weapon that secretly decapitates the unworthy who dishonor it; and the time has also come to overthrow those who do not represent us, even though we have elected them. Abstentionism is not an option; we need those who have not used democracy to use it to wrest from the dictatorships that false democracy they crow about. We have misused this two-edged sword of freedom against ourselves; through lack of maturity, young and old do not go to the polls. When in the electoral lists almost all the candidates are from the same family or from the same mafia, we can use the blank ballot, that other edge of the sword that decapitates the contenders who in no way can run again in the next election. In the ambiguous power struggle, good and evil have always been a dichotomy in the eternal reason of human existence, and democracy is perfect to resolve this issue. Democracy costs, but it is of NO use if it is given away and is a sterile seed that does not sprout.

In spite of the Cuban Adjustment Act or "wet foot, dry foot" that the United States applied for fifty-one years, the result was the individual desire of thousands of Cubans to set foot in Florida, which was stronger than the breath of freedom that only grew in the martyrs and anonymous heroes silenced by the Castro regime on the island. It only remains to overcome the fear of more than half a century of regime, because the generations of indoctrinated people, none of them illiterate, destined to survive without living, badly reciprocated by the regime, do not deserve it. From Cuba, the north points out to them the illusion of feeling that freedom is impossible for them, alien to those who live on the other shore in exile, ninety miles away, who live a magnificent dream in Little Havana, and do not notice that their longing for sovereignty has blinded the heart of their homeland;

a reflection that, unwittingly, causes that longing to be free to languish in their brothers in their own territory. On the island, intellectuals, scientists, artists, musicians, poets, peasants are all educated people submerged in frustration, who since birth have seen the light that does not belong to them and manifest their pain on their way home when they count their steps on a timeless boardwalk. Only the sea consoles them, speaks and tells them: "Courage, friend, yes you can; it is the same courage that others of you also had when, hidden in the night, they launched their raft onto the swaying waves, with a fixed course to their destination. Without the slightest fear, look up, and if those who watch you notice that slight smile of complicity, as they will, and someone asks, in a nice moment of sharing, look up and blame it on the full moon, and you will find the perfect excuse to smile with them, who also hide their longing to meet their own again, some day; who dream of redeeming the pride they lost because of others who also lost theirs, who dishonored it and who do not expect any grace other than that which could give them the love and humble forgiveness of their now ragged, noble and sad mother, the stunning Cuba".

Democracy is not for cowards either. Dear Venezuela, you are like this because of decades of paternalistic governments — with more of the same —, that during the oil bonanza did little or nothing to educate you and that, at the point of subsidies, with everything imported, Daddy Government fostered in you the indifference for agriculture and that is why even today you want everything for free. Do you think that it is fair taking from those who have more, when you thought you had little? Don't fool yourself, Venezuela, there is nothing to eat, and your natural resources are being taken by others. A few bandits have stolen everything from you, and also the State's money; put paid to them and that corrupt dictatorship which, on a stupid whim and ignorance when oil had value, was not able to raise its head properly — its shame did not allow it to — and really look north, to the right, to countries like Norway, which cared more about educating the people, which is the first thing to do; or Sweden and Finland, which have tried everything. In the 90's, for example, Sweden went to the extreme: it tried to build an immense State and nationalized too many assets, but when it was about to go bankrupt, it was able to realize the virtue of free enterprise: healthy ambition encourages and fosters development. Venezuela, now to you, who have less, I say: the most that has been stolen from you is the power you have to decide, which does not consist of stealing from your neighbor; it is to fight so that we all have what is fair according to our work and sacrifice and to be able to live in peace. The instrument for that is, and will always be, true democracy. Venezuela, my friend, go for your freedom now!

Ultimately, morally and economically, plagues such as single thought, final solution, extermination, annihilation, genocide, modern slavery, repression, concentration camps, guerrilla warfare, subversive attacks, all have in common the great corollary of the elimination of the other as a solution: "As you are of no use to me, do not get in my way because, either way, I am going to annihilate you; I am going to kill you". Democracy is that pure thing that has been the reason for wars and the perfect excuse to declare them. This is not necessary, when they are avoided at the right and precise moment because of the clamor of the people, whose voice achieves great things: that is the greatness of democracy. This does not mean that decisions are made by a crowd permeated by thieves and bandits. When the people allow themselves to be manipulated and decide without information, no State, good or bad, elected in democracy, can allow ochlocracy,[174] the degradation of power and the degeneration of democracy.

---

[174] https://en.wikipedia.org/wiki/Mob_rule

It is the worst political system; it feeds on rancor and ignorance, decides, takes power and rules! What a pity, Venezuela, first it happened with the dictatorship, and now again with the recent illegitimate elections.

The most mature multiparty democratic societies tend to highlight the ethical and intellectual qualities of individuals who choose to avoid extremes; to achieve social justice, they propose to take the best of the right and free enterprise — regulated so that it adapts to the center and does not favor predation — and the best of the left, the obligation of the State to provide a broad, open and free education, without indoctrination of any kind, and universal quality health for all, including those who are just passing through. To achieve greater success, it must be done with the support of honest societies which, before defending the principles of the "party", prioritize the being, and before having too much, moderate themselves so as not to go crazy with excesses. We have had enough of hatred and speculation. We can blur the extreme capitalists' belief that to be a socialist is to be a communist and that everyone who has that social approach is a communist; communists assume that every socialist must be a communist. And both are wrong, because clarity is found in the center, never in the blindness of the extremes.

Wisdom is "more" than ethics; it is not just about moral behavior, but about the "center," the place from which moral perception and behavior flow.

MARCUS JOEL BORG (1942-2015)

In his search for nirvana — to free himself from suffering and the cycle of rebirths —, Siddhartha Gautama stopped eating and almost died of starvation, until he observed a teacher telling his pupil that the string of the zither should not be too taut, because it could snap, nor too slack, because it would not emit any sound. Simon Bolivar (1783-1830) was right in his last proclamation: "If my death contributes to the cessation of parties and the consolidation of union, I will go down to the grave in peace", because given the proximity to the center in ideas, things are naturally resolved with the evolution of thought. It is time for this to happen with a simple majority, we will achieve the change that will not come from one side or the other. We will achieve the balance with what we needed to build something different, which neither Marx (1818-1883) — with his absurd communism — nor Ronald Reagan (1911-2004) and Margaret Thatcher (1925-2013) — with their neoliberal policies that led to the expansion of modern slavery — could have imagined. Therefore, if we turn to the inner self to focus and concentrate on correcting errors of all kinds, with the awakening of the intelligent consumer, who knows that in education is the pillar that will allow us to face fear, ignorance and corruption, the true enemies of humanity, I am certain — from experience — that a movement will grow in us that will allow us to live in fullness, and that it will also allow an educated environment for a just society to live in peace in the midst of an honorable, social democracy. For this, it is urgent, — this is how we see it in various parts of the world, — and the recent gasoline cuts show how, and how much, dependence on fossil fuels can affect us; it is time for us to ride the fourth wave of free and clean energy. The post-industrial society, with a different educational model, which leaves behind the obsolete education of the industrial era with its comparisons and labels. That's how, since we were little, we learned to hate: "That person is not like you; I think that family is black; that person is not in the club; I think he is a communist; he is gay; he likes to hang out with the poor; don't you see he is a Catholic?; he's not a Lakers fan; and how, if she's an immigrant woman who lives in Madrid, she's a "sudaca"[175]; and many more.

In the age of knowledge, scientists will share information. If we manage to get knowledge and information to the farthest corners of the Earth and enter fully into clean energies — which do not require wires and poles — we will soon be able to make our way into outer space and thus enable the expansion of our species to other habitable planets. Otherwise, it will remain a pipe dream, even in the long term. Let's not swallow stories. This world already let us know that nothing would happen — unless it is a cataclysm — that could affect us immediately; we had the opportunity to prepare for the COVID-19 pandemic, but we did not do it. In spite of that, more and more of us are beginning to change things day by day; when you go out, in bars, restaurants, stores, supermarkets or on the street, you will notice that the intelligent consumer does not echo the news, turns off the TV, comes out of his drowsy state and prefers to enjoy his family, reading, cooking, studying, listening to music and chatting with friends. If you think this is not the case, in the morning, when you wake up and hesitate, because it doesn't matter, think that "current education continues to produce sick people for a sick society", as Augusto Cury, a psychiatrist and writer at the University of San José do Rio Preto, in Brazil, says. Cury also says that knowledge must be humanized and establishes some principles for the age of knowledge:

> We are committing an intellectual crime with children, adolescents and university students, because we are making them believe the false truth that producing knowledge is only

---

[175] A derogatory term commonly used in Spain to refer to people from Latin America.

the task of superheroes and giants, and it is not so, because the great producers of knowledge have also gone through crises, suffered dilemmas and were rejected; classrooms should change their configuration and students should be placed in a semicircle before the teacher, with classical music that slows down thinking and strengthens the imagination: knowledge must be humanized and the key is to enhance its tools.

In relation to the brain, it is estimated that, with the capacity to think, 95% of the human mind works from the unconscious and what is conscious in "one" only about 5% is what is known as life. The truth is, with the power of one, which lies in you more latent than ever, connected with yourself and with the cosmic mind that some call the collective unconscious, that 95% unconscious is what you can change things with. When — with knowledge — you begin to bring light in the darkness of the unconscious, the mind begins to become conscious, it begins to grow, you have more awareness of things, of what you do, and you begin to know yourself and the universe. That conscious 5% that grows is your intelligence, which is getting bigger; your potential is at its maximum, and the universe, which always aims at its maximum expression, at some point enlightens you. Suddenly, you think you know everything, and it is because, in those moments, very close, you have almost all the conscious knowledge that constantly increases and renews itself. When you learn some of the knowledge of the world, you add information that is not new to your brain, because it was already in the whole of the mental aspect of the collective unconscious in the universe. Your brain is just an antenna that connects you with the macrocosmic mind, enters into that mental aspect and becomes conscious of that new thing when you learn it. When you open your mind, enlightenment occurs as a logical process. In the depths of your unconscious, which then asks you to consciously resolve your greatest glooms, doubts, ghosts and demons, knowing every aspect of your unconscious becomes a microcosmic process that, when it is resolved by the human being, on many occasions, it is possible that it is creating a blockage to the cerebral subconscious, which disconnects it from the universal mind with what happens: "It sees what it wants to see, and only believes in that". However, when that creative force is at its maximum expression, the cosmic mind tries to reach you to illuminate your unconscious, to let you know its truth and make itself known. It is enough to open your heart.

You may say I'm a dreamer, but I'm not the only one. I hope someday you'll join us, and the world will be as one.

JOHN LENNON (1940-1980)

Final reflection

In 2019, NASA scientists found ribose in meteorites that bombarded the Earth in its formative period. Ribose — crucial for ribonucleic acid, RNA, which copies the explicit instructions of DNA — the oldest sugar involved in protein synthesis along with the other amino acids indispensable for life that they had previously found in those same meteorites, suggests that life may have originated first by chemical and then biological processes and reinforces the idea that life may have come from outer space. Another dilemma is the hominid evolutionary lineage. Since apes have twenty-four chromosomes and we have twenty-three. The other big question is the spontaneous appearance of a sharper intelligence that set modern humans apart in such a short time, which suggests that the DNA in *Homo sapiens* may have been "manipulated" at some point. Science that "manipulates" and edits DNA without measuring the consequences does not deny that we are doing wrong by playing God. The container in which we live has only 43% of purely human genetic composition and the remaining 46%, the genes of microbes, fungi, viruses, bacteria, and other microorganisms constitute — like a fingerprint — the microbiota that differs in each body. The microbiome is unique to each human individual and that is why there are people with glorious bodies who seem to be unaffected: nothing they eat makes them fat. Even so, regardless of this biological response, in the remaining mix of genes, the secret of life is and will continue to be that gene of LIGHT that we carry within us. And what about life? From the first cell to the second, from there to four more, to eight, and so on, including that energetic *quantum* — which we have forgotten to include in the concept — ; the purpose of life itself has always been to share knowledge.

The universe is composed mostly of hydrogen and helium. The set of creative forces includes gravity, electromagnetism, strong and weak nuclear forces. In 2019, scientists confirmed the theory of a fifth force:[176] helium which, when disintegrating, projects a light with particles of different mass at an angle that is uncommon, and it is believed that it could be the key to connect the visible world with the dark matter of the universe. With this fifth force, if we take into account the merger of antimatter with matter — the residue of this implosion is perhaps dark matter —, the creative forces could be six, seven, eight, or even more. But in the instants in which they conjugate to find their own balance, we have forgotten to include the creative force that is born of us and that with its energetic polarity, from the feelings, affects

---

[176] https://www.cnn.com/2019/11/22/world/fifth-force-of-nature-scn-trnd/index.html.

our destiny and the universe itself. Everything starts primitive. An unconscious cosmic mind that, as it evolves, acquires consciousness, and knows itself. The same happens with us. We have already seen how the macro and the micro in the cosmos are connected — the mental aspect of the collective unconscious and the cerebral subconscious — and that consciousness is not an intrinsic quality of the mind; intelligence comes after millennia or millions of years of evolution. According to this evolutionary aspect, in order to respond to unexplainable natural facts, we created circumstantial gods, and yet the vision of a single God was a purely spiritual act conceived 'instinctively' by the 'mind' over time. The highest product, the ultimate evolution at which the universe arrives, is that omega point of the great cosmic mind, the divine matrix, which at will knows itself in its totality. The universe is teleological: *Telos* (in Greek, τέλος) means 'end', 'goal', or 'purpose'. And in that sense, GOD — the end and the beginning —, creation and evolution have in common that same teleological aspect. With my contribution, I intend no disrespect; so, again, I apologize if I offend anyone with my approaches and my less egocentric and more real position regarding God, which could fully satisfy cultures.

When we look at existence, the way genes adapt to the environment or the self-regeneration of particles and cells, for example, it is evident that behind the physical there is an intelligence that directs creation and evolution towards its maximum potential, the omega point. Thus, the term itself, the final point at the end of the objective: evolution — which constantly adds up to change — is not a random act. Like yin and yang, mind and matter are sides of the same coin that coexist as two aspects that cannot be separated; the universe is dimensional and dimensionless energy. Mind has that same dimensional — physical — aspect that controls what we know, what we can see around our lives and in the same way, is connected to humanity, life itself and the universe. Matter also has a mental, non-local, dimensionless aspect that directs our evolution. Intelligence — in the mental aspect of physical matter — is outside of time and space; we cannot study it, nor see it, nor describe it, but science and quantum physics give proof that it exists. Since it is outside of the dimensional — that is, omnipresent —, it is everywhere at the same time and nowhere at the same time: in the human universe, in every atom that exists, the only God capable of performing miracles, who constantly hangs on to us and on himself, who is about to be resolved or finished because the simple dynamics of his paradox requires it, and because it is his own nourishment. God is the Love that, from the beginning, out of feelings, consists in the eternal sum of all the energies emanated by the living, and released by the dead, but not before, because otherwise we would not exist to be thinking about these questions. In the universe, the Love emanated and released by the 108 billion *sapiens*, and the other beings with some trait of intelligence that have walked this earth, is so great and powerful that, at the moment, it is consistently capable of governing the other forces; it is expanding and identifies the unique trace of the human presence in the universe.

In particular, we humans are a very powerful tiny particle, a toroid; a dynamo connected to the universe that, in itself — from feelings —, has the capacity to receive, transmute, create and emit infinite energy at the same time. May we learn in unison how to use it. The surrounding whole works like this: that which we call divine destiny or punishment — catastrophes, even luck or good fortune — is the answer to the message of negative, neutral, or positive polarity that we have always been sending to the divine matrix, which, with its own laws, constantly checks the balance of things. COVID-19 hit hard, and it was just a simple threat; in moments like that, paradoxes are unleashed, and the whole tells us that the prophecies that others wrote in times when God was "Who" and they did not know that He is Love, call our attention. Fear and ignorance have always reigned. And it is time for us to change the negative message that we carry because we really owe it to the young people: to our children.

There is neither any need to fear God, nor changes, nor a change of path. On the contrary, whenever faced with the vicissitudes of destiny, the intelligent consumer knows and counts on the fact that Love will always be on his side. And in the present circumstances, in order to give way to the positive, it is time to recognize that the present economic model of "extract, produce and waste" has reached the limit of its physical capacity. For the time being, the alternative is the circular economy,[177], which is based on eliminating waste and pollution by design; keeping products and materials in use — no more programmed obsolescence, which is disastrous for the expansion of our species —, and most importantly: it reduces the impact on the preservation of resources and ecosystems and fully complies with the goals of sustainable development. For all this, it is essential that the devices we have been postponing since the 1980s — inspired by Tesla's theory of radiant energy — are brought to light, developed, and marketed, which will open up that immense range of business possibilities, jobs and professions. In this 21ST CENTURY, it is high time that China, Russia, and the United States — the countries with the least scruples —, instead of continuing to dispute over the world's natural resources — for example, bidding for Greenland or buying land in Africa —, adopt the real changes that humanity requires. In this way, the trauma of change will pass more quickly than in previous waves. Each wave brings its own, and the reality is that the truths exposed

---

[177] Circular Economy, ellenmacarthurfoundation.org.

were not convenient for the elites' usufruct; by disregarding warmongers and the use of fossil fuels — coal, oil and gas —, the fourth wave gives us the possibility of correcting the mistakes of the past; as a society, it is up to us to turn the page and leave behind the way we used to transport ourselves or produce food: no matter how many we are, the planet would breathe again.

Scientific, economic, and financial studies are already on the table for politicians. In the United States, at least, it is estimated that, starting in 2021, over the next fifteen years, clean energy as a whole could provide sixty million jobs. This is not counting the jobs demanded by the infrastructure of roads, bridges, and railways for high-speed trains — which are so badly needed —, plus the 5X factor, which would generate an optimized local agribusiness. I forgot to say that, in the ecological transition, there are plans to increase the number of high-efficiency superchargers for electric vehicles at gas stations that take advantage of the solar panels that accumulate energy on their terraces. The reflection for the world would be such that the fourth wave, with spare capacity, would absorb and support the job losses from the hangover of the previous wave, which was exacerbated by the pandemic in 2020. Real leaders could begin to build a new dream: a world at peace and without borders that would consider having a single currency across the 'globe' that would once again be supported by gold, which is the patrimony of all; under the protection of the State and with new methods to produce clean energy, extractive mining would be controlled, and the earth would no longer be scratched. The unbacked money left to countries after paying off their sovereign debt, and that which is not regulated by banks in the volatile environment of stock exchanges, such as the electronic and weightless dollar, could be supplied by the cryptocurrencies that today attract investors of all kinds: the people in general would participate in stock exchanges all over the world. If this equity is achieved, the opportunity for everyone would be a huge *reset*: a new beginning. But never forget that you should never risk the money you need to live on or your roof over your head for any reason, least of all in the stock market. There is still a lot to learn, a lot to study, a lot of science to share so that in a bright world we can actually speak less of globalization — not as the growing economic relationship between countries — and more of a globalization that positively facilitates social mobilization between countries and so that the trend is then to complement each other from scientific and technological integration, with investment policies and trade reforms that allow education to promote environmental protection with the support of the media and information technology. Thus, by speaking of globalization without the rhetoric of patriotism, flags will only serve to identify the regions of the world in sporting events.

Not long ago, Abraham Lincoln said, "This is the last, best hope of the earth, either we save ourselves or we lose." In the present circumstances, America's last chance to fulfill that dream of defending democracy and, if it really wants to lead the world, it should take advantage of what is coming and evolve.

The first time a president was elected on the North American continent, between contenders of different political parties with multiple candidates, was in the United States in 1796: John Adams, of the Federalist party, won against Thomas Jefferson, of the Democratic-Republican party. Because of the immensity of its territory and the difficulty in communications, once optimal, now obsolete, the electoral college system does not elect fairly: it has been proven that at the end of the process, at least five times already, it has confirmed persons "NOT anointed by the supreme popular vote" for the most important office of the nation. In this bipartisan system, which seems more like a dogma that gives way to hypocrisy, you hand over your electoral faith to others, who are called to blindly follow a color, a flag. The old rather paternalistic idea of "everything for the people, but without the ignorant people", who must delegate power to a wise ruling class, corresponds in the United States, to a representative democracy based on the use of the federal electoral college system, which is very rough on democracy. For example, when a third party appears that is more in tune with one of the two major parties, by subtracting votes from them, the interest they have in common ends up affecting them both and the friendly party could cost it the loss of a state and even the presidency. The people know it: enlightened despotism is an old rusted concept supported by an obsolete and undemocratic system. To approach the center is not to lose, but to strangle capitalism, in the midst of its fear and hatred for socialism, and the other hatred which injects communism, not understanding that, with this movement, the extreme left naturally also tends to disappear: hatred is what drives them mad. The other thing is *lobbying*, which is not the same as *making a lobby*, because it corrodes just like the millionaires' donations to electoral campaigns do. The whole system must be reviewed.

In the United States, the pension fund for Social Security contributions has been depleting: Social Security can only support seventy-nine cents for every dollar and the State has been assuming this enormous debt that grows over the years. Recently, when I mentioned the idea of an honorable social democracy to an ex-military friend of mine, so that, for example, in the United States, the rich could rescue the pension fund and Social Security, since they could perfectly well renounce their contribution from Social Security in exchange for a lifetime rebate on their taxes, and it would be the best way for humanity to focus on living in peace; thinking of Colombia, he — who is very right-wing —, very annoyed, answered me: "OK, get a grip! We are uneducated Indians, and we like everything that is given away, here privilege prevails and corruption is the law; privilege is valid here, where a politician is worth more than a doctor and a soccer player is worth more than a professional; we are lazy, there is extreme poverty, in short, everything evil is in this land".

My message in response to Latin America is that the intelligent consumer — which is all of us — should not continue to support the sort that claim to be the socialists of the 21ST CENTURY (as in Venezuela) that never knew that the true social approach works with zero corruption; and with the money stolen by that corrupt caste of bandits, who never wanted to know how socially advanced countries work, supposedly because that was too much for us. The populism they promulgate, which at the end of the day is just another "-ism" that entails hate, no matter where it comes from, takes power by inciting your fears and, when it succeeds, it tries to impose, at any cost, its philosophy and implement its destructive agenda: "Take away everything, starve them to death so they just focus on surviving".

Language is no longer an excuse, and, without disintegrating, America is one from Alaska to Patagonia; however, it is inconceivable that Latin America, which for the United States has always been its backyard, is already being fertilized by a distant overseas power. But we all decided! It is America's turn to be great: No more Trumps,[178] no more Petros[179] and no

---

[178] Former 45th president, ultra-right-wing U.S. Republican Party member who will go down in history for inciting the mob that stormed the Capitol on January 6, 2021, in response to the 2020 presidential election, which Joe Biden — 46th president — won by a margin of more than seven million votes in a legitimate and democratic manner.

[179] Colombian politician and current president of Colombia, promoter in Latin America of the extreme left-wing socialism model of the 21ST century, established in Venezuela by dictators Hugo Chávez Frías and Nicolás Maduro.

more Bolsonaros![180] Ignorant egomaniacs with demagogic and inflammatory speeches, who only think of themselves so as to get more power, or stay in power, and destroy democracy. It should be noted that, in Spain, Pablo Iglesias[181] had a dignified exit: "When one realizes that he no longer contributes anything, he should retire". In spite of the stupidity, violence and looting, in America maturity seems to be coming: the social uprising highlighted that our neighbor is not the enemy and that we cannot expect, neither more nor less, from the politicians of the day with their totalitarian delusions that continue to divide us and make us live in their extreme world. In North America, from the economic point of view, for years, financial institutions have been setting a great example by leaving behind the overcharges for bank account users. The United States set a political example in the 2020 presidential election: a people who are already protesting constantly against the systemic and racist actions of sectors of their society, in the face of the pandemic and the obstacles that many are trying to impose, voted massively. In Central America, in spite of the repression and disappearances, the discontent with the dictatorship in Nicaragua is manifest; and in the south, Chile, three years after the social uprising, works to reduce the size and expense of Congress — Italy did the same — ; I hope that Chile does not fall into decadence and the reforms of Constitution don't fail. This is what happened in

---

[180] President of Brazil. In his extreme right-wing denialist government, his country reached the second largest number of deaths by pandemic in the world and the Brazilian Amazon rainforest — since he took office on January 1, 2019 — until July 2020, had lost 20 500 km², almost two thirds of Belgium or half of Switzerland, which has 41 285 km².

[181] Spanish ex-politician and co-founder of the political party Podemos, which is situated between the left and the extreme left, founded in 2014, in which he acted as secretary general until announcing his retirement in May 2021.

Colombia with the 1991 Constitution, which, in spite of being modern and inclusive, has ended up gutted by corruption and manipulated by the governments in office; more than fifty-six reforms have left it like a sieve, which makes it vulnerable for those to come and calls into question the consistency of the original text. Nor do the prisons deserve those "seventh heads"; and the "corrupt" judges had better resign, because it would be very easy, and this is no joke, that their identity card, passport, or driver's license could be marked diagonally in bright red and well crossed with "666", the number of the beast of the Apocalypse, whose name is corruption. All that remains is for the young people who protest to go out and vote. Statistics clearly show that they do not. Organize your ideas, draw conclusions, mature, and fulfill your mission, because it is valid to protest peacefully for what is right, but never, never, never ever feel tempted to vote for a totalitarian, and even less for a crooked one. Check their resumes well and, if you want peace, choose among your own — there are some without stain — real leaders, worthy, honest, and willing to approach the center, which is where morality and balance are born.

I believe in humanity, in Love and in Jesus as our spiritual guide. In Jesus it is God who speaks to make his will felt; for Christians, Ash Wednesday marks the beginning of Lent: "Dust thou art and unto dust shalt thou return" and your energy will be released. If they do not want to disappear, religions will also have to make reforms and abandon the extremes so as to unify criteria. It is undeniable how machismo — which also affects religions — has demeaned women. For example, in some marriage rituals, they are still placed lower or at the back to serve and please the man. Depending on the religion, machismo dictated the precepts that forced them to cover certain parts of their body, or from head to toe. Among other things, in China or Japan, when women get married, they totally lose their surnames; as the "male" is supposed to take care of the household, it is still the custom in most parts of the world for children to bear their fathers' surnames. By nature, having XX or XY chromosomes is not even a sufficient reason to justify it. Things are changing, for example, in Sweden, if the parents do not reach an agreement, the child is registered with the mother's surname;[182] sons are born to women and having children is a right that should be shared. The important thing is what it implies socially and to the conscience: that we are really responsible for "our actions". But, above all, sexism is that other great hatred that we must eliminate. Those were other times and other customs, let's stop with the "witch hunt". As a basis for fair judgment, harassment can be subtle and is sometimes an extremely vague concept; I hope we understand that, as children, we were all victims of a simultaneous machismo that flowed from pulpits, desks, and home as we grew up. Women, although it is valid for you to protest and denounce rapists when there is concrete evidence, it is not to gossip about them before they are judged; we all, and I say all, must recognize that this extreme thinking of feminism that points to 3 750 million men as rapists — the male world population —, by shouting "the rapist is you!", unjust and absurd, is certainly equivalent to what we have heard in the other extreme and in religions with machismo: "The temptation is you!".

Although it seems to have gone unnoticed, our history presents another prophecy that was fulfilled. Among its relics, Christianity preserves a text that was made known in Venice in 1595. The prophecy of St. Malachy (1094-1148) consists of 112 opuscules involving the next 111 popes — who would rule the Catholic Church — and Francis. The motto *The Glory of the*

---

[182] https://www.rtve.es/noticias/20101104/asi-cultura-apellidos-mundo/367438.shtml.

Olives (*De Gloria Olivae*), which would correspond to the last pope, is no longer a mystery; despite the somber circumstances surrounding the retirement of the previous popes, in this case, the olive tree — which is a symbol of achievement, victory, honor and peace — refers to the honorable and peaceful retirement of Joseph A. Ratzinger, Benedict XVI, and Francis — the current Pope. Ratzinger, Benedict XVI — last pope and last Peter of a specific doctrine in the Catholic Church — ; the prophecy and the sentence say: "In extreme persecution, in the Holy Roman Church Peter the Roman will reign, who will feed his flock among many tribulations, after which, the city of the seven hills will be destroyed and the Terrible Judge will judge his people. The end."

In the world, people refer to Rome as the city of the seven hills and the popes, which today is actually the Vatican City. If we take into account that for a thousand years — east of the Tiber River in Rome, from Constantine in the 4TH CENTURY until the 14TH CENTURY — the Lateran Palace was the papal seat and NOT the Vatican, which did not yet exist at the time of the saint in the 12TH CENTURY, therefore, the city "destroyed" in Malachi's vision, the city of the seven hills, corresponds in modern times to the Vatican City in Rome: the city of the popes. With the emergence of ISIS or Islamic State group and after Ratzinger's retirement, never before in history had the atrocious way of massacring Christians been recorded with videos, and in countries such as North Korea, China, Egypt, Iran, Iraq, Nigeria, Sudan, Eritrea, Syria, Saudi Arabia, Turkey, India, Pakistan; the worldwide merciless, social and bureaucratic harassment had a peak that worsened between 2015 and 2017 in at least a hundred more countries. [183]

---

[183] https://www.christianitytoday.com/news/2021/january/christian-persecution-2021-countries-open-doors-watch-list.html

Other popes had already resigned in 1045, 1294 and 1415, but in different ways and for grotesque reasons: Benedict IX, in the midst of corruption, for economic and sentimental interests, occupied the papal chair three times and married after his last retirement; Celestine V was not even a bishop, but a hermit monk of eighty-five years of age with the reputation of a saint; it is said that his goodness was abused, he was manipulated and, after his retirement, he was poisoned; Gregory XII was involved in what was perhaps the darkest passage of the Church — as far as corruption was concerned up to that time —, though he was good, he was involved in the Western Schism, in which there came to be three obediences: the Roman — to which he belonged — ; the Avignonese with Benedict XIII and the Pisan with the antipope Alexander V: three popes at the same time. In the 21ST CENTURY, the city of popes, shaken by financial scandals and by the fall of the reputation of the Church due to the outcry produced by the pederasty cover-ups worldwide; the Vatican, since the departure in 2013 of Pope Benedict XVI, who had tried almost daily to appease the crowds, faced the collapse and the verdict of the terrible judge — from the Latin. *terribilis*, 1. adj. That causes terror — : "I am the beginning and the end". The end of a doctrine, led by Joseph Ratzinger — although German, the last Roman Peter, hence the symbolism —, built on the basis of always venerating a deified and distant Jesus, dead and nailed to a cross, to whom we had to constantly beg and ask forgiveness for our faults; and the beginning, according to the report, of a Jesuit doctrine, incarnated in Jorge Bergoglio — the first Jesuit pope — who, feeling the risen Jesus, founded on gratitude, announced the arrival of a human Jesus who will always vibrate in the hearts of men. And so, it was. From that first day, March 13, 2013 — another sign —, the new hierarch, who was of a renewed Catholic Church, refused to take possession of the pontifical apartment — the traditional enclosure destined for previous popes — ; for he assures that, within himself, he felt a "NO" and preferred — for a personal act of humility — to stay and live in room 201 of the Santa Marta residence. And in honor of Francis of Assisi — the saint of the poor —, he asked to simply be called Francis.

In numerology, among other things, 201, $2 + 0 + 1 = 3$, the number three, symbol of expansion, signifies passion: the striving to accomplish and culminate things. No wonder. It is also no coincidence that Nikola Tesla was obsessed with the number three: he spent his last years in the New Yorker Hotel in New York, in room 3327: $3 + 3 + 2 + 7 = 15$; $1 + 5 = 6$, a multiple of three. Ah, I almost forgot, speaking of entities and numbers, let's avoid having a chip implanted with personal information that goes against our privacy.

Now, the outlines of the economy have been blurred; companies in general, in order not to go bankrupt, will have to reduce their costs, but recovery is on the way. It is remarkable that pollution has been reduced during the pandemic; this shows the way forward, not only in the spiritual: before picking up the pace of things, it is the ideal time for countries to implement or increase train systems to interact with high-speed lines connecting their cities, which would create a more dynamic, economical, and planet-friendly infrastructure. We have already seen that the important thing is direct access to clean energy that does not depend on distribution networks: instead of going back to the same thing, the automakers should bring out the models they have that run on river or sea water, or hydrogen and other renewable energy sources, and if they do not have them, they should look for them, because these inventions have already been on the street for some time. Several countries, such as Spain or Germany, have been extending the benefits offered by the State to acquire an electric car and encourage "the leap" and are already exploring the financial viability of these other models. Things do not just happen; when you are afraid, it is very difficult to glimpse the solutions. In the face of the foolish who lead the retreat to the third wave, Angela Merkel rightly prevailed and Europe is undoubtedly at the forefront of political intentions for change.

Meanwhile, in America, energy companies should continue to promote talent contests like the one won in 2016 in the United States by thirteen-year-old Maanasa Mendu for creating a device capable of generating renewable energy that costs only five dollars. Producing clean energy is no mystery; one of the guidelines for universities in cutting-edge countries is to openly teach models that serve to produce renewable energy. It is ironic that, in the United States, energy from NON-renewable resources and nuclear plants is still just over 60%, while in Iceland it is 0%. The whole of America is full of volcanoes. In that sense and in the management of CO_2 waste, the Icelanders have a lot to teach us, because there producing clean and renewable energy — not only geothermal — is a simple matter of common sense, as engineer Albert Albertson — pioneer of the environmental movement in the industry, director of the Blue Lagoon Park in Grindavik, Iceland — rightly comments in an interview with Zac Efron in the first chapter of the 2020 Netflix documentary *Down to Earth*. To this club of countries powered 100% by renewable energy belong Portugal, Norway, Costa Rica, Uruguay, Lesotho, which have made a short-term commitment to never again consume fossil fuels. And, for God's sake, the countries that have them should close down their nuclear power plants for good. The only thing that Russia, China and, especially, the United States need is attitude, attitude, and attitude, because this was the word that made them grow; remember, the planet would breathe again.

We hope the environment shall continue to become clearer, and it seems that way because the mainstream is already beginning to agree with the second lane reasoning. For example, it is pleasing to realize that for "establishing the basis for understanding how oxygen affects cellular metabolism and physiological function favorably" the Nobel Prize in Medicine was awarded in 2019 to the Americans, William Kaelin and Gregg Semenza, and the Briton, Peter Ratcliffe, whose discoveries ratify the original idea that the German physiologist Otto Heinrich Warburg (1883-1970) — Nobel Prize in Physiology and Medicine in 1931 for discovering the nature and mode of action of respiratory enzymes — had at the beginning of the last century. The health outlook in the United States is not very flattering. A 2019 report warns that, instead of improving, the average life expectancy in men decreased in the previous three years (2016 to 2018); a report by Steven Woolf reveals that, due to overdoses, suicides, alcoholism, and diseases such as cancer, death is increasing among young people at an alarming rate: 33 000 deaths that should not have happened since 2010. In addition, he mentions that the average weight of women has increased and is now equal to the average weight of men fifty years ago: humanity is letting the serious and silent weight problem pass.

Even before, democratic ideals succeeded in liberating most nations from the "communist axis"; let us not forget that, in relative calm and peace, nothing could prevent the fall of the Berlin Wall. Communist China evolved into a weird capitalism in which the government only plays with an elite of reliable civilians and insists on its arbitrariness; and although its leaders do not recognize it, the Chinese people do know what it is to be militarized at all times. And they would not have to be if they encouraged their neighbors Cambodia, Laos, Vietnam, North Korea to rescue the basic principles of what their leaders despotically called nationalism: civic education inclusive of all ethnicities, democracy, and social welfare. China shows the world its successful upper class but hides the shame of its immense popular base: an "exploited and battered underclass". To avoid an internal disaster, China could surprise the world with a show of will: give full freedom to the Himalayan peoples who, once autonomous and rejoicing, would welcome back their Dalai Lama.

What about the wars? The reasons are already more than discussed. I read that the best religion is to be a good person. Many think that this will be another end of the omens, and this is, without a doubt, the right time to propose to live in peace. Human arrogance has always believed that it is licit to quickly and violently crush the small enemy, and it is naive to think so because there has never been an investment in weapons, defense or intelligence that has been able to eradicate, or stop in a short time, an ideological advance, much less so if it is religious. A thousand years ago, after invading Spain, the Muslims had already been chased in the crusades to Jerusalem in a never-ending war. Only five centuries ago, they were expelled from the Iberian Peninsula and, from then until today, Jews, Christians and Muslims have lived intermingled; but what we have not visualized is that — just as rivers pierce the rock to widen their channel — sabers, swords, cannon shots, bullets, stones or insults, the "holy" wars have only managed to widen the borders in the mental gaps of men. Today it remains for us to realize that only with an education that gathers prudence and wisdom, Love — the one and only true God — will succeed in appeasing the hatreds that exist without reason among the brothers and sisters who have always been the children of Abraham. There are no physical limits that can stop an ideology, much less if it is of a religious nature. All religions as they are, with all their schisms — Revelation 7: "Next I saw four angels, standing at the four corners of the earth, holding back the four winds of the world to keep them from blowing over the land...." — tend to disappear. But in the ark of the covenant, the truth of its power, which is the covenant itself, will be the perfect weapon that will defeat the very reason — common enemy and inseparable companion of fear — that divides us: the latent doubt that persists regarding the best kept secret: the true name of God. And if we have all been equal in the eyes of God, was it so difficult to realize that the real power that the ark of the covenant possessed, consistently in its name, is the covenant of the churches of the world around Love, the one and only true God?

Love is NOT to be feared!

Lord, forgive all those who without knowing His Name — the name of Him who creates all and makes all things possible; who sees all, though we cannot see Him, but we can feel Him and is everywhere; GOD, who is not Who, for that would be too small, but LOVE is His true name — have sown doubt in the ignorant more unfortunate than themselves; with no more ado, turn aside from the path to teach hatred instead of love, and with the power of their sign, misinterpreting wise words, install the fear of God in the subconscious of people:

> ...and gave him [Jesus, son of Mary] the Gospel containing guidance and light, which corroborated the earlier Torah, a guidance, and a warning for those who preserve themselves from evil and follow the straight path.

QUR'AN 5:46

I remember the inquisitive face of the adults when someone mentioned the word Koran, and I suppose that today it is the same in a Muslim family if someone dares to ask about the Bible, because if they ask about the Talmud or the Torah, I am almost sure that the slap is delivered. If this answer to a child sounds familiar: "Don't mess with that because you wouldn't understand it!", the same would be true of: "Only here — in the Bible or the Koran — will you find the answers you need!".

It is possible, very possible, that Jews and Christians did not know of the love and respect that Muslims have in the Koran for the Holy Family, so much so that among its 114 surahs — the chapters into which it is divided, only eight of which have someone's name as a title — the prophet gave the title Mary (Maryam) to sura 19, and also mentions her as the unique and relevant woman that she is:

"The angels said: '*Oh, Mary, indeed God has favored you and made you immaculate, chosen you from all the women of the world*'."

QUR'AN 3:42

It is sad that, of the little that remained within the reach of Jewish, Christian, and Muslim scholars — who promulgate the same faith in a single god —, they preferred **not to** make known details of our history together; to remain silent and to ignore everything that binds us. The "sacred" texts are the compendium of written testimony about extraordinary events, some healthy, others chaotic, and although they are also reference books, some believe that they say it all. Researching the history of Islam on the internet and scrutinizing — because it was not easy —, I have gone back fourteen centuries and practically stumbled on a document so old that, when I read it, I understood that because it was beautiful and honest, at some point it could have affected the very particular "basic" interests in certain sectors of Islam and Christianity. Because of the "fear of on each side" of losing followers, it was never openly made public knowledge. I could say that for these institutions it was much more valuable to protect the idea they had in common: the contempt, hatred, or indifference for the Jewish people, which transcended and is not recent. The text exposes the truth and the welcoming kindness of the Muslim people, which favors Christians and Jews as well as other peoples. This is the authentic message of the Prophet Mohammed — addressed to St. Catherine of Alexandria, an illustrious and wise woman —, which was jealously preserved for 1,400 years under the protection of the Muslims in the Monastery of the Transfiguration, the oldest Christian monastery in the world, located at the foot of Mount Sinai. In Spanish, the Islamic pages of Chile and Mexico present it as follows:

Prophet Muhammad's fraternal message to Christians

The proclamation transcribed below is one thousand four hundred years old. It is practically unknown in the West, and it is a faithful translation that we offer to Spanish-speaking readers. It is the bearer of the spirit of Islam, of its tolerance, of its mercy towards all beings. Its universality lies in love, understanding and knowledge, and it is a call to fraternity among human beings. Islam, which was and is unjustly accused of implanting the faith by the sword, categorically rejects this accusation and in response offers this eloquent message that is a testimony until the end of time. This valuable historical document **was dictated by the prophet Muhammad** (B. P., Great Prophet) and in it are printed the legal norms that were to regulate the coexistence between Christians and Muslims. Muhammad (B.P.) was unlettered. He subscribed his letters, treaties, proclamations with his personal seal. On this occasion, his secretaries forgot him, and the beneficiaries demanded that he endorse it with his rubric, as the other Islamic peoples did. **Without hesitation, he impressed his thumb digit on the pad and printed it at the bottom of the document:** "Here is **the signature. Like this there is no other like it**." He then exclaimed:

"This promise, formulated by Muhammad, sent by God to all peoples, as announcer, interpreter and promoter of the laws that He imposes on His creatures, is addressed to all the followers of the Christian religion, whether Arabs or of other races, whether near or far, whether known or unknown."

"In issuing this message, after a rigorous examination of conscience, I bear public witness that it is inspired by divine justice and, therefore, Muslims who observe it meticulously will strictly comply with the postulates of Islam, standing out as its most excellent co-religionists; and whoever flouts the rule that I establish, leading himself along paths forbidden to austere believers, will simply be a traitor and a despiser of his creed, whether he is a sultan or any of the Muslims."

"I formalize this solemn promise in my name and in the name of the good believers who constitute my people, offering myself with them and for them to the general judgment."

"I give the pledge of God and His blameless Word, invoking the conscience of His Prophets, of His Messengers, of His undefiled Messages, of the faithful of the Almighty, of believers and Muslims past and present. On the basis of the agreement that God has concluded with the prophets and by which He imposes on them obedience to His Precepts and faithful fulfillment of the duties contracted with Him, I give my indeclinable and precise word":

"That I will protect the refugees in my ports, with my cavalry and infantry, with my guards of order and my civilian subjects, wherever they may be found, far or near, both in times of peace and in times of war."

"That, in addition to a tranquil life, I guarantee them their own defense, that of their temples and convents, their chapels and abbeys, the collective or particular residence of their monks and the security of the roads for their tours, wherever and in whatever form they may be, in the East and in the West, on mountains or in the bosom of valleys, in caves as in villages or in deserts, on flat or broken land, and in every place where they dwell."

"That I will defend their religion and their property wherever and however they may be, in the same degree I would do so for myself, for my religion, for my relatives and their belongings, and that I will likewise protect them against any harm, displeasure, unlawful imposition or illegitimate liability, shielding them against any foreign force that would seek to attack them with my own person and mine, whether they be soldiers or civilians, without regard to the potential of the enemy."

"That from now on I consider them under my protection and safeguard, in such a way that no harm will touch them, without previously reaching my dignitaries, in charge of the national defense".

"That I exempt them from the tax burdens that the nomads pay, in accordance with the existing agreements, asking them to contribute with the sum that would be to their liking, without such contribution being considered an unavoidable tribute".

"That, henceforth, no Christian priest shall be compelled to renounce his investiture, nor any individual to abandon his worship, as likewise monks shall not be hindered in the exercise of their profession, nor shall they be forced to vacate their convents, to suspend their missionary tours."

"That not even a small part of their temples shall be demolished, nor shall their acquisition be permitted for mosques or Muslim residences; for whoever would do so would break the solemn promise given in the name of God, disobey the prophet, and openly betray the happiness of his conscience."

"That, as for the tax on revenues, derived from large maritime or terrestrial business, determined by the extraction of metals, pearls, precious stones, gold or silver, coming from considerable capitals belonging to Christians, it shall in no case exceed twelve drachmas annually if these reside and remain in the same place in which they exercise their trade."

"That no tribute shall be demanded of persons, whether domiciled or not, who live on the beneficence of others, with the exception of those who inherit taxed with taxes, in which case they shall continue to pay them without any increase, being able, however, to partially fulfill this obligation in case of difficulties in paying the canon previously fixed to the testator."

"That if any of them should acquire movable or immovable property for the purpose of benefiting from its exploitation or lease, they shall not pay higher taxes than those paid by their peers".

"That the Christians will be considered, as for the rights of conscience, equal to ours, without being obliged to go out with the national armies to meet the enemy or to join them, since the defense corresponds exclusively to the Muslims. Nevertheless, the Christians will be able to contribute voluntarily to the provisioning and remounting of the army, genuinely Muslim, with arms and horses, which will be remembered with benevolence and gratitude".

"That no Christian shall be compelled to convert to the religion of Islam, nor shall his belief be discussed with him, but on affable terms, and he shall be treated by all Muslims with mercy and affection, protecting them against all injury or prejudice wherever they may be and in whatever situation they may find themselves."

"That if any Christian should be led to commit a grave fault or crime, it is the duty of the Muslims to induce him to the right path by means of exhortation and good advice, and, if he has done so, to serve his defense to the extent of repairing the damage done, striving to make peace with the offended Muslim subject, to assist in the pursuit of these ends".

"That the Muslims will not contribute to any failure of the Christians, nor will they be denied the necessary collaboration, nor from the bosom of the nation".

"That by means of this divine promise I grant them the same guarantees enjoyed by Muslims, assuming, consequently, the obligation to protect them against all inconveniences and provide for their benefit so that they may be true citizens, solidary in common rights and duties."

"That, as regards marriage, a Christian woman shall not be obliged to marry a Muslim, nor shall she be grieved if she resists the engagement, her prior consent being indispensable; And that, in the event of such a union, the husband shall leave the wife free to practice her worship according to the guidance of her spiritual leaders, from whose norms she shall take example, without obliging her in any case to abjure her religion or to oppose it if these were her wishes, for any act contrary to these postulates would place him among the fallacious, violators of the promise of God and of the word of His Prophet."

"That if Christians need to build or refurbish their temples, chapels or holy places, or any other realization of interest for their worship, the corresponding technical or financial collaboration will be provided at their request, considering such an act as a simple charity, in accordance with the promise given by the prophet and in accordance with the norms that God imposes on all Muslims".

"That they shall not be compelled, in case of war, to serve as emissaries, guides, or observers over the enemy camp, nor to any activity of a warlike character; and that if anyone should require them, either individually or en masse, to do otherwise, he shall be held in contempt of the prophetic word and in disobedience to their testimony."

"These conditions were imposed by Muhammad, the envoy of God, in favor of the followers of the Christian religion, without exception."

The only duties established in their regard, under the aegis of their good conscience and the postulates of their creed, are the following:

"That they will not aid the enemy in war with the Muslims, publicly or secretly, nor will they give shelter or refuge to the adversary in their houses, holy places or regions, nor will they second him with troops, arms, horses or men, nor will they constitute themselves as depositories of their property, nor will they maintain communication with them."

"That they will not refuse to lend a lodging of three consecutive days to any of the Muslims nor to their horses, wherever they may be or direct, without this obliging them to provide extraordinary food, which would mean an increase in their usual expenses."

"That if any of the Muslims in distress should be forced to take refuge in their homes or regions, they will treat him cordially, helping and encouraging him in his misfortune and concealing his whereabouts from the enemy without omitting any effort to fulfill this duty."

"Whoever violates the prefixed conditions will be considered a renegade from God and from the solemn promise given by the prophet to the Christian priests and monks, with the testimony of the nation."

"This is an inescapable command contracted by the Prophet on his own behalf and on behalf of all Muslims, and to the observance of which they are strictly bound until the day of the Resurrection and completion of the world."

ISLAM MEXICO, 2016

The time is fulfilled; the time of the advent has come: With the blessing of Abraham, the first patriarch of faith in God, father of the Arab peoples descended from Ishmael and of the Jews descended from his half-brother Isaac, father of Jacob or Israel, let reconciliation take place and Muslims and Jews alike, with reforms in the temples, synagogues and mosques of the East and with the evolution of the churches of the West and the others of the world, will welcome us Christians and all alike in the name of the Love and the acting of Jesus Christ.

For the good of humanity, religions will set their affairs straight: they will tear down the walls that divide us, they will extend the bridges of reconciliation recognizing Love as the one and only true God; an unsolvable dogma solved in good part by science. The Jesuits have been expelled many times by different States, alleging economic reasons and criticisms for always promoting education and proposing free thinking, which curiously supports "conscience"; but the energies of the universe, in search of their own balance — God's timing is perfect — Jesuit thought is favored on this occasion, and divine inspiration to initiate the doctrine with a new era of hierarchs founded on gratitude and Jesus, who beats in the hearts of men, represented in Francis, your humble servant, who with his renewed Church will guide us on the path to dignify the Church for what the Church is.

We are creators and, therefore, it is human to know how to ask for forgiveness and to forgive, and common to people who live in peace, love will emerge as the reason to coexist. Therefore, we must support, with what is within our grasp, those who thinking of others do not expect anything in return: pastors, imams, abbots, nuns and monks, rabbis, priests, lay sisters and brothers who extend their labors and their hands, more than you and I would do, to the helpless: the homeless; the little old people left to their own devices; the poor; the sick; the orphaned children who hunger and thirst; for the unhinged; the prisoners in jails; the abused women; the raped children, ragged, without toys and without school; for the immigrants without shelter, without food; and the mothers who, without a breath of hope, abandon their children at the doors of the temples. All of them, with humility, sharing even their plate of food, are worthy of respect and are sacred entities. Not so — we always misunderstood it — the buildings: churches, temples, synagogues, and mosques are just landmarks — sacred or not —, meeting places of the institutions that enable these people to fulfill their mission. The risen Jesus beats in our hearts and is the light that illuminates the path of awakening.

It is time to get to know John again — the most persevering *influencer* in the last two thousand years —, to understand his words and to follow the greatest of all, Jesus, who already walks among us. And if only at the end of the text you try to find innovation in my words, I can bring you some Hindu wisdom. If you have read the book from the beginning, I can assure you that having reached this page, and even more so when your body — the one you inhabit — asks you: "What are we eating today?", you will know that the innovator here has been you and that aware of your "being" you will do your part to build the new history of humanity.

"Things are when they are meant to be, not before or after" and all the graces are contained in a beautiful word:
Namaste!

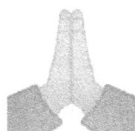

JOHANN CAROLUS

www.ingramcontent.com/pod-product-compliance
Lightning Source LLC
Chambersburg PA
CBHW020531030426
42337CB00013B/797